T0373185

Benign Cerebral Glioma, Volume I

AANS Publications Committee
Michael L.J. Apuzzo, MD, Editor

Neurosurgical Topics

American Association of
Neurological Surgeons

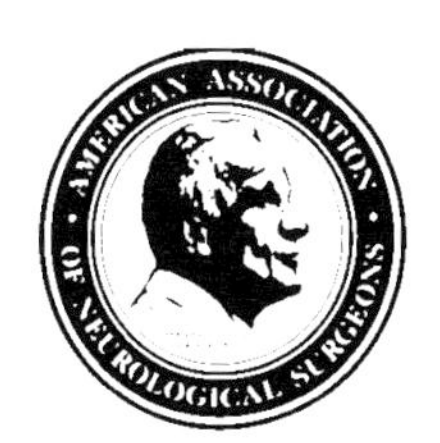

Library of Congress Catalog
ISBN: 1-879284-31-6

Neurosurgical Topics ISBN: 0-9624246-6-8

Printed in U.S.A.

American Association of Neurological Surgeons
22 South Washington Street
Park Ridge, Illinois 60068-9924

This publication is published under the auspices of the Publications Committee of the American Association of Neurological Surgeons (AANS). However, this should not be construed as indicating endorsement or approval of the views presented by the AANS, or by its committees, commissions, affiliates, or staff.

Daniel L. Barrow, MD, Chairman
AANS Publications Committee

Gay Palazzo, AANS Staff Editor

AANS1.75M395

Neurosurgical Topics SERIES

FORTHCOMING BOOKS

1995

Benign Cerebral Glioma, Volume II
Edited by Michael L. J. Apuzzo, MD

Endovascular Neurological Intervention
Edited by Robert J. Maciunas, MD

Neurosurgical Aspects of Pregnancy
Edited by Christopher Loftus, MD

COMPANION BOOKS

Malignant Cerebral Glioma

Neurosurgical Aspects of Epilepsy

Neurosurgery for the Third Millenium

DEDICATION

to
Gwyneth Carpenter

Eine herausragende und dramatische charakter voller gegensätze und extreme

Inbegriff einer zeitgenössischen Heldin

Contents

CONTRIBUTORS vii

PREFACE xiii

VOLUME I

PART I: THE INTELLECTUAL SETTING

Chapter 1 Evolving Dimensions at the Frontiers of Human Cerebral Surgery 1
Michael L. J. Apuzzo, MD

PART II: DEVELOPMENT, PATHOLOGY, AND MOLECULAR BIOLOGY

Chapter 2 The Developmental Biology of Glial Cells and Its Relation to the Study of Glioma Biology 13
Mark E. Linskey, MD

Chapter 3 The Pathology of Benign Cerebral Astrocytomas 55
Michael L. Rodriguez, MBBS, FRCPA, and Parakrama Chandrasoma, MD

Chapter 4 The Pathology of Oligodendrogliomas 83
M. Beatriz S. Lopes, MD, Scott R. VandenBerg, MD, PhD, and Bernd W. Scheithauer, MD

Chapter 5 The Pathology of Benign Ependymomas 95
Ignacio Gonzalez-Gomez, MD, and Floyd H. Gilles, MD

Chapter 6 The Pathology of Ganglion Cell Tumors 115
Mahlon D. Johnson, MD, PhD

Chapter 7 Patterns of Tumor Growth and Problems Associated with Histological Typing of Low-Grade Gliomas 125
Catherine Daumas-Duport, MD, PhD

Chapter 8 Growth Factors and Proliferation Potential 149
David R. Hinton, MD, FRCP(C)

Chapter 9 Molecular Genetic Basis of Cerebral Gliomas 163
David N. Louis, MD, Bernd R. Seizinger, MD, PhD, and Webster K. Cavenee, PhD

Chapter 10 Malignant Progression in Gliomas 181
Thomas C. Chen, MD, David R. Hinton, MD, FRCP(C), and Michael L.J. Apuzzo, MD

CME QUESTIONS FOR VOLUME I 189

ANSWERS TO CME QUESTIONS 210

CUMULATIVE INDEX FOR VOLUMES I AND II I-1

VOLUME II

PART III: CLINICAL ASPECTS OF BENIGN GLIOMA

Chapter 11 The Natural History of Low-Grade Gliomas 213
Michael Salcman, MD

Chapter 12 Congenital Syndromes Associated with Benign Gliomas 231
Corey Raffel, MD, PhD, and Marvin D. Nelson, Jr., MD

Chapter 13 Imaging Features of Benign Gliomas 247
Chi-Shin Zee, MD, Peter Conti, MD, Sylvie Destian, MD, David C.P.Chen, MD, Leonard Petrus, MD, and Hervey D. Segall, MD

Chapter 14 Role of Stereotaxis in the Management of Low-Grade Intracranial Gliomas 275
Patrick J. Kelly, MD

Chapter 15 Role of Surgery In Diagnosis and Management 293
Mitchel S. Berger, MD

Chapter 16 Radiotherapeutic Aspects 309
Zbigniew Petrovich, MD, Gary Luxton, PhD, Gabor Jozsef, PhD, and Michael L. J. Apuzzo, MD

Chapter 17 Application of Focused Beam Principles 329
Zbigniew Petrovich, MD, Gary Luxton, PhD, Gabor Jozsef, PhD, Chi-Shin Zee, MD, and Michael L.J. Apuzzo, MD

Chapter 18 Epilepsy and Benign Gliomas 347
André Olivier, MD, PhD, and Daniel Lacerte, MD

Chapter 19 Surgical Aspects and General Management of Astrocytomas 381
Edward R. Laws, Jr., MD, FACS

Chapter 20 Surgical Aspects and General Management of Oligodendrogliomas 397
Dennis E. Bullard, MD, FACS

Chapter 21 Surgical Aspects and General Management of Ependymomas 413
John A. Duncan III, MD, PhD, and Harold J. Hoffman, MD, BSc(Med),FRCS(C), FACS

Chapter 22 Surgical Aspects and General Management of Ganglion Cell Tumors 427
Robert J. Maciunas, MD

EDITOR'S POSTSCRIPT 445

CME QUESTIONS FOR VOLUME II 447

ANSWERS TO CME QUESTIONS 474

Previously Published Books in the *Neurosurgical Topics* Series 475

CUMULATIVE INDEX FOR VOLUMES I AND II I-1

List of Contributors
Volumes I and II

Michael L. J. Apuzzo, MD
Edwin M. Todd/Trent H. Wells, Jr. Professor
Department of Neurological Surgery
and Radiation Oncology
University of Southern California
School of Medicine
Director of Neurosurgery
Kenneth R. Norris Jr. Cancer Hospital and
Research Institute
Los Angeles, California

Mitchel S. Berger, MD
Associate Professor of Neurological Surgery
American Cancer Society Professor of
Clinical Oncology
University of Washington
School of Medicine
Seattle, Washington

Dennis E. Bullard, MD, FACS
Chief of Surgery
Department of Surgery
Rex Hospital
Raleigh, North Carolina

Webster K. Cavenee, PhD
Director
Ludwig Institute for Cancer Research
Center for Molecular Genetics and
Department of Medicine
Professor of Medicine
University of California, San Diego
San Diego, California

Parakrama Chandrasoma, MD
Associate Professor of Pathology
University of Southern California
School of Medicine
Chief of Anatomic Pathology
Los Angeles County and University of
Southern California Medical Center
Los Angeles, California

David C. P. Chen, MD
Associate Professor of Radiology
Nuclear Medicine Section
University of Southern California
School of Medicine
Los Angeles, California

Thomas C. Chen, MD
Clinical Instructor
Department of Neurological Surgery
University of Southern California
School of Medicine
Los Angeles, California

Peter Conti, MD
Assistant Professor of Radiology
PET Imaging Center
University of Southern California
School of Medicine
Los Angeles, California

Catherine Daumas-Duport, MD, PhD
Department of Pathology
Hopital Sainte-Anne
Paris, France

Sylvie Destian, MD
Associate Professor of Radiology
Neuroradiology Section
University of Southern California, School of Medicine
Los Angeles, California

John A. Duncan III, MD, PhD
Chairman, Department of Pediatric Neurosurgery
Hasbro Children's Hospital
Providence, Rhode Island

Floyd H. Gilles, MD
Burton E. Green Professor, Pediatric Neuropathology
Department of Pathology
Neuropathology Section
Children's Hospital Los Angeles
Professor of Pathology (Neuropathology), Neurosurgery, and Neurology
University of Southern California,
School of Medicine
Los Angeles, California

Ignacio Gonzalez-Gomez, MD
Research Associate
Department of Pathology
Neuropathology Section
Childrens Hospital Los Angeles
Los Angeles, California

David R. Hinton, MD, FRCP(C)
Associate Professor
Pathology, Neurology & Neurological Surgery
University of Southern California,
School of Medicine
Neuropathologist,
University of Southern California
University Hospital
Los Angeles, California

Harold J. Hoffman, MD, BSC(Med), FRCS(C), FACS
Division of Neurosurgery
University of Toronto
Chief of Neurosurgery
The Hospital for Sick Children
Toronto, Ontario Canada

Mahlon D. Johnson, MD, PhD
Assistant Professor of Pathology
Vanderbilt University Medical School
Nashville, Tennessee

Gabor Jozsef, PhD
Assistant Professor
Department of Radiation Oncology
Kenneth Norris Jr. Cancer Hospital and Research Institute
University of Southern California,
School of Medicine
Los Angeles, California

Patrick J. Kelly, MD
Professor and Chairman
Department of Neurosurgery
New York University Medical Center
New York, New York

Daniel Lacerte, MD
Resident, Department of Neurosurgery
Montreal Neurological Hospital - Institute
Montreal, Quebec Canada

Edward R. Laws, Jr., MD, FACS
Professor of Neurosurgery
Professor of Medicine
University of Virginia
Health Sciences Center
Charlottesville, Virginia.

Mark E. Linskey, MD
Visiting Instructor
Department of Neurological Surgery
University of Pittsburgh
Pittsburgh, Pennsylvania
van Wagenen Fellow, American Association of Neurological Surgeons
Park Ridge, Illinois
International Exchange Fellow,
National Cancer Institute
Bethesda, Maryland and European Organization for the Research and Treatment of Cancer
Brussels, Belgium
Ludwig Institute for Cancer Research
University College London
London, England

M. Beatriz S. Lopes, MD
Assistant Professor of Pathology
Department of Pathology
(Neuropathology)
University of Virginia
School of Medicine
Charlottesville, Virginia

David N. Louis, MD
Assistant Professor of Pathology
Assistant Neuropathologist
Co-Director
Molecular Neuro-Oncology Laboratory
Neurosurgical Service and Department of Pathology (Neuropathology)
Massachusetts General Hospital and Harvard Medical School
Boston, Massachusetts

Gary Luxton, PhD
Associate Professor & Head of Division of Radiation Physics
Department of Radiation Oncology
Kenneth Norris Jr. Cancer Hospital and Research Institute
University of Southern California
School of Medicine
Los Angeles, California

Robert J. Maciunas, MD
Associate Professor of Neurological Surgery
Vanderbilt University Medical Center
Nashville, Tennessee

Marvin D. Nelson, Jr., MD
Department of Radiology
University of Southern California
School of Medicine and
Director of Neuro Imaging
Children's Hospital, Los Angeles
Los Angeles, California

André Olivier, MD, PhD
Chief, Department of Neurosurgery
Montreal Neurological Hospital - Institute
Chairman, Division of Neurosurgery
McGill University
Montreal, Quebec, Canada

Zbigniew Petrovich, MD
Albert Soiland Professor and
Chairman of Radiation Oncology
Kenneth Norris Jr. Cancer Hospital and Research Institute
University of Southern California, School of Medicine
Los Angeles, California

Leonard Petrus, MD
Neuroradiology Fellow
University of Southern California
School of Medicine
Los Angeles, California

Corey Raffel, MD, PhD
Associate Professor
Department of Neurological Surgery
Childrens Hospital, Los Angeles
University of Southern California
School of Medicine
Los Angeles, California

Michael L. Rodriguez, MBBS, FRCPA
Research Assistant Professor
University of Southern California
School of Medicine
Los Angeles, California

Michael Salcman, MD
Clinical Professor of Neurosurgery
George Washington University
Towson, Maryland

Bernd W. Scheithauer, MD
Consultant in Pathology
Department of Laboratory Medicine and Pathology
Mayo Clinic
Rochester, Minnesota

Hervey D. Segall, MD
Professor of Radiology
Director
Neuroradiology Section
University of Southern California
School of Medicine
Los Angeles, California

Bernd R. Seizinger, MD, PhD
Oncology Drug Discovery
Bristol-Myers Squibb Pharmaceutical Research Institute
Princeton, New Jersey

Scott R. VandenBerg, MD, PhD
Professor of Pathology and Neurological Surgery
Director of Neuropathology
University of Virginia
School of Medicine
Charlottesville, Virginia

Chi-Shin Zee, MD
Professor of Radiology
Neuroradiology Section
University of Southern California
School of Medicine
Los Angeles, California

AANS Publications Committee

The American Association of Neurological Surgeons is accredited by the Accreditation Council for Continuing Medical Education (CME) to sponsor continuing medical education for physicians.

The American Association of Neurological Surgeons designates the continuing medical education activity as 15 credit hours in Category I of the Physician's Recognition Award of the American Medical Association.

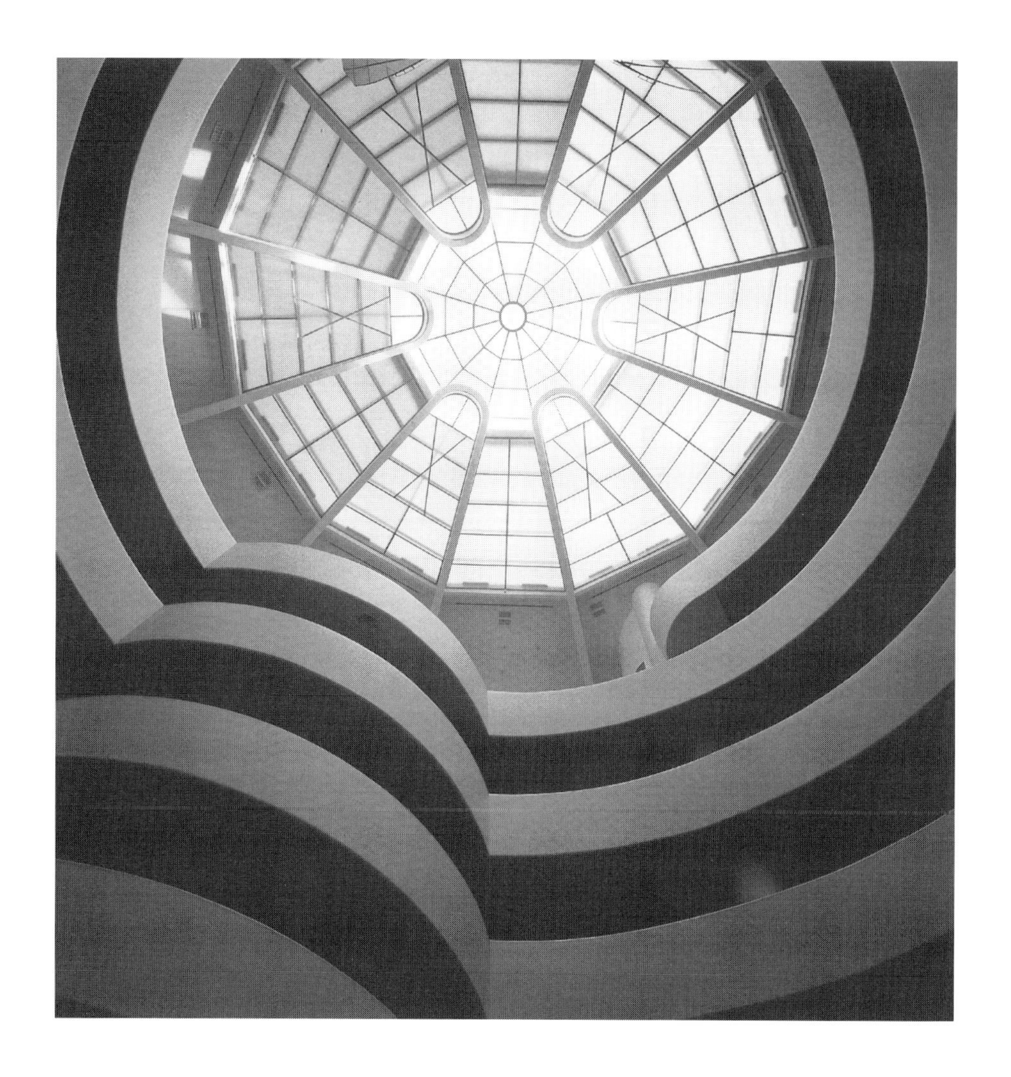

The Solomon R. Guggenheim Museum of Frank Lloyd Wright:
a view of the skylight of the rotunda.

A concept born in 1924, conceptually finalized in 1944, and practically realized in 1959.

As the third millennium approaches, it remains a monument to the avant garde and an inspirational testimony to foresight and human genius.

Preface

At the Edge of the Millennium: A Kaleidoscope Unfolds

"Cogito ergo sum"

—**René Descartes**
Discours de la Methode pour bien
Conduire la Raison, et Chercher la
Verite dans les Sciences.
Leyden, 1637 AD

Perhaps nowhere in the spectrum of human affliction is a histologically benign neoplasm more potentially devastating or refractory to satisfactory management or less predictable in clinical behavior and timing of impact on the person than in the human cerebrum.

The enigma of the "benign" intrinsic cerebral glioma continues to elude adequate comprehension; however, following a century of neurosurgical frustration, fruit is being born from multifactorial effort and data accumulation on many fronts. New disclosures from disciplines focused on glial development, molecular biology, molecular genetics, and pathology are augmenting rigorous data collection in clinical sectors; these have been bolstered by the new complex imaging methodologies, stereotactic, microsurgical, and radiotherapeutic advances, and consideration of expanded comprehensive data pools available during this computer age. A concatenation of bits of understanding is providing apertures of comprehension within this unsolvable puzzle, promising significant advances in our ability to offer patients more satisfactory management in the near future.

This monograph is designed to present a succinct and focused presentation of the major investigational areas which are representative of a bright kaleidoscope of activity and the "pieces of the puzzle" that are currently in position as the equation's solution is established and the circle is closed.

Additionally, practical guidelines for contemporary clinical management within the framework of currently available knowledge is presented. As the new millennium approaches, the fruit of progress is being born as a product of intellectual creativity, energy, and persistence.

Michael L. J. Apuzzo, MD
Los Angeles, California

CHAPTER 1

Evolving Dimensions at the Frontiers of Human Cerebral Surgery

Michael L. J. Apuzzo, MD

"Aut viam inveniam aut faciam" (Where there's a will, there's a way) — Roman proverb

Milieus and Developments

A combination of social, economic, and scientific developments have provided neurological surgeons with a creative and unusually robust quarter-century. As we approach the third millennium, a concatenation of developments have initiated unusual highs and lows within the human element and key developments within the scientific sector. These developments have been far-reaching in terms of changing the attitude of man toward his nature, environment, and his own personal capabilities for achievement within dimensions of science. At no time was this more strikingly apparent than in the 1976 Mars Expedition, when robotic vehicles landed on the Martian surface and the planet's landscape was appreciated in the nearest sense as the soil of the surface was analyzed and experienced by man-made machines.

The spectacular achievement in robotics, signal transmission, and signal processing that was apparent in the first pictures transmitted to the Jet Propulsion Laboratory in Pasadena, California, from the Martian surface gave evidence of striking capability in terms of the computer analysis and signal amplification competency that were developed during this period (Figure 1). This was a robust period in the development of the computer as an essen-

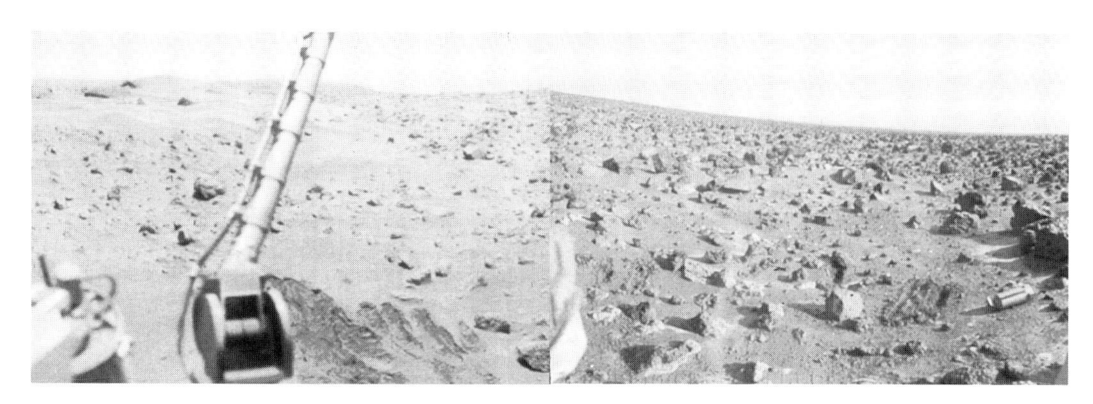

Figure 1: Images transmitted from the surface of the planet Mars by the Viking Lander. The robotic arm for soil sampling methodology is seen to the left.

tial and very viable tool in man's accomplishments. Achievements in manned space flight were no less spectacular, with developments in this sector permeating science and humanity with a "can-do" attitude that promoted advancements in other areas.

The period from 1965 to 1990 showed very dramatic changes in the discipline of neurological surgery, changes and promises that were documented in the monograph *Neurosurgery of the Third Millennium*, published in 1992.[4,5,17] In this monograph, the developmental trends in the technical neurosurgical discipline were noted. These included: 1) refinement of preoperative definition of structural substrate, 2) minimization of operative corridors, 3) reduction of operative trauma, 4) increased effectiveness at the target site, and 5) incorporation of improved technical adjuvants as physical tools.

Concurrently, historical analysis indicates that neurological surgery has enjoyed a recent series of highly productive operative eras. These may be appreciated as an initial period from 1965 to 1985, in which *surgery of the cisterns and perineural areas* was the primary area of focus, with the introduction of the operating microscope, related operative techniques, and increased diagnostic capability with advanced image processing and the availability of computed tomography (CT), magnetic resonance imaging (MRI), and high-resolution angiography of various forms. The next period, from 1986 to 1994, was a time when *surgery of the cranial base* and related structures received major attention. Various windows and new dimensions of knowledge as well as key early developments within the sectors of neuroscience point to the current emergence of a new era in which *surgery within the structure of the nervous system and the neuraxis* will be the primary area of targeted interest from 1995 through and beyond the year 2000. This being the case, the surgery and management of the intrinsic benign glioma deserve special attention. This will be an important period, with the development of new perspectives and capabilities that will lead us into a period of *advanced surgery of the human cerebrum*.

A perspective of the opportunities for ultimately shaping the elements and approaches to the discipline of advanced cerebral surgery may be gained by considering a number of current, innovative concepts as they will impact in a concatenation of developments and events to add energy and potential to the possibilities and capabilities for surgery within the human brain. These include: 1) imaging, sensors, and visualization; 2) localization and navigation within the cerebral content; 3) refined capabilities for target point action; and 4) concepts related to the development of sophisticated operative venues.

Cerebral Imaging, Sensors, and Visualization

Striking advances have been made in biomedical imaging from the perspective of sophisticated signal generation and signal processing to define structural elements of the neural complex by CT, MRI, and ultrasound. Capabilities for functional definition are now possible through special forms of MRI, positron emission tomography (PET), and magnetoencephalographic and optical imaging.

Structural Definition

From the viewpoint of structural definition, it is obvious that hundreds of thousands of data points may be combined to develop three-dimensional concepts of the cranium-brain composite with strikingly refined definition of gyral-sulcal patterns, ventricular contours, and even components related to nuclear groups within the brain substance.[13] The generation of three-dimensional forms and composites allows for rehearsal of operative procedures within the cranium exclusive of the in vivo situation (Figure 2).

Functional Definition

The concept of functional imaging provides more intellectual excitement and stimulates the imagination as one considers the possibilities of superimposing a strict functional definition of cerebral processes upon a refined structural foundation. We are now entering a continuum of realizing this refinement. The July 30 1993, edition of *Science* considered the major scientific innovation of 1993[2,3,10,20] to be medical

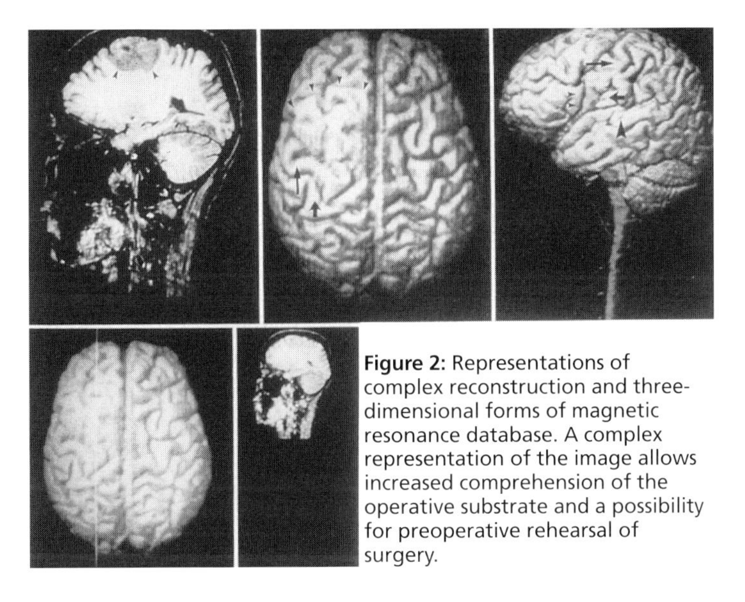

Figure 2: Representations of complex reconstruction and three-dimensional forms of magnetic resonance database. A complex representation of the image allows increased comprehension of the operative substrate and a possibility for preoperative rehearsal of surgery.

imaging with particular attention being devoted to concepts of *echo-planar MRI,* imaging in a fraction of a second. This MRI methodology requires only one nuclear spin excitation per image and has the capability for mapping an organ blood pool, organ perfusion, blood flow dynamics, and cerebrospinal fluid dynamics. Given changes in these parameters with function, the early stages of the development of a science for precise measurement of both physiological and cognitive functions of the brain are established. The early development of this concept was presented in *Science* by Belliveau et al,[8] in which the functional mapping of the human visual cortex by MRI was eloquently presented.

Magnetic source imaging allows the noninvasive recording of magnetic field changes induced by peripheral stimulation from the cerebral cortical region.[9,11,14,19] Multichanneled recording devices allow the measurement of changes in magnetic flux on the cortical surface related to either peripheral stimulation or generation of fields by activities within the cortical regions (Figures 3 and 4). This methodology allows the physiological determination of cortical regions that may then secondarily be superimposed on three-dimensional CT or MRI representations of structural contours.

The concept of *optical imaging* requires critical exposure. This imaging method allows the identification of functional regions based on optical interpretation of changes in tissue. This technique is thought to be based on a number of possible physiological changes in the region, which include: 1) the flow of ionic currents, 2) oxygen delivery, 3) blood volume changes for potassium accumulation, and 4) glial swelling. The methodology was reported by Haglund et al[12] in 1992. The technique was utilized to demonstrate clearly the presence of epileptiform activities and changes in the human cerebral cortex as well as the presence of activity within functional area in the exposed cortex.

The importance of the imaging capabilities that are evolving, particularly from a standpoint of functional reference, should be obvious to all who are involved in surgery in and around the brain, and has striking significance for the future of transcerebral and intracerebral operations and corridors.

Cerebral Navigation and Localization

The concepts of localization and navigation have been greatly facilitated by the wedding of imaging methods to stereotactic instrumentation during the course of the past 15 years. The evolution of stereotaxy in terms of structural navigation has been expanded beyond the platform of linked systems using base rings to nonlinked systems, which currently include various forms of digitizers that allow for navigation

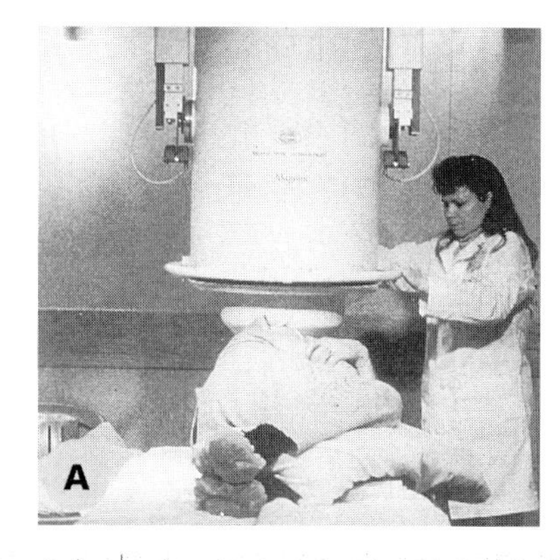

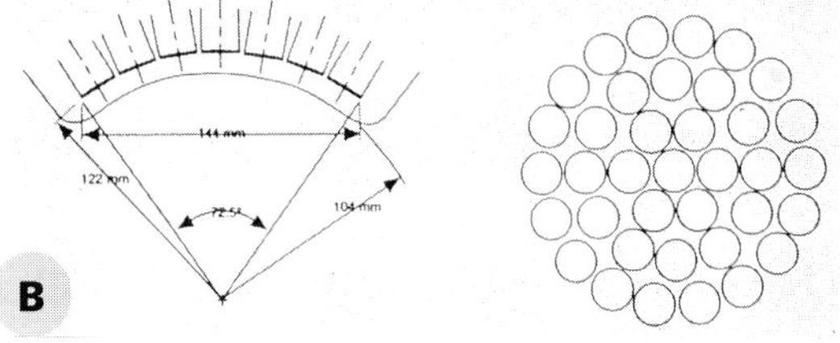

Figure 3: A) Photograph showing a technician operating a scanner array over a lateral patient cranium. **B)** Representation of multiple source recorders for magnetic source imaging.

within the brain. These approaches in association with methods of "mapping" for functional guidance in a pre-procedural setting include utilization of grids, MRI, magnetoencephalographic imaging, and evoked response testing. Intraoperatively, evoked response testing and optical imaging can be and are being used as functional adjuvants for localization.

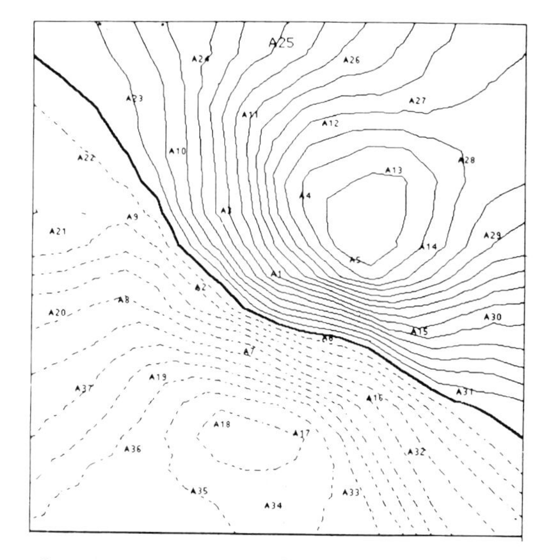

Figure 4: Representation of magnetic source gradients demonstrating magnetic field flux from cortical regions generated by peripheral stimulation.

Stereotaxy

The stereotactic era employing imaging-directed techniques has evolved rapidly, especially during the past decade. Initially, stereotaxy was a "*point*"-oriented method in which a point was approached with minimal consideration of structures in the line of cerebral transit. The capability for developing detailed three-dimensional images and using these images as a whole in a navigational substrate has expanded stereotaxy into what might be considered the "*volume*"-oriented mode. This has been eloquently discussed and developed by Morita and Kelly[16] originally in Buffalo, New York, then in Rochester, Minnesota; multiple imaging plane slices were obtained in "line of site" and "line of transit" to develop a regional corridor locked into a stereotactic space and then utilized as a reference guide for resection of intracerebral lesions.

The concept of *nonlinkage stereotaxy* was imaginatively presented in 1986 by Roberts and a group at Lebanon, New Hampshire.[18] They used a sound-based system in which an amalgam was effected with the patient's cranium, the operating microscope, and brain images so that images could be projected through an operating microscope that had a reference point to the

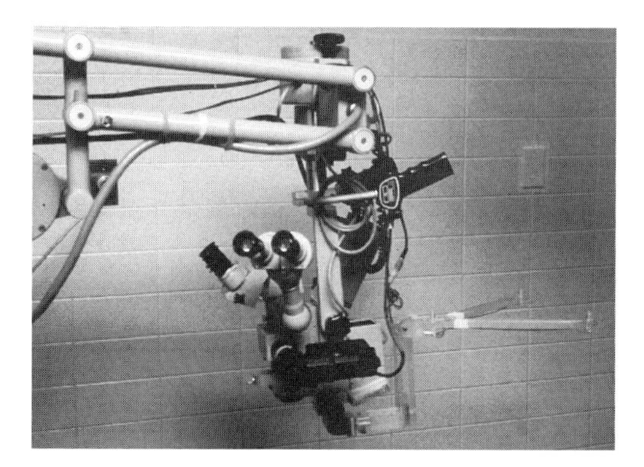

Figure 5: An operating microscope used in the non-linked system described by Roberts et al.[18] Note the spark gap array microscope attachment for orientation of the plane of microscope position with respect to microphones in the operating room ceiling. Photograph courtesy of David Roberts.

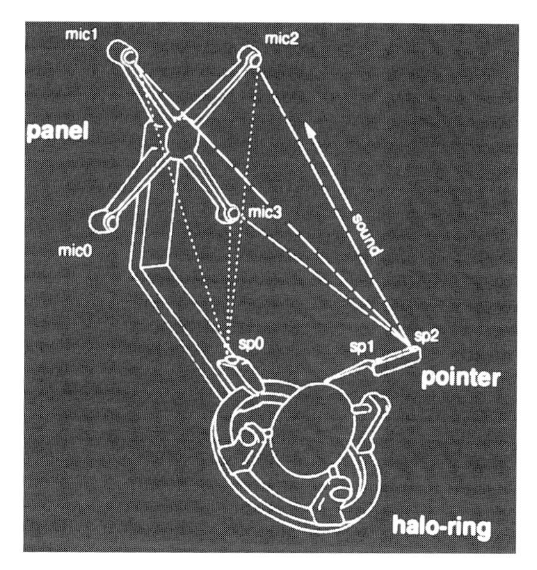

Figure 6: Schematic representation of forceps-based sound orienting system developed in Basel, Switzerland, for intracranial localization.

focal plane of the microscope at a given time (Figure 5). The so-called "nonlinkage system" was achieved by the utilization of fiducials on the patient's scalp, which were used as a reference point for images, and a series of spark gaps in the single plane that were placed on the operating microscope. An amalgam was made between images, the patient's cranium, the microscope, and the focal plane via a computer system in which the location of the microscope position was recorded by spark gap sounds and microphones in the ceiling of the operating room. This innovative concept was employed to orient the surgeon using the microscope and to produce a visual reference point for intracerebral resection of glial tumors and intracerebral orientation in a system of stereotactic space in which the operating room became, in fact, a stereotactic instrument.

Three-dimensional digitizers were introduced in the later portion of the 1980s. Watanabe and his group[22,23] from the University of Tokyo presented their concept of the three-dimensional digitizer (the neuronavigator). In essence, this system used an articulated arm with a pointer that was oriented in space in relation to the patient's head; the point of the wand provided a localization factor that could be related to images that were secondarily projected on a screen. A number of variations on this theme have been presented, one of the more elegant of which was that of Reinhardt and the group in Basel, Switzerland (Figures 6 and 7). This particular system used sonic digitizers to achieve a point of reference with a forceps from which the surgeon could precisely localize his position intracranially in relation to previously obtained images. Currently, optical and other methods related to a forceps-type base are also under development.[15]

The capability for intracranial navigation and localization is critical. It is very apparent that the amalgam of structural and functional

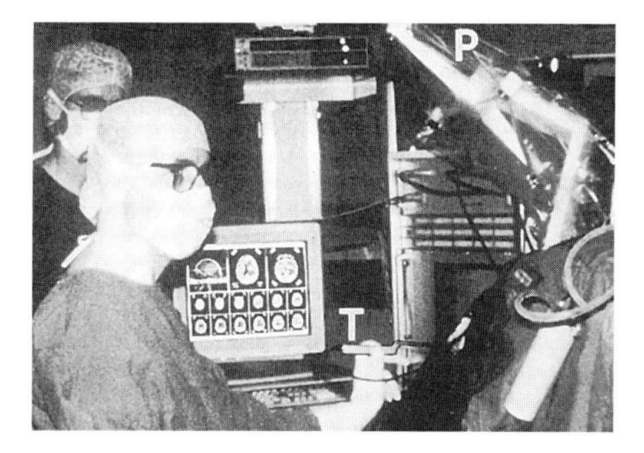

Figure 7: Forceps-based orientation system in use in the Swiss operating room setting. Note the screen panel providing images for localization at the forceps tip site (T).

imaging and ability to navigate and to localize within this defined framework is important for the entire equation of increased sophistication of cerebral surgery.

Target Point Action

Of critical importance in consideration of the new dimensions in cerebral surgery is the concept of action at the target point. This may be divided into two major subsections: *ablation* and *functional restoration*. Ablation methods may be considered as comprising microdissection techniques and application of high-energy forms to achieve an end, and functional restoration as utilizing conceptually autografts, fetal grafts, or genetic molecules and genetically altered cells—the so-called "molecular neurosurgery."

Ablation

The ablative techniques of *microdissection* are well established and need little comment. The application of *high-energy forms* is a more critical and evolving field. The concept of *stereotactic radiosurgery* was introduced by Leksell in the 1950s; however, it is perhaps of benefit to categorize this concept under the rubric of "application of high energy forms" for ablation within the nervous system. High-energy forms include particle radiation and the various components of the electromagnetic spectrum.

Particle radiation requires complex units for delivery (Figure 8); proliferation of these units is currently prohibited because of expense. However, the concept of utilizing these high-energy particles is attractive because of the ability to model and contour the radiation delivery precisely to a lesion's configuration through the application of filters and taking advantage of the Bragg peak absorption character of the energy. A relatively large number of particles are available for such treatments, with given dose distribution advantages and biological effect at the target (Figure 9).

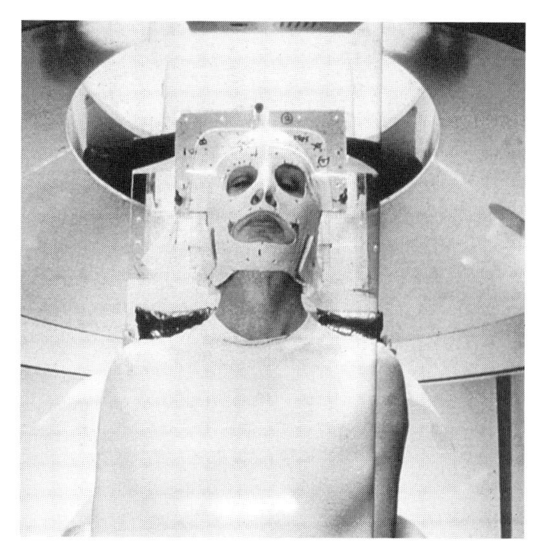

Figure 8: Patient undergoing heavy-particle radiation treatment at the Lawrence Berkeley Laboratories in Berkeley, California.

The *conventional (photon) forms* of stereotactic radiosurgery are delivered by either fixed beam collimator or rotational systems. The current model of the Leksell gamma unit represents the epitome of the *fixed collimator system* with 201 cobalt-60 sources in individual collimators wedded to an arc-centered frame system and augmented by a sophisticated software package that allows the delivery of multiple "shots" to achieve optimum isodose configurations in respect to neural elements that require preservation (Figure 10).

The *dynamic devices* utilize standard hospital-based linear accelerators and are predicated on the rotational concepts of the couch and gantry, with variation of collimator size (Figure 11). Such systems require sophisticated support from radiation physics personnel within house; however, appropriate software packages are being developed to mitigate the need for intellectual resources of a high order to facilitate safe treatment.

Medical lasers represent a high-energy form; however, limitation in wavelength availability and cost has hampered the use of these devices in the mode that would seem to be optimum for the basic concept. The *free-electron laser* represents a device that may provide neurosurgery with an element of substance in pressing the envelope of laser utilization within the nervous system. The *free-electron laser* is based on a concept in which electrons are accelerated through multiple magnetic fields. As the electron is accelerated, it is possible to vary the magnetic field strength, thus "wiggling" the electron in its course of acceleration. This process creates monochromatic light in coherent form (i.e.,

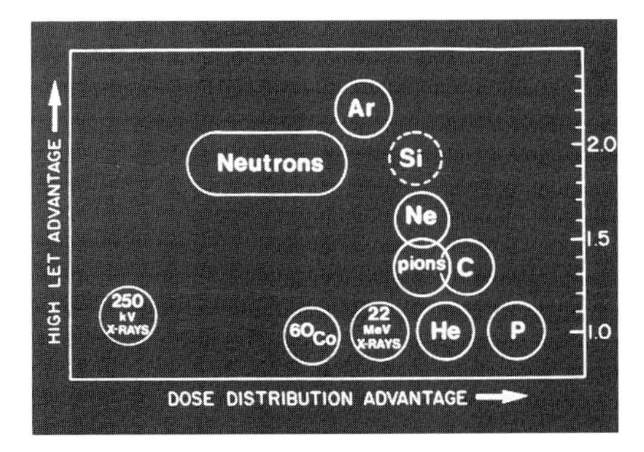

Figure 9: Representation of particle schema with dose distribution and biological advantage depicted for various available heavy particles.

laser energy). The variation in magnetic field produces various wavelengths of energy; therefore, a large portion of the electromagnetic spectrum may be reproduced, thus creating what is, in fact, a tunable laser over many wavelengths. The result is a laser of multiple frequencies that can produce ultra-short pulses at ultrahigh intensity—desirable features for a surgical laser. Such devices are currently quite substantial in size and expense; however, progress in biomedical engineering has resulted in reducing the size and expense of such instruments, making more practical their potential application within neurosurgery (Figure 12).

Photodynamic therapy, the utilization of intravascular dyes that have an affinity for certain lesions and the subsequent activation of these dyes within the lesions, presents a conceptually promising technique for the treatment of intracerebral processes, both neoplastic and infective. Problems relate to the purity of dye, biochemical affinity of dye for the process at hand, and the potential complicating effect of photosensitization of the host with the intravenous injection of the dye. The use of new dyes that create a better "capture net" with the potential utilization of the free-electron laser and its spectrum of laser energies provides a promising combination for action at the target point for ablative purposes. The possibility exists that a coherent light that could act as an activating energy source can be achieved with a very low coefficient of absorption, with the result that absorption within normal brain tissues would be minimal. However, at the capture point within the net of dye, the coefficient absorption could be tuned, thus exacerbating the target effect.

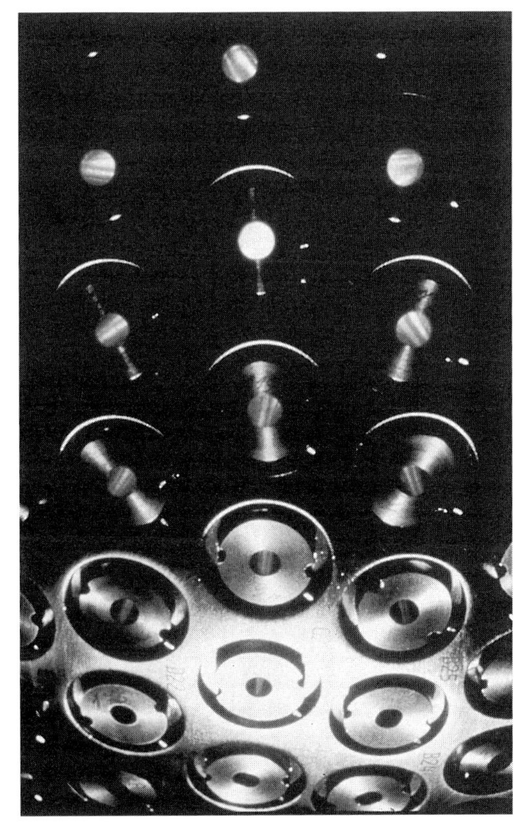

Figure 10: Magnified view of the ports of a collimator helmet of the Leksell gamma unit. These ports of the carefully oriented helmet are the entry points for gamma source radiation and direct its convergence to the target region.

It is possible to visualize that a combination of stereotactic methods, high-energy sources such as the free-electron laser, and photodynamic dye methodology could be combined to produce a sophisticated ablative source that would allow for treatment without craniotomy.

Functional Restoration

The concept of functional restoration within the nervous system is a reality that may be achieved within the course of the next few decades. Regeneration and restoration of function within the nervous system have attracted various levels of enthusiasm over a 100-year pe-

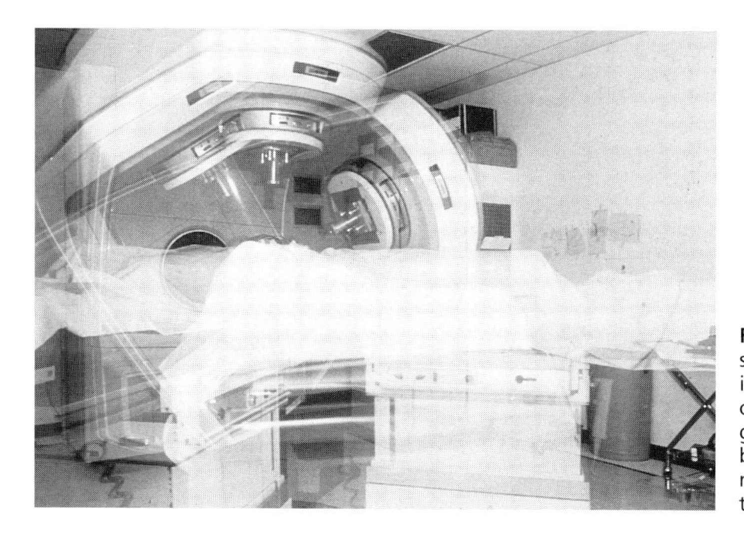

Figure 11: Dynamic single-source stereotactic radiosurgical unit taking advantage of the rotational components of the couch and gantry to provide an infinite number of entry points over the cranium with beam convergence at the target site.

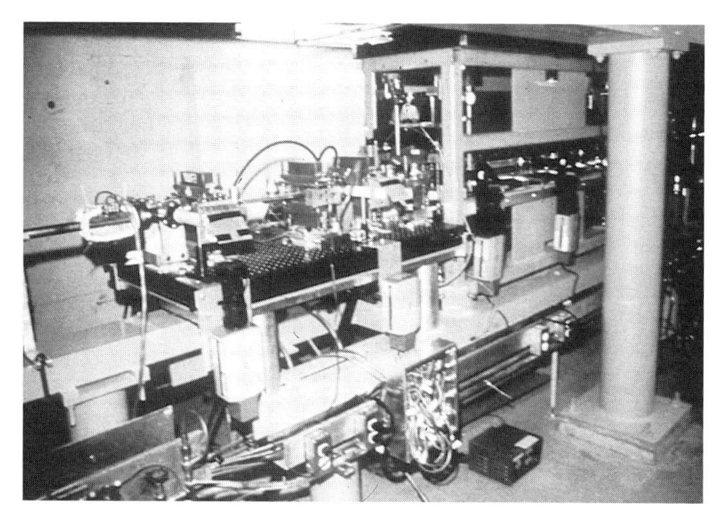

Figure 12: A free electron laser unit is shown in operation at Stanford University.

riod. The use of *autografts* has encouraged a recent explosion of investigative effort and has fueled interest in the concept.[1,7] The development of the term *"molecular or cellular neurosurgery"* during the course of the past 5 years represents the surgical introduction of *genetic information or genetically modified cells* for functional augmentation and restoration within the nervous system.[21] In addition, the concept of cellular or molecular neurosurgery could also be used for ablation (Figure 13). This concept represents a primary ongoing research effort in many sectors of the globe, and it is apparent that utilization of vectors or cells that are genetically determined will be an important element of human cerebral surgery in the future. The application of molecular neurosurgery for the management of brain tumors has been investigated over a 2- to 3-year period in the laboratory and a highly controlled clinical setting. Practical problems with this technique are being addressed, with the current belief that this is an important and very viable research area.

Operative Venue

Considering the developments in imaging, stereotactic procedures, and microsurgery as well as the arrival of the computer as a neurosurgical tool, the current operative venues will be largely inadequate to optimally apply the technology that is emerging for the new concepts in cerebral surgery. At the University of Southern California (USC) it was our belief that

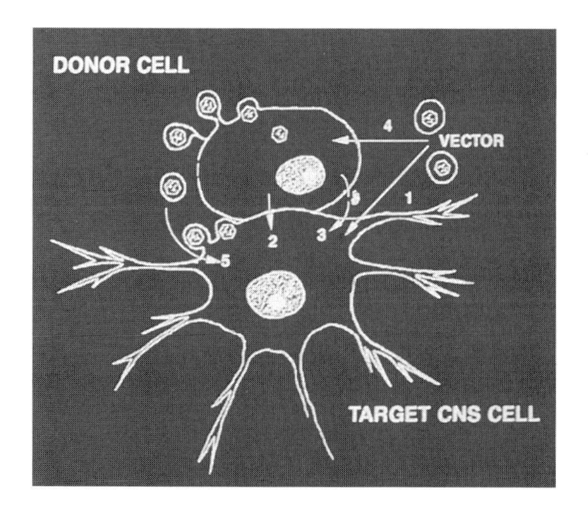

Figure 13: Representation of potential utilization of genetically engineered principles for engineering cellular action within the central nervous system (CNS).

a dedicated self-contained operating suite that allowed for full computer support, visualization packages, and integration of all micro-operative and stereo-operative methodologies was a necessary element in the development of neurosurgery for the 21st century. The concept was conceived in 1978 and reached physical fruition in 1992.[6] This idea was supported by expertise from the Jet Propulsion Laboratory (a subsidiary of the National Aeronautics and Space Administration) and the California Institute of Technology as well as the School of Cinema which provided practical knowledge essential in the development of the operating site. The program was developed with the USC School of Engineering, Computer Science, and Electrical Engineering as well as the School of Medicine with its Department of Neurological Surgery and Medical Imaging and the School of Cinema with support from its Television Laboratory.

Modern neurosurgery has grown beyond the limited confines of the medical school; we believe that it requires the support of science, engineering, and technical individuals from both the general university and the industrial sector. Because of this, a complex program was developed entitled "New Windows on the Human Brain" in which studies for data acquisition, signal and image processing, and visualization were simultaneously undertaken with the direction of all members of the research team as noted (Figure 14).

The concept of *visualization,* or the visual presentation of mental and concrete images, was introduced as an important element of the new operative venue, taking full advantage of trends in computer graphics, image processing, computers, video displays, and software. The *practical objectives of design* of the visualization system within the operating venue were: 1) realization of the stereotactic point and volume planning and procedure; 2) realization of microstereotactic volume planning and procedure; 3) a nonlinkage microscopic image integration; 4) complete graphics rehearsal of stereotactic and microscopic procedures; 5) an operative team integration through presentation of im-

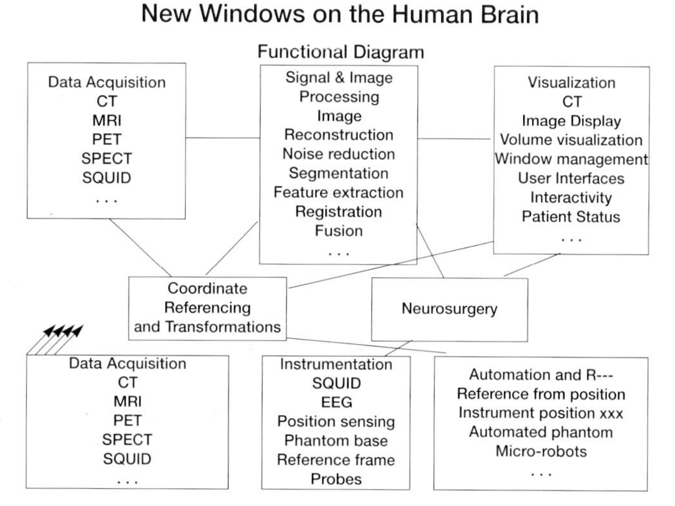

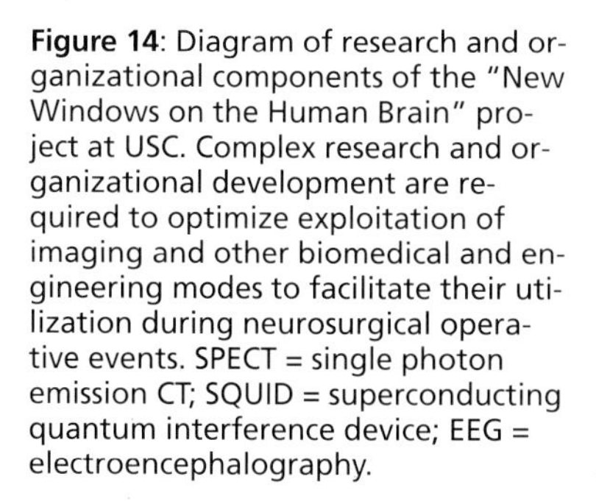
Figure 14: Diagram of research and organizational components of the "New Windows on the Human Brain" project at USC. Complex research and organizational development are required to optimize exploitation of imaging and other biomedical and engineering modes to facilitate their utilization during neurosurgical operative events. SPECT = single photon emission CT; SQUID = superconducting quantum interference device; EEG = electroencephalography.

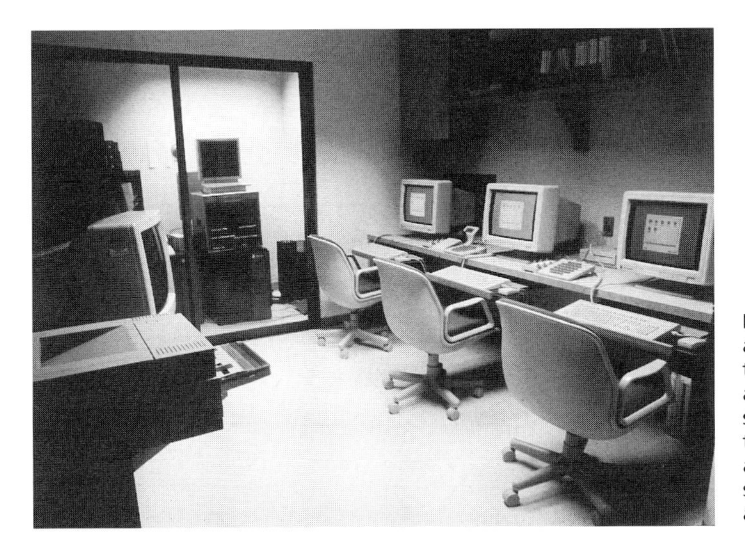

Figure 15: The neurosurgical visualization/rehearsal laboratory at the USC University Hospital. The area is used as a computer resource for data storage, manipulation, and processing. Full rehearsal and graphics capabilities are present within the three workstation areas to the right.

ages within the operative venue; 6) display of reference data and retrieval in the presentation of scientific and practical information for the performance of any given procedure; 7) real-time presentation of physiological monitoring parameters throughout the operating room; 8) real-time presentation of operative structural staging; 9) multiparameter recording of all operative events; 10) complete storage of a nursing catalog of the individual case and surgeon's setup, instrumentation, and idiosyncratic preferences; and 11) the enhancement of the educational experience and the database.

The *operative venue* was physically developed with a *visualization/rehearsal laboratory* that was immediately adjacent to but separate from the operating room (Figure 15). This area is electronically in concert with imaging base instrumentation and the *operating room.* It is a locale for data storage and for rehearsal and graphic development as well as software development to support the operating room itself. It is the site for remote observation of operative procedures and, in fact, acts as a neurosurgical graphics laboratory.

The operating room measures in excess of 700 sq ft and is virtually totally self-contained (Figure 16). The operating microscope and track are overhead. Multiple cabinetry spaces are present. A flexible video wall comprises six to seven large monitors, two recording devices, and a control console for good viewing by all members of the operative team (Figure 17). In addition, two 35-in. monitors are suspended diagonally at either end of the room and one other portable monitor is available for presentation of visual data. To optimize floor transit, all lines are ceiling-suspended. The room is designed to allow for the visualization presentation over two major walls and work in progress utilizing the other two major walls.

Computer support and visualization presentation is dependent upon development of complex software. Therefore, the major effort following the physical installation of elements of the system after architectural design discussions related to software development and has proved to be one of the most difficult and costly components of the enterprise. Currently the visualization system and operative integration functions are designed for: 1) multidimensional presentation of the micro-operative field, imaging data, patient physiological parameters, and an atlas of technical reference data; 2) the capability for the complex recording of all that has been noted; 3) stereotactic data processing and simulation; 4) complex imaging, three-dimensional data presentation; and 5) organization sensitive to surgeon preference and case requirements.

Currently evolving *software development* includes: 1) microscope tracking and image and atlas integration into heads up and general displays; 2) complete and flexible image fusion of CT, MRI, digital subtraction angiography, PET, and magnetic encephalography; 3) full instrumentation graphics integration; 4) real-time

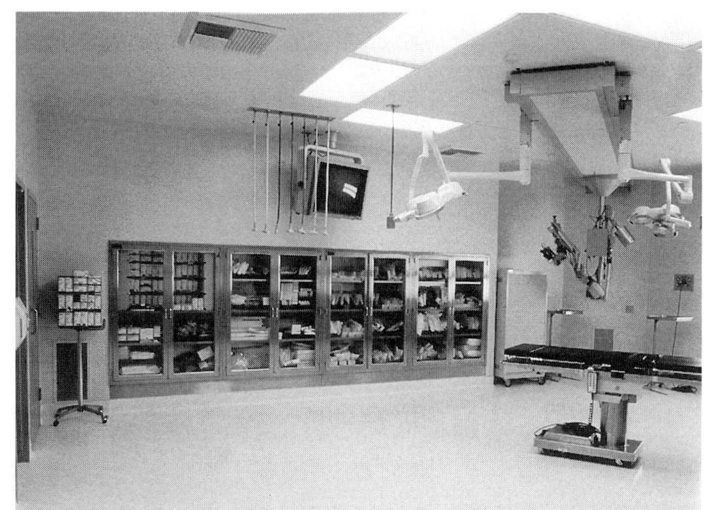

A

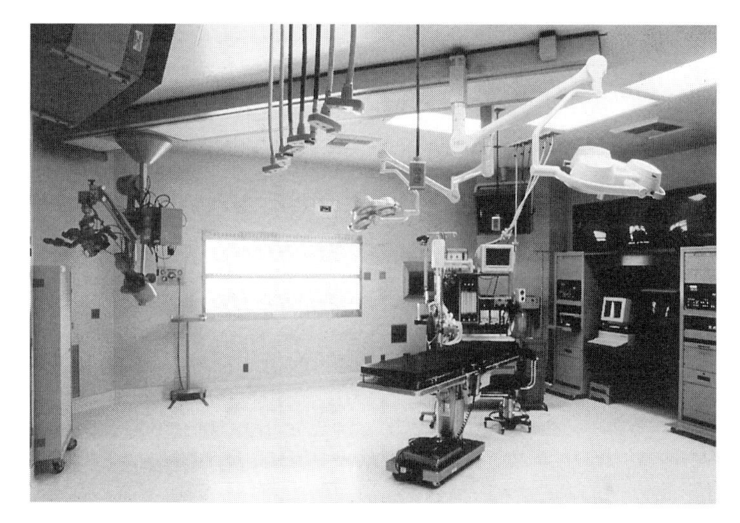

B

Figure 16: A) View from the entry door of the microstereotactic operating theater. The unit is completely self-contained with computer support for performing both stereotactic and microsurgical procedures. The operating room space is approximately 700 sq ft with care taken to optimize transit within the area by overhead positioning of the microscope and power and support conduits. **B)** A second, angular view of operating room area. Note the video wall to the right.

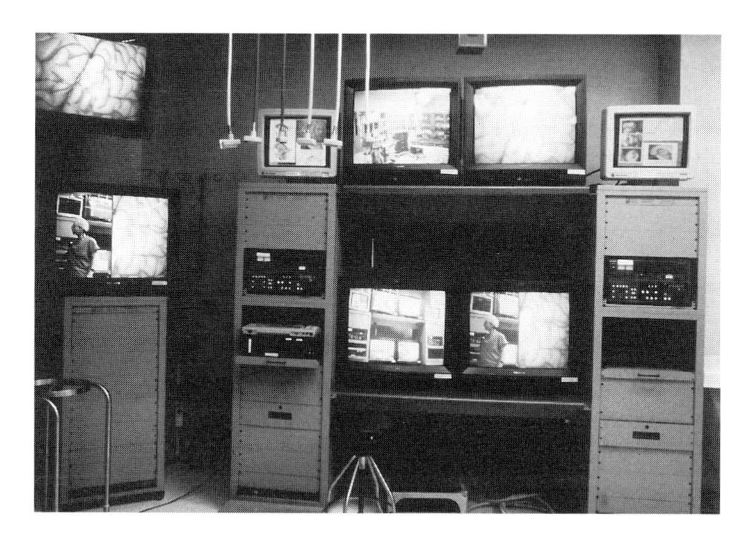

Figure 17: A multiple compartmentalized video wall offering several screens for large image reproduction and complex recording of operative events. Two 35-in. overhead monitors and one 33-in. portable monitor augment this instrument panel. All components of the system are interfaced and related to visualization laboratory facility features.

sensor integration; 5) full microsurgical preoperative simulation; and 6) full intraoperative stereotactic simulation.

The requirements of software development for support of the complex system and needs of a highly sophisticated and futuristic neurosurgical operating venue are enormous. This is compounded by the potential integration of sensory emergence to employ concepts of virtual reality or cyberspace for the surgeon in the appreciation of individual patient anatomy and pathological distortions.

Conclusions

The rapid evolution of stimulating new dimensions at the frontiers of the discipline of human cerebral surgery is real. Its frontiers provide an exciting promise for the future. Applications of imaging, sensors, visualization, localization and navigation, complex target point action, and expansion of the idea of the operative venue all provide a concatenation of windows of development and opportunity that will make surgery of the human cerebrum one of medicine's and surgery's most exciting endeavors for the 21st century.

The application of all of these concepts to the treatment of benign cerebral glioma is not only important but key as one approaches the current body of knowledge in relation to this topic.

References

1. Ahlskog JE: Cerebral transplantation for Parkinson's disease: current progress and future prospects. **Mayo Clin Proc 68:**578-591, 1993
2. Alper J: Echo-planar MRI: learning to read minds. **Science 261(5121):**556, 1993
3. Alper J: EEG + MRI: a sum greater than the parts. **Science 261(5121):**559, 1993
4. Apuzzo MLJ (ed): **Neurosurgery for the Third Millennium. Neurosurgical Topics Series.** Park Ridge, Ill: American Association of Neurological Surgeons, 1992, 211 pp
5. Apuzzo MLJ, Chin LS, Chen T, et al: Neurosurgery: a futuristic prospectus, in Apuzzo MLJ (ed): **Neurosurgery for the Third Millennium. Neurosurgical Topics Series.** Park Ridge, Ill: American Association of Neurological Surgeons, 1992, pp 11-23
6. Apuzzo MLJ, Weinberg RA: Architecture and functional design of advanced neurosurgical operating environments. **Neurosurgery 33:**663-673, 1993
7. Bakay RAE, Allen GS, Apuzzo M, et al: Preliminary report on adrenal medullary grafting from the American Association of Neurological Surgeons graft project. **Prog Brain Res 82:**603-610, 1990
8. Belliveau JW, Kennedy DN, McKinstry RC, et al: Functional mapping of the human visual cortex by magnetic resonance imaging. **Science 254:**716-719, 1991
9. Benzel EC, Lewine JD, Bucholz RD, et al: Magnetic source imaging: a review of the Magnes system of biomagnetic technologies incorporated. **Neurosurgery 33:**252-259, 1993
10. Crease RP: Biomedicine in the age of imaging. **Science 261(5121):**554, 557-558, 561, 1993
11. Gallen CC, Sobel DF, Waltz T, et al: Noninvasive presurgical neuromagnetic mapping of somatosensory cortex. **Neurosurgery 33:**260-268, 1993
12. Haglund MM, Ojemann GA, Hochman DW: Optical imaging of epileptiform and functional activity in human cerebral cortex. **Nature 358:**668-671, 1992 (Letter)
13. Hu XP, Tan KK, Levin DN, et al: Three-dimensional magnetic resonance images of the brain: application to neurosurgical planning. **J Neurosurg 72:**433-440, 1990
14. Kamada K, Takeuchi F, Kuriki S, et al: Functional neurosurgical simulation with brain surface magnetic resonance images and magnetoencephalography. **Neurosurgery 33:**269-273, 1993
15. Koivukangas J, Louhisalmi Y, Alakuijala J, et al: Ultrasound-controlled neuronavigator-guided brain surgery. **J Neurosurg 79:**36-42, 1993
16. Morita A, Kelly PJ: Resection of intraventricular tumors via a computer-assisted volumetric stereotactic approach. **Neurosurgery 32:**920-927, 1993
17. Rabb C, Levy M, Couldwell WT, et al: Protection and retrieval of the neuronal pool during ischemia, trauma, and surgery, in Apuzzo MLJ (ed): **Neurosurgery for the Third Millennium. Neurosurgical Topics Series.** Park Ridge, Ill: American Association of Neurological Surgeons, 1992, pp 117-147
18. Roberts DW, Strohbehn JW, Hatch JF, et al: A frameless stereotaxic integration of computerized tomographic imaging and the operating microscope. **J Neurosurg 65:**545-549, 1986
19. Sobel DF, Gallen CC, Schwartz BJ, et al: Locating the central sulcus: comparison of MR anatomic and magnetoencephalographic functional methods. **AJNR 14:**915-925, 1993
20. Stehling MK, Turner R, Mansfield P: Echo-planar imaging: magnetic resonance imaging in a fraction of a second. **Science 254:**43-50, 1991
21. Suhr ST, Gage FH: Gene therapy for neurologic disease. **Arch Neurol 50:**1252-1268, 1993
22. Watanabe E, Mayanagi Y, Kosugi Y, et al: Open surgery assisted by the neuronavigator, a stereotactic, articulated, sensitive arm. **Neurosurgery 28:** 792-800, 1991
23. Watanabe E, Watanabe T, Manaka S, et al: Three-dimensional digitizer (neuronavigator): new equipment for computed tomography-guided stereotaxic surgery. **Surg Neurol** **27:**543-547, 1987

CHAPTER 2

The Developmental Biology of Glial Cells and Its Relation to the Study of Glioma Biology

Mark E. Linskey, MD

We are fortunate to be witnessing a veritable explosion in our understanding of the developmental biology of glial cells over the last 10 years. Renewed interest and progress in this field is very timely when one considers that, despite continued advances in surgical tools and techniques, neuroimaging, and radiation technology, our clinical ability to control or cure gliomas has remained relatively static over the last 15 years.

Most malignant gliomas are not surgically curable due to their diffusely infiltrative nature and occasional multicentricity, while even the subset of "benign" or "low-grade" gliomas that are not diffusely infiltrative may not be amenable to surgical excision due to critical location. Unfortunately, the only nonsurgical treatment modalities currently available involve various forms of radiotherapy and/or chemotherapy. Both of these modalities solely exploit a difference in proliferation rate between tumor and normal cells for their effectiveness. As a result, their therapeutic index (the ratio of effectiveness to treatment-limiting toxicity) is low, and improvement in survival is often achieved at the expense of distressing and sometimes dehumanizing central nervous system (CNS) toxicity.

Since neoplasia tends to "pervert" or deregulate pre-existing mature as well as dormant developmental cellular mechanisms as a way of tumor initiation and maintaining preferential tumor growth, the simultaneous study of normal glial neurobiology and glioma biology offers the advantage that discoveries in one field should lead to discoveries in the parallel field (and vice versa). We can only hope that a more in-depth understanding of the cellular and molecular biology of glial cells will lead to new "molecular targets" and more selective strategies for treating patients with gliomas.

The goals of this chapter are: **1**) To trace the early history of the study of glial differentiation; **2**) to introduce the modern cell biology and molecular biology tools now available, which continue to lead to advances in the field; **3**) to describe the individual glial cell types currently distinguishable in the CNS and to enumerate their distinguishing features; **4**) to outline our current understanding of the progression and control of gliogenesis, stressing the role of cell signaling via both cell-cell contact and diffusable signaling molecules as well as the intracellular signal transduction pathways associated with these processes; **5**) to discuss the implications of findings from the study of gliogenesis for the study of neuro-oncology; and **6**) to point out ways that the study of glioma biology can be improved through the application of developmental glial biology principles and techniques.

In-depth description and discussion of these same molecules and processes as they relate to the parallel field of glioma biology can be found in Chapters 8 ("Growth Factors and Proliferation Potential") and 9 ("Molecular Genetics"). Maximum benefit can best be achieved by reading these three chapters as a group. Further information on the developmental biology of glial cells can be obtained by referring to one or more recent reviews on the subject.[48,104,165,179,205,228,273,274]

Descriptive Morphology and Histology: Initial Inroads

Early studies of neuroembryology and gliogenesis were based almost exclusively on light microscopic examination of organs and cells of whole embryos and tissue sections of embryonic CNS. Specimens from many different animals could be serially examined at successive stages all the way through maturity. New stains were developed to accentuate different cytological organelles and to visualize the intricately entwined cell processes within the neuropil, allowing better distinctions between cell types. These techniques established the basic structural progression of CNS development.

CNS Organogenesis

CNS organogenesis begins with the mesodermally derived notochord inducing the overlying ectoderm to form neuroectoderm. These cells respond by forming taller columnar epithelium and then involuting along a longitudinal axis to form the neural tube. This "neurulation" begins at two points—the cervical-hindbrain junction and the midbrain-forebrain junction—and then continues in both rostral and caudal directions. The dorsal edges of the neurulating tube break away from the fusion line to form the neural crest, which will ultimately give rise to the peripheral nervous system (including contributions to both the autonomic and somatic nervous system), the enteric nervous system, several cranial nerves, portions of the branchial arches, and melanocytes. Up to the point of closure of the neural tube, there do not appear to be any differences between individual neuroectodermal cells. It is at the point of closure that neuroectodermal cells begin to differentiate from one another.

In the portion of the neural tube destined to become the spinal cord, the lumen gradually shrinks in size until, in the adult, it only persists as the vestigial central canal. In the portion of the neural tube destined to become the brain, the lumen dilates to form three segmentally arranged vesicles (the prosencephalon or forebrain, the mesencephalon or midbrain, and the rhombencephalon or hindbrain) separated by two annular constrictions. In the brain, the neural tube lumen persists as the ventricular system. The adult brain develops from the differential growth of the three primary vesicles, the emergence of four flexures (the cervical and the mesencephalic flexures, which are concave ventrally, and the pontine and the telecephalic flexures, which are concave dorsally), and a series of complex three-dimensional foldings.

CNS Histogenesis

Despite major external differences between the rudimentary spinal cord and brain at this early stage, the cellular organization of tissue between the internal and external limiting membranes in both areas remains remarkably similar right up to the point of active glio- and neurogenesis (Figure 1). As the tall columnar epithelium transforms into pseudostratified columnar epithelium, the lateral walls of the neural tube thicken while the dorsal and ventral surfaces thin to form the roof and floor plates, respectively. Each cell has a process in contact with the internal limiting membrane lining the neural tube lumen and another process extending out to the external limiting membrane surrounding the neural tube. Early in development, all cells in the neural tube divide through a process of interkinetic nuclear migration where the nucleus travels to-and-fro within the cell cytoplasm, and where the nucleus position at any given time is determined by the stage in the mitotic cycle (actual cell division occurs close to the internal limiting membrane).[263]

Initially, the pseudostratified columnar ep-

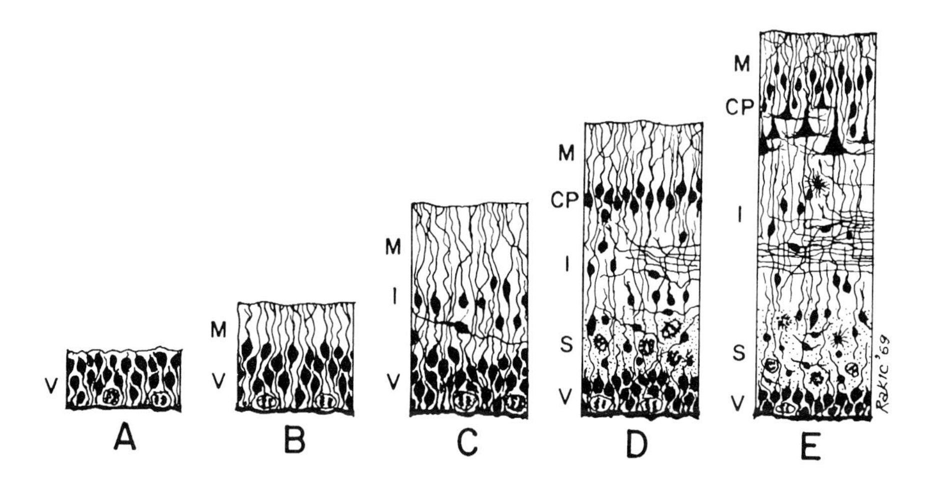

Figure 1: Schematic drawing of the five stages **(A-E)**, and subsequent five layers, in the development of the CNS as described in the text. M = marginal zone; V = ventricular zone; I = intermediate zone; CP = cortical plate; S = subventricular zone. (Photograph of original drawing courtesy of Pasko Rakic; reprinted from the Boulder Committee[43] with permission.)

ithelium forms three zones.[43] The layer nearest the lumen is the ventricular zone (formerly known as the matrix or matrix layer, medulloepithelial layer, neuroepithelial layer, maternal layer, or primitive ependyma), which is defined as the space to which the to-and-fro nuclear movement during interkinetic nuclear migration is confined. The layer nearest the external limiting membrane is the marginal zone, which is relatively acellular, consisting mostly of the outer cytoplasmic extensions of the ventricular cells. The layer in between the two is the intermediate zone (formerly known as the mantle layer), which is composed of the first cells that cease interkinetic nuclear migration; these cells release from the internal limiting membrane and migrate outward to form this intervening layer. A little later in organogenesis (and predominantly in the brain), these three layers are joined by a fourth and then a fifth layer.[43] The subventricular zone (formerly known as the subependymal layer or the subependymal germinal matrix) is the fourth to form and is located between the ventricular and intermediate zones. It is an extremely cell-dense zone composed of a morphologically homogeneous population of small round cells with a high proliferative rate. Unlike ventricular cells, they remain stable in position (do not rely on interkinetic nuclear migration) and are not attached to the internal limiting membrane. The last zone to form is the cortical plate, which arises between the intermediate and marginal zones and consists of cell bodies that eventually form the cortical gray matter.

A morphological description and categorization of mature glial cell types was gradually worked out over approximately a 60-year period, thanks in large part to the efforts of del Rio Hortega[70] and Ramon y Cajal.[242] According to their work, microglial cells were not considered to be of neuroepithelial origin and macroglial cells were divided into oligodendrocytes, ependymal cells, fibrous astrocytes, protoplasmic astrocytes, and specialized glial cells (e.g., Bergmann glial cells and Müller cells). However, the morphological description and categorization of neuronal and glial precursors eluded definition. Most neuronal and glial precursors appeared to arise from the subventricular and ventricular zones. Cells in these layers are so homogeneous that they could not be reliably distinguished by morphology or standard histochemical stains. Theories concerning the origin of mature neuronal and glial cell

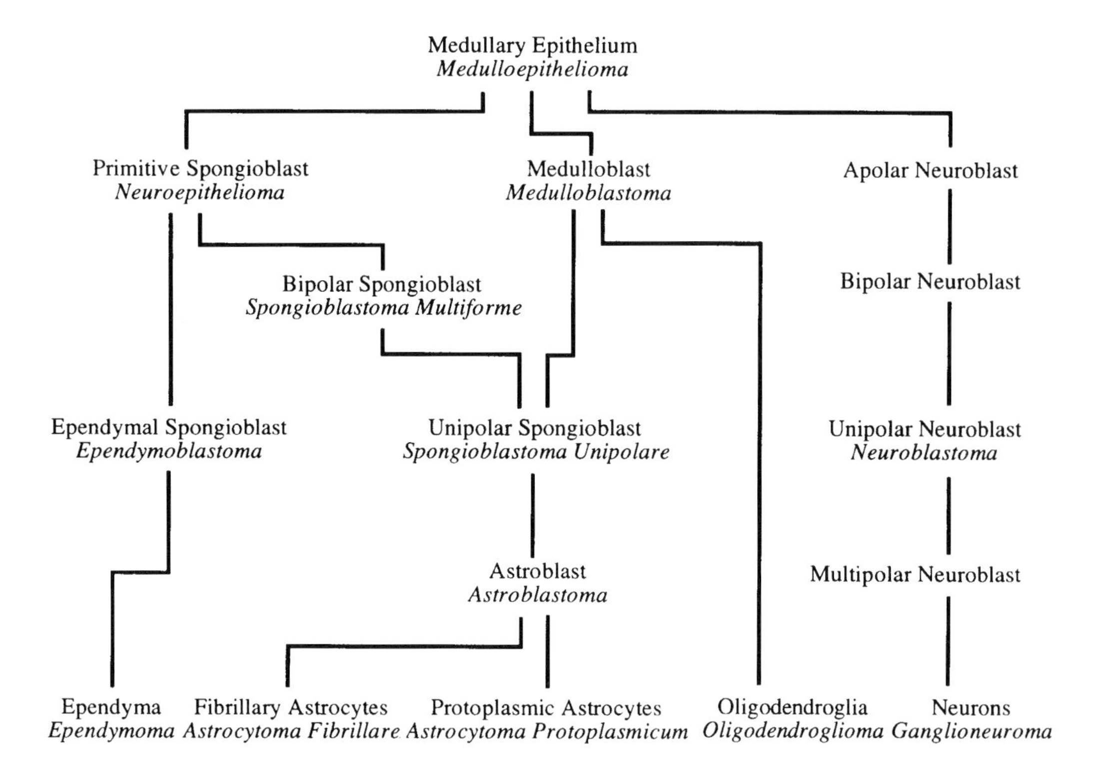

Figure 2: Schematic flow chart showing the stages and progression of neuroglial differentiation as envisioned by Bailey and Cushing[13] in 1926. The neoplasm presumed to arise from each stage of development is listed in italics.

types became a matter for speculation and conjecture.

There were two basic theories. The first, proposed by His,[122] speculated that neurons and glia arose from two separate classes of precursor cells (Keimzellen and Spongioblasten, respectively). The second, espoused by Schaper,[265] suggested that neurons and glia arose from a single homogeneous precursor cell population. Despite the inability to prove their hypotheses with the tools available at the time, some investigators managed to formulate extremely detailed and complex theories. An example of such a theory is the differentiation schema proposed by Bailey and Cushing,[13] which tried to reconcile the then-current thinking about neuronal-glial differentiation with their classification system for neuronal-glial malignancies (Figure 2). Many of these terms have found permanent homes in medical terminology, which led Russell and Rubinstein[256] to comment in the most recent edition of their popular neuropathology textbook that "the prevailing name 'medulloblastoma' given by Bailey and Cushing (1925), is unfortunate because there is no embryonal cell that has been identified as a medulloblast."

Modern Tools for the Study of Glial Developmental Biology

Since morphology and conventional histochemistry proved inadequate to advance our understanding of the progression, control, and stages of glial differentiation, the field remained relatively static until the development of new scientific tools allowed investigation to proceed. Some of these tools required further advances in already established fields (e.g., physics, biochemistry, electrophysiology, and physical chemistry),

TABLE 1

DISTINGUISHING NEUROGLIAL CELL TYPES ACCORDING TO METABOLITE CONCENTRATIONS AND METABOLITE RATIOS AS DETERMINED BY ^{1}H NMR SPECTROSCOPY*

Metabolite/Metabolite Ratio	Neurons	O-2A Progenitors	Oligodendrocytes	Type-1 Astrocytes
β-Hydroxybutyrate	High	Barely Detectable	Barely Detectable	Barely Detectable
N-acetyl-aspartate	High	High	Absent	Absent
Glycine	Low	High	High	Low
Choline:aspartate ratio	Low	Low	Low	High
Choline:glutamate ratio	Low	Low	Low	High
Choline:glycine ratio	Low	Low	Low	High

*Adapted from reference 298.

while other tools awaited the development of whole new fields including in vitro cellular biology, immunology, and molecular biology.

Key Advances in Established Fields

Physics

Advances in physics led to the development of electron microscopy, which provided much higher resolution for the study of subcellular structure. Initial studies using this technique tried to distinguish "astroblasts" and "oligodendroblasts" by differences in cytoplasmic organelle number, density, and morphological structure (differences most pronounced in the endoplasmic reticulum).[276] Later studies combined electron microscopy with immunolabeling in order to better distinguish cell types by antigenic phenotype.[273] Electron microscopy could also be combined with ^{3}H-thymidine autoradiography to study cell proliferation.[276,277]

Biochemistry

Key biochemistry advances centered around major strides in protein chemistry including the development of Western blot techniques, two-dimensional isoelectric focusing, and automated protein sequencers and synthesizers. New biochemical assays which could functionally distinguish glial cells from one another included assays for the activity of 2', 3'-cyclic nucleotide 3'-phosphohydrolase (CNP), a myelin-associated enzyme (oligodendrocytes),[184,237] and glutamine synthetase (astrocytes).[82] The identification and purification of cytokines and growth factors[8,106,264] was a major achievement that allowed the exploration of the control of differentiation through soluble mediators and the development of serum-free media for in vitro cell studies.

Electrophysiology

An important advance in electrophysiology was the emergence of microelectrophysiology, which included the development of microelectrodes for sampling both the intracellular and extracellular ionic environment, and the development of patch clamp techniques to identify and distinguish different transmembrane ionic channels. These new tools provided another functional means of distinguishing glial cell types.[15,16,19,20,36,40,125,142,173,244,282]

Physical Chemistry

Within physical chemistry, proton nuclear magnetic resonance (^{1}H NMR) spectroscopy has recently emerged as a new noninvasive way of examining cells either in vivo or in vitro. This technique holds great promise for being able to distinguish different neuronal and glial cell types by examining a wide range of cellular metabolites (Table 1 and Figure 3).[298,299]

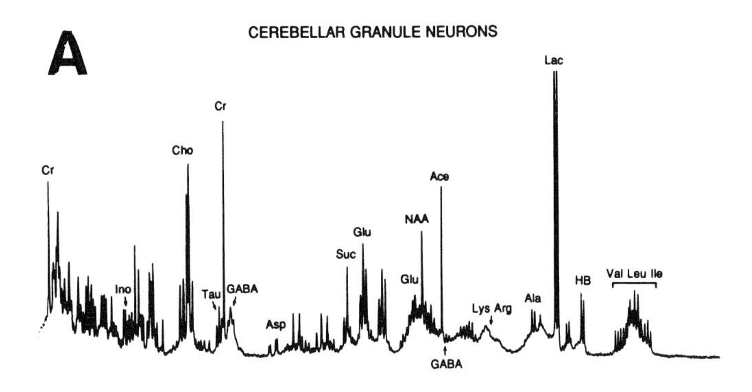

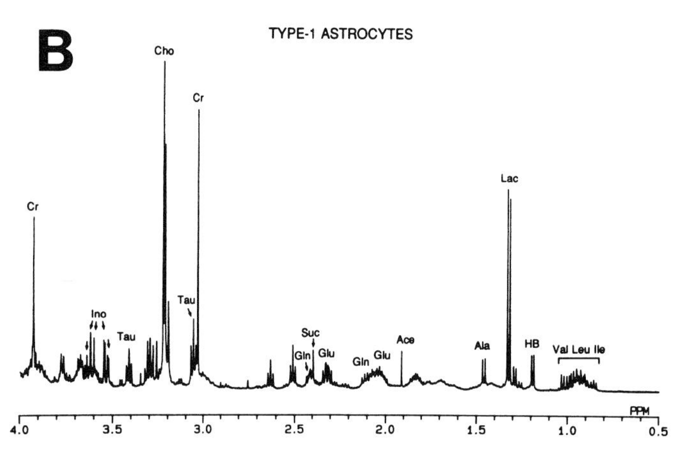

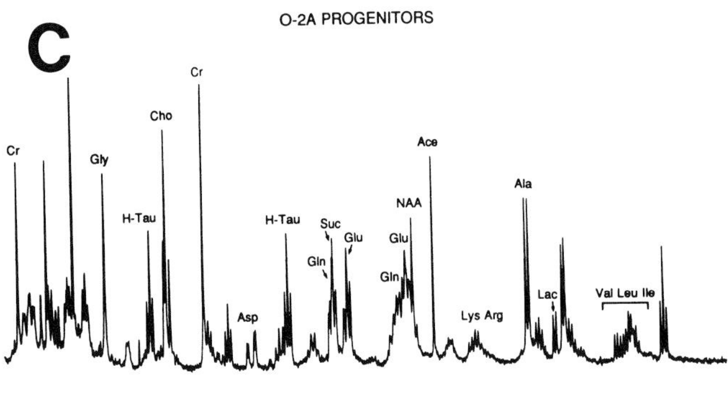

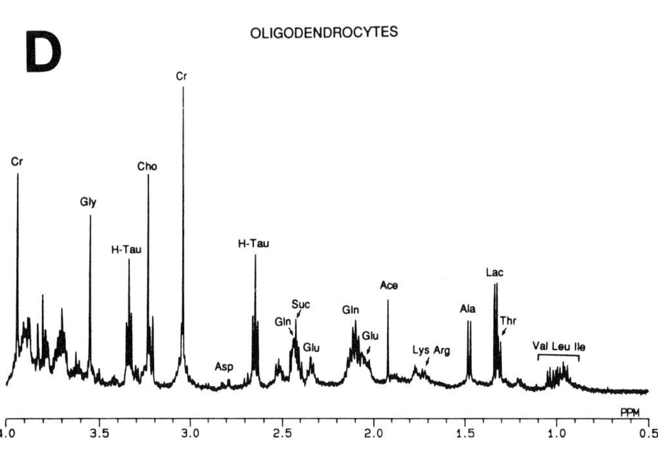

Figure 3: Representative ^{1}H NMR spectra obtained from extracts of cultured cerebellar granule neurons **(A)**, T1As **(B)**, perinatal O-2A progenitor cells **(C)**, and oligodendrocytes **(D)**. Perchloric acid extracts of each cell type contained 4.5, 17.4, 1.0, and 1.5 mg of protein, respectively. Immunostaining showed that the cell purity was approximately 90% for neurons, and >95% for the remaining three cell types. Analysis was performed at pH 8.9 with 512 scans recorded at 500 MHz. Spectra, referenced to 3-trimethylsilyl-tetradeuterosodium propionate (0 ppm), are displayed between 0.5 and 4.0 ppm. The amplitude of each peak is proportional to the number of hydrogen atoms resonating at that frequency.

Identified signals include (from right to left): valine (Val), leucine (Leu), isoleucine (Ile), β-hydroxybutyrate (HB), threonine (Thr), lactate (Lac), alanine (Ala), lysine (Lys), arginine (Arg), gamma-aminobutyric acid (GABA), acetate (Ace), N-acetyl-aspartate (NAA), glutamate (Glu), glutamine (Gln), succinate (Suc), hypotaurine (H-Tau), aspartate (Asp), creatinine (Cr), taurine (Tau), choline-containing compounds (Cho), glycine (Gly), and inositol (Ino).

Note that the ^{1}H spectra of neurons and perinatal O-2A progenitor cells show high signals of NAA, that those of perinatal O-2A progenitor cells and oligodendrocytes demonstrate high Gly signals, and that the amplitude of the Cho signal is greater, and the Asp, Glu, and Gly amplitudes are lower for T1As than for the other three cell types. Distinguishing metabolite concentrations and ratios for each cell type are outlined in Table 1.

(Reprinted from Urenjak et al[298] with permission)

Important New Fields

In Vitro Cellular Biology

One of the most influential new fields to develop was in vitro cellular biology. The evolution of cell culture techniques had a major impact on the study of glial developmental biology. Individual cells, as well as groups of cells, could be studied over significant periods of time under controlled conditions. For the first time the whole three-dimensional structure of any given cell could be visualized without having to worry about "the plane of section." In addition, cells could be studied while they were still alive, allowing the dynamic investigation of cellular processes. Cells could be studied in isolation or in co-culture constructs which allowed the examination of cell-cell interactions.[118,119,208,279] Medium conditioned by one cell type could be used to grow cells of another cell type in order to assess cell-cell interactions mediated by diffusible factors.[1,4,209,252]

Initial work in cell culture focused primarily on the goal of cell survival, leading to the development of many different types of media. Most successful media recipes required the addition of animal serum (usually fetal calf serum (FCS)). To some extent this early reliance on animal serum was unfortunate. Once the blood-brain barrier forms, serum proteins are for the most part excluded from the extracellular space, meaning that in vitro conditions that include serum do not resemble the in vivo situation in the CNS. However, it probably did not affect the validity of extrapolation of in vitro results to the in vivo situation for early neuronal and glial cells prior to the formation of the blood-brain barrier.

As we shall see later in this chapter, serum (especially serum of fetal origin) contains many "factors" that specifically affect glial development and behavior (both normal and neoplastic glial cells). The more recent development of glial-compatible, chemically defined, serum-free media,[42] as well as astrocyte-conditioned media (CM)[1,4,164,209,231,236,315] (since astrocytes are the cells primarily responsible for maintaining extracellular fluid homeostasis in the CNS), has provided a much more accurate in vitro environment for studying in vivo CNS cellular biology.

TABLE 2

USEFUL ANTIBODIES FOR DISTINGUISHING CNS CELL TYPES AND STAGE OF MATURATION*

Antibodies Against Cell Surface Gangliosides, Sulfatides, and Cerebrosides
- mAb LB1/mAb R24 (both anti-GD3)
- mAb A2B5
- mAb O4
- anti-sulfatide
- anti-galactocerebroside
- mAb O1

Antibodies Against Intracellular Cytoskeletal Proteins
- mAb rat-401/anti-nestin
- anti-vimentin
- anti-glial fibrillary acidic protein
- anti-neurofilament
- anti-Class III β tubulin

Antibodies Against Intracellular Membrane-Bound Proteins
- anti-myelin basic protein
- anti-proteolipid protein
- anti-myelin associated glycoprotein
- anti-2',3'-cyclic nucleotide 3'-phosphohydrolase

Antibodies Against Cell Surface Proteins
- mAb RAN-2
- anti-platelet derived growth factor receptor
- anti-growth associated protein-43
- anti-tetanus toxin receptor
- anti-fibronectin
- anti-Fc receptor
- mAb OX-42

Antibodies Against Antigens of Uncertain Location and/or Nature
- mAb RC1
- mAb RC2
- mAb A4

* Antibodies are listed according to the category of antigen recognized.

While cells could be grown as dissociated suspensions,[231,315] the most common form of study involved growing cells attached to a two-dimensional surface. Another innovation involved the study of the individual cell's fate using clonal analysis.[105,231,233,249,250,288,289] Recently, three-dimensional cell culture systems have been developed which not only allow the study of developing glia in a controlled three-dimensional setting,[33,35,124,149,268,294] but also provide an ideal in vitro substrate for studying glioma invasion (Figure 4).[34,80,81,171]

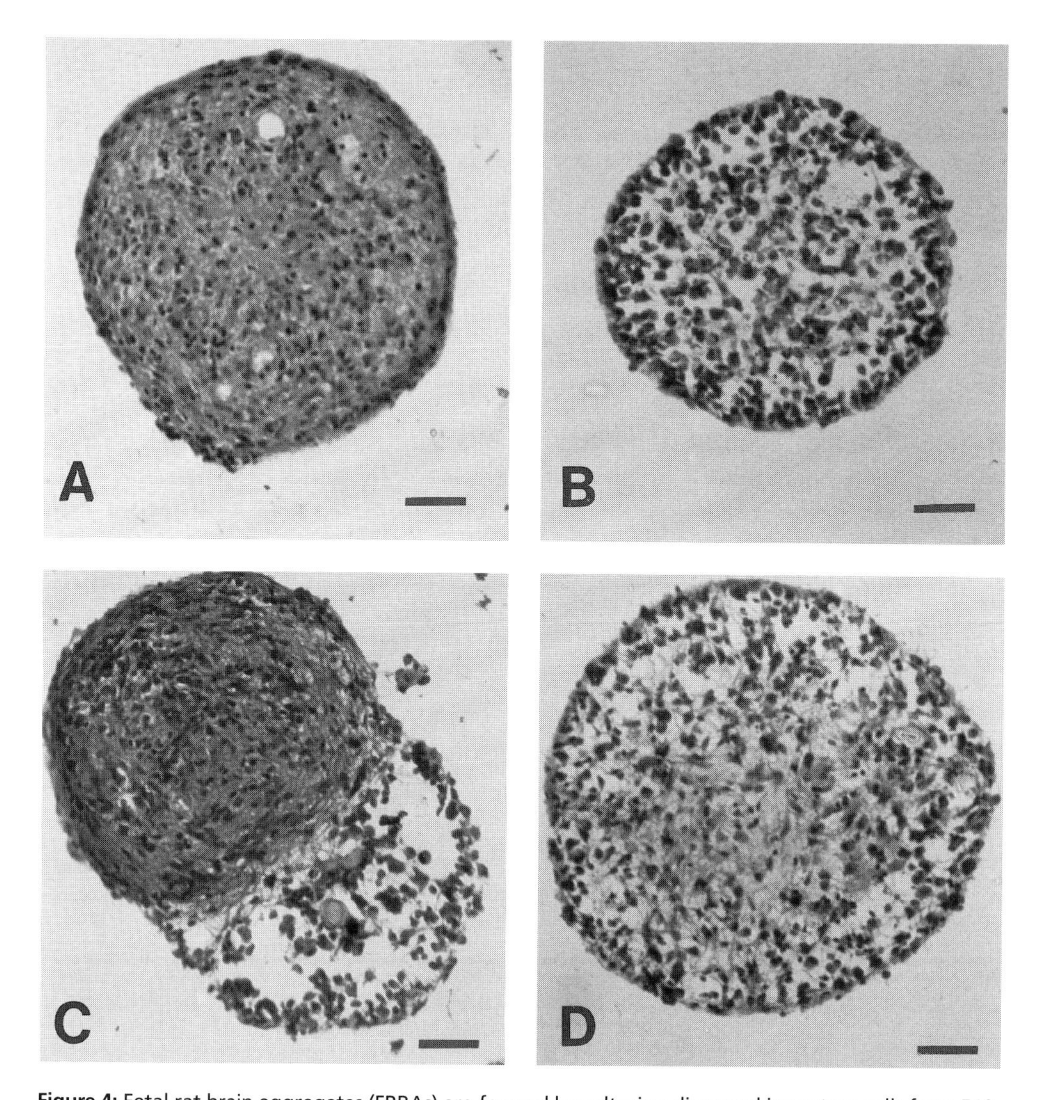

Figure 4: Fetal rat brain aggregates (FRBAs) are formed by culturing dispersed immature cells from E18 rat cerebrum under nonadherent conditions using agar-liquid media overlay techniques. These cells reaggregate over several days to form FRBAs, which by 20 days in culture contain mature astrocytes, oligodendrocytes, and neurons, as well as a tightly packed neuropil containing myelinated axons and synaptic structures. **A)** A 24-day-old mature FRBA is shown. FRBAs provide useful substrates for studying CNS invasion in vitro. **B)** A three-dimensional multicellular tumor spheroid (MTS) which was produced by culturing Hu-O-2A/Gb1 human glioma cells (a human glioblastoma cell line of O-2A lineage; cf Figure 11) under nonadherent, agar-liquid media overlay conditions.
The in vitro CNS invasion assay involves confronting the MTS with a mature FRBA under the same nonadherent, agar-liquid media overlay conditions. **C)** Two days after confrontation, the MTS has attached itself to the FRBA over an arc consisting of about 120° of the FRBA circumference. The surface of the FRBA where the MTS is attached has become irregular and the immediately underlying neuropil is becoming looser in density. **D)** Seventeen days after confrontation, glioma cells have migrated to completely cover the surface of the FRBA. The majority of the FRBA has been destroyed, while the remaining portion demonstrates a loose, disrupted neuropil and evidence of individual glioma cell invasion. *A-D* are 12 mm-thick sections of 4% paraformaldehyde-fixed specimens. (hematoxylin-eosin, original magnification $\times$ 20; scale bars = 50 μm)

Immunology

Combining antibodies with fluorescent conjugates or peroxidase reagents permitted the staining of individual cells in culture (immunocytology) as well as cells in tissue section (immunohistology or immunoelectron microscopy). Table 2 provides a selected (and by no means complete) outline of some of the more useful antibodies and antigens for distinguishing various glial cell types at various stages of development. Many of the early useful antigens were intracellular proteins[31,79,214] which were robust in the sense that they remained stable in many types of chemical fixation or tissue embedding. Most of the useful antigens were either cell-surface gangliosides, sulfatides, and cerebrosides, or the carbohydrate moieties attached to them.[76,228, 235,243,281] While this is an advantage since they are resistant to the trypsin digestion used for passaging cells in vitro, it means that they are best detected on live cells or freshly frozen tissue sections. Formalin fixation or paraffin embedding of tissue are suboptimal conditions for most of these antigens.

Antibodies were the first tool that could be used to examine the status of gene expression in any given cell by determining its antigenic phenotype. Two cells that looked similar morphologically (or the same cell at two different points in time, the second occurring after it had progressed to a more advanced stage of maturation) could now be distinguished by differences in antigenic phenotype. Combined with cell culture, this tool was primarily responsible for advancing glial developmental biology beyond the boundaries previously established by the study of cellular morphology alone.

Another important use of antibody technology was in assessing the chemical dynamics of cellular interactions. Antibodies directed against selected proteins could be used to effectively block the function of those proteins in cell culture. This allowed scientists to assess the effect of loss of function for any given protein on in vitro cellular biology.[84,131,210,233]

Molecular Biology

The final new field with major implications for the study of glial developmental biology was the field of molecular biology. While antibody technology provided the first glimpses into the genomic state of the cell by determining its antigenic phenotype, molecular biology provided an even better handle on the genomic state of the cell by allowing the examination of both the deoxyribonucleic acid (DNA) present in the nucleus (Southern blotting) and the activated genes of a cell through its messenger ribonucleic acid (RNA, Northern blotting). The development of polymerase chain reaction technology provided the means to amplify even small amounts of genomic nucleotides or artificial nucleotides, which greatly facilitated study.[257,258]

Advances in molecular biology led to the development of retroviral gene transfer techniques, whereby individual cells could be infected in vivo with a defective retrovirus containing the β-galactosidase gene.[221-224,261,297, 3,09, 310,316] In this way, all progeny of this infected cell could be detected by a histochemical stain utilizing the chromogen X-gal later in development. This technology performed the same function in vivo as clonal analysis did in vitro. Molecular biology also led to the development of in situ hybridization techniques where cells expressing a desired gene could be identified in vivo by incubating tissue sections with a complementary ("anti-sense") oligonucleotide probe.[25,120,225,226,291] Like retroviral gene transfer, in situ hybridization was another tool that could be employed at earlier stages in development, when anatomical and cell type-selective primary neuroglial cell culture was technically more difficult.

Glial Cell Types

For developmental glial biology, the most extensively studied nonmammalian systems are the insect *Drosophila melanogaster*, and the avian quail and chicken systems. The most extensively studied mammalian system is the rat. While both in vitro and in vivo studies have been performed using rat whole brain, cerebellum, isolated corpus callosum, and spinal cord, the simplest model to study has been the rat optic nerve since it contains astrocytes and oligodendrocytes but no neuronal soma or

TABLE 3

GLIAL CELL LINEAGE AND STAGE OF MATURATION DEFINED BY ANTIGENIC PHENOTYPE

Cell Type	GD3	A2B5	RAN-2	O4	GalC	O1	Vimentin	GFAP	NF	Class III β Tubulin	RC1	Rat-401	Fibronectin	OX42	FC Receptor
T1A precursor	?	–	+	–	–	–	+	–	–	–	?	?	–	–	–
Mature T1A	–	–	+	–	–	–	+	+	–	–	–	–	–	–	–
Perinatal O-2A progenitor	+	+	–	–	–	–	+	–	–	–	?	?	–	–	–
Adult O-2A progenitor	+	+	–	+	–	–	–	–	–		?	?	–	–	–
Immature oligodendrocyte	+	+	–	+	–	–	±	–	–	–	?	?	–	–	–
Mature oligodendrocyte	–	–	–	+	+	+	–	–	–	–	–	–	–	–	–
Mature T2A	–	+	–	–	–	–	–	+	+	–	–	–	–	–	–
Radial glia	–	–	?	–	–	–	+	–*	–	–	+	+	–	–	–
Ependymal cell	–	–	+	–	–	–	+	–	–	–	+	?	–	–	–
Meningeal cell	–	–	+	–	–	–	–	–	–	–	–	–	+	–	–
Neuron	–	+	–	–	–	–	–	–	+	+	–	–	–	–	–
Microglia/ macrophage	+	–	–	–	–	–	–	–	–	–	–	–	–	+	+

*Radial glial cells are GFAP$^+$ in primates but GFAP$^-$ in all other mammals.

ependymal cells. As there appear to be at least some differences in gliogenesis between nonmammals and mammals (structural radial glia persist into adulthood in nonmammalian cortex[49]), this chapter will restrict discussion to data obtained using the rat mammalian system unless specifically stated otherwise. Table 3 and Figure 5 provide outlines to assist in organizing the description of normal glial antigenic progression and lineage direction that follows.

Type 1 Astrocyte Lineage

Antigenic Phenotype and In Vitro Morphology

Cells of the type-1 astrocyte (T1A) lineage are characterized phenotypically by being monoclonal antibody (mAb) RAN-2$^+$ [1,232,313] and mAb A2B5$^-$.[189,230,232] T1A precursors are mAb A2B5$^-$, mAb RAN-2$^+$, and glial fibrillary acidic protein (GFAP)$^-$, while mature T1As are mAb A2B5$^-$, mAb RAN-2$^+$, and GFAP$^+$.[1,189,230,232] Morphologically, T1As appear broad and flat ("fibroblast-like") with few, if any, processes in cell culture (Figure 6).[230] However, as previously stated, morphology is a poor indicator of cell lineage since morphological changes in cell culture depend on cell density, and because increased cyclic adenosine monophosphate (cAMP) can cause T1As to adopt a process-bearing morphology.[230]

Other Distinguishing Features

Glia have been shown to possess both voltage-dependent ion channels (Na$^+$, K$^+$, Cl$^-$, and Ca^{++}) and neurotransmitter-gated ion channels,[17,141] although their channel density is not large enough to allow for the generation of a self-sustaining action potential. In vitro, T1As

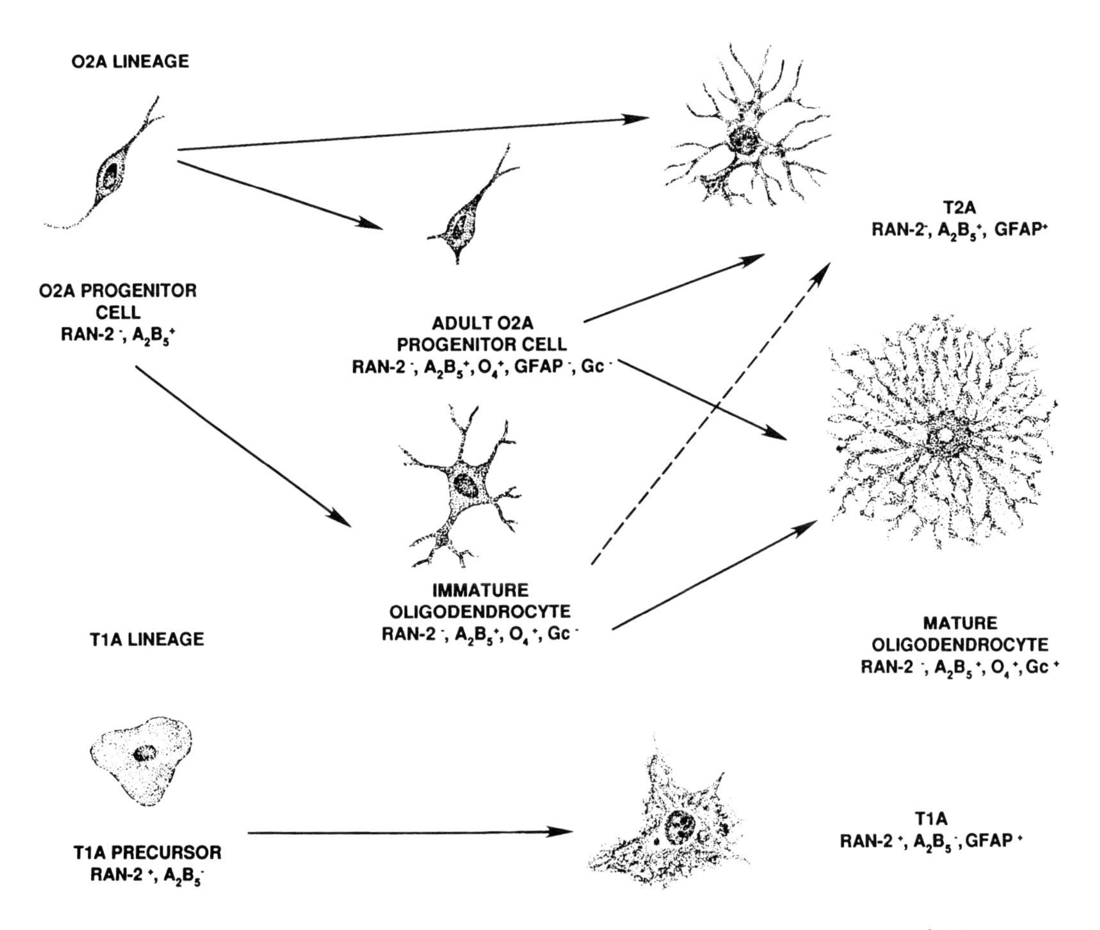

Figure 5: Summary of the potential course of differentiation for both T1A precursors and O-2A progenitor cells in vitro, listing their major distinguishing antigenic features, and demonstrating their typical in vitro morphologies. This figure should be used along with Table 3 to assist with organizing the outline of glial differentiation presented in the text.

demonstrate a delayed rectifying K^+ current (K_D), as well as gamma aminobutyric acid (GABA)-gated Cl^- channels.[40] In addition to these channels identified in vitro, T1As also demonstrate an inwardly rectifying K^+ current (K_{IR}) and a slow voltage-dependent Na^+ channel in vivo.[36,193] T1As do have voltage-dependent Na^+ channels in early cell culture, but go on to lose them over 1 to 3 days.[192,193] Some researchers speculate that the difference between T1A ion channel expression in vitro and in vivo is due to up-regulation of glial ion channels by neurons in vivo.[62,192]

By means of ^1H NMR spectra, T1As can be distinguished from other neuronal and glial cells by their extremely high ratio of choline-containing compounds to amino acids and their low overall glycine concentration (Table 1 and Figure 3).[299]

Oligodendrocyte-Type-2 Astrocyte Lineage

Glial cells of the oligodendrocyte-type-2 astrocyte (O-2A) lineage (so called because both oligodendrocytes and type-2 astrocytes (T2As) arise from a common progenitor cell in vitro) include perinatal O-2A progenitor cells, oligodendrocytes (the myelin-producing cells of the CNS), adult O-2A progenitor cells, and T2As. While the existence of O-2A progenitor cells and oligodendrocytes has been confirmed in vitro and in vivo, there is a great deal of controversy as to whether T2As exist in vivo. This section will present the data distinguishing T2As from other glial cell types in vitro. The controversy surrounding the existence of T2As in vivo will be discussed in the next section ("Progression and Control of Gliogenesis").

Antigenic Phenotype and In Vitro Morphology

Cells of the O-2A lineage are characterized by being mAb A2B5$^+$ and mAb RAN-2$^-$.[232] Perinatal O-2A progenitor cells are mAb A2B5$^+$, Galactocerebroside (GalC)$^-$ and GFAP$^-$ (Figure 7).[5,26,234,236] Most perinatal O-2A progenitor cells are bipotential precursor cells, which can give rise to either oligodendrocytes or T2As.[26,234,236,315] In vitro T2As are mAb A2B5$^+$, GalC$^-$, and GFAP$^+$ (Figure 8),[156,189,230,236,315] while oligodendrocytes are mAb A2B5$^-$, GalC$^+$, and GFAP$^-$ (Figure 9).[189,235]

The antigenic progression from a perinatal O-2A progenitor cell to a mature oligodendrocyte involves at least four stages. The perinatal O-2A progenitor cell (first stage) which is mAb O4$^-$, acquires mAb O4 expression and becomes mAb A2B5$^+$, mAb O4$^+$, and GalC$^-$ (second stage).[185,261] Cells in this second stage are still bipotential precursor cells, which can be induced in vitro to form T2As.[101,102,296] During the very brief third antigenic stage, cells become mAb A2B5$^+$, mAb O4$^+$, and GalC$^+$. However, once they express GalC, they very quickly lose mAb A2B5 expression to become mAb A2B5$^-$, mAb O4$^+$, and GalC$^+$ mature oligodendrocytes (stage four).[2,155] The point where they begin to express GalC appears to mark the point where O-2A lineage cells are committed to become oligodendrocytes.

A subset of perinatal O-2A progenitor cells are tripotential since in addition to oligodendrocytes and T2As, they appear to be able to give rise to adult O-2A progenitor cells (Figure 10), which persist throughout life in rats.[207,320,322,324] Adult O-2A progenitor cells may provide a continual source for oligodendrocytes (and possibly T2As) throughout life. While perinatal O-2A progenitors are mAb O4$^-$ and vimentin$^+$, adult O-2A progenitor cells are mAb O4$^+$ and vimentin$^-$ after 1 day in vitro.

Morphologically, perinatal O-2A progenitor cells are bipolar in vitro (Figures 3 and 7). In contrast, adult O-2A progenitor cells have multiple tiny cell processes in vitro but usually have a single, large, dominant process, and thus are often described as "unipolar" (Figures 3 and 10).[320] T2As appear "neuron-like" with multiple cell processes (Figures 3 and 8). Immature oligodendrocytes demonstrate several fine processes in vitro, while oligodendrocytes have little cytoplasm but a complex arborization of fine, branched processes (Figures 3 and 9).

Other Distinguishing Features

Electrophysiologically, perinatal O-2A progenitor cells demonstrate three different K$^+$ currents (K_D "A-type" (K_A), and a Ca^{++}-activated K$^+$ current)[282] and both "glial-" and "neuronal-type" voltage-gated Na$^+$ channels.[20] While no voltage-gated Ca^{++} channels have been identified in rat perinatal O-2A progenitor cells,[20] two different Ca^{++} channels have been identified in mouse O-2A progenitor cells.[304] In addition, perinatal O-2A progenitor cells have been shown to express non-NMDA (N-methyl-D-aspartate) glutamate-gated ion channels,[20,300] and GABA-gated Cl$^-$ channels.[307] While some researchers have noted three types of K$^+$ currents in mature oligodendrocytes (K_{IR}, K_D, and K_A),[16,20] others have shown that, as perinatal O-2A progenitor cells differentiate into oligodendrocytes, they down-regulate their voltage-gated Na$^+$ channels and most K$^+$ channels while up-regulating the K_{IR} channel.[141,142,282] Mature oligodendrocytes continue to express GABA-gated Cl$^-$ channels.[307] T2As appear to express both "glial-" and "neuronal-type" voltage-gated Na$^+$ channels, two types of Ca^{++} channels, and three types of K$^+$ currents (K_{IR}, K_D, and K_A) in vitro.[15,16] Like perinatal O-2A progenitor cells, T2As appear to possess non-NMDA glutamate-gated ion channels in vitro.[300] T2As can also be distinguished from T1As in vitro by the fact that they demonstrate GABA accumulation via a high-affinity transport system,[100,137,156,157] have excitatory amino acid receptors (e.g., glutamate) coupled to amino acid transmitter release,[99,100,328] and synthesize chondroitin sul-

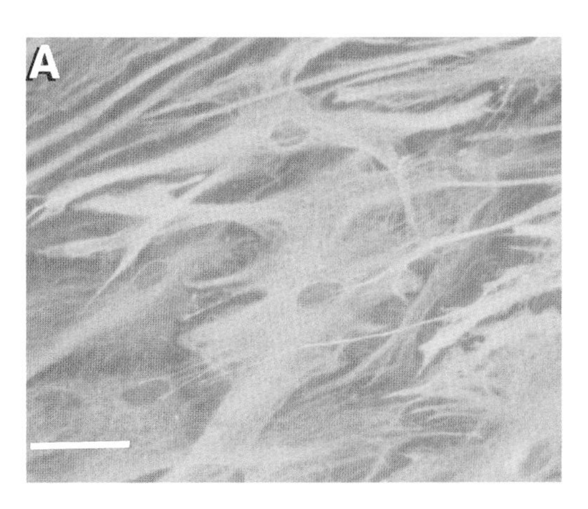

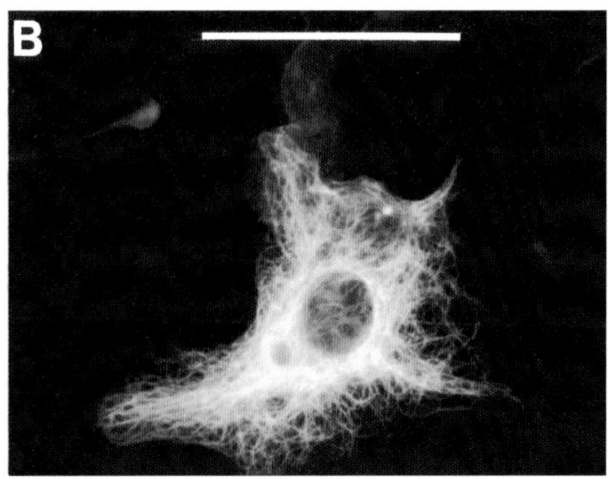

Figure 6: In vitro fluorescein fluorescence micrograph utilizing anti-GFAP primary antibodies and fluorescein-conjugated secondary antibodies, demonstrating a monolayer of T1As **(A)** and a more magnified view of a single T1A **(B)**. Note the paucity of cell processes, the flattened appearance, and the generous amount of cytoplasm. Monolayers of the type demonstrated in *A* are useful for producing serum-free astrocyte-conditioned medium. (original magnification under oil × 40 [A], × 100 [B]; scale bars = 50 μm)

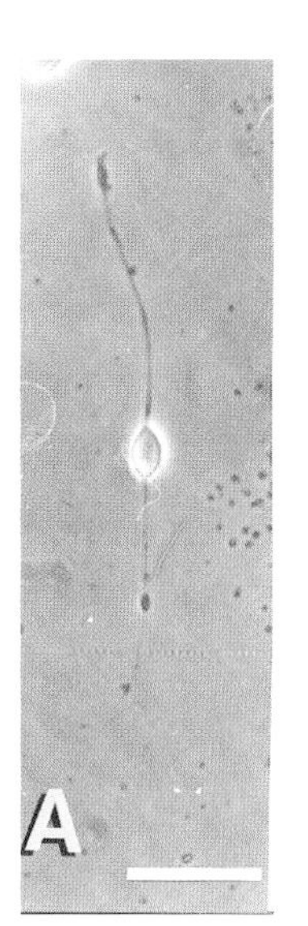

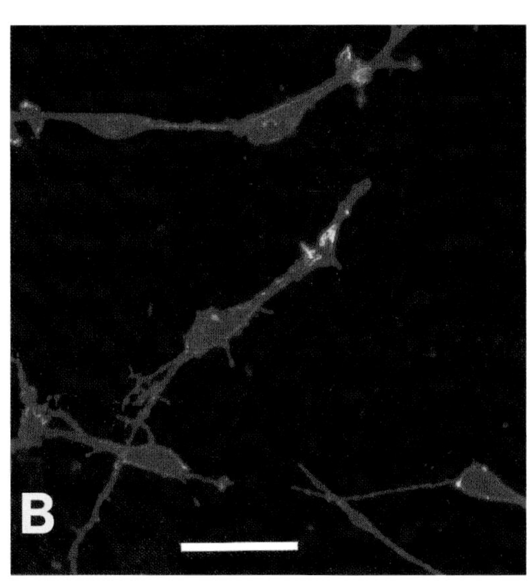

Figure 7: Perinatal O-2A progenitor cells in vitro. **(A)** A live perinatal O-2A progenitor cell viewed with inverted phase-contrast microscopy. (Photomicrograph courtesy of Guus Wolswijk.) **(B)** A group of perinatal O-2A progenitor cells stained with mAb A2B5 and a rhodamine-conjugated secondary antibody viewed with fluorescence microscopy using rhodamine optics. Note the characteristic bipolar morphology of the perinatal O-2A progenitor cells and compare this morphology with the "unipolar" morphology of the adult O-2A progenitor cells in Figure 10. (original magnification × 30 [A], × 40 [B]; scale bars = 50 μm)

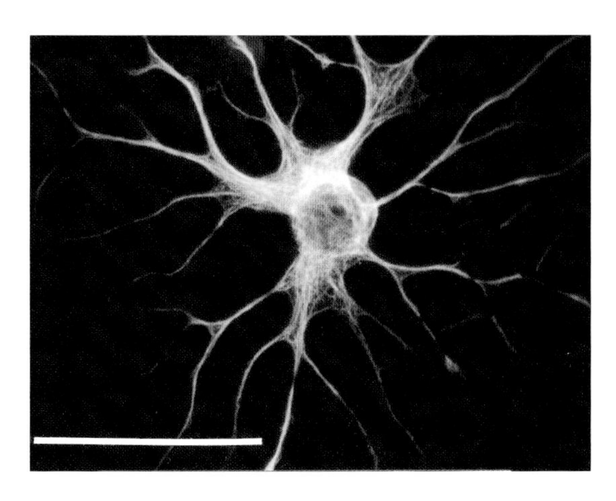

Figure 8: In vitro fluorescein fluorescence micrograph utilizing anti-GFAP primary antibodies and fluorescein-conjugated secondary antibodies, demonstrating a T2A with multiple cell processes. (original magnification under oil × 100; scale bar = 50 μm)

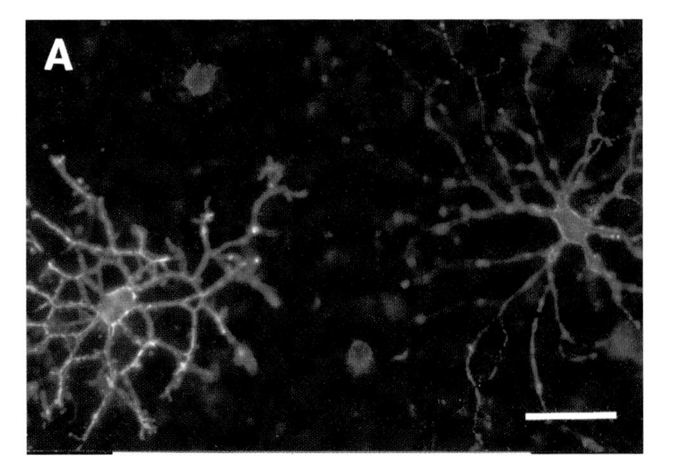

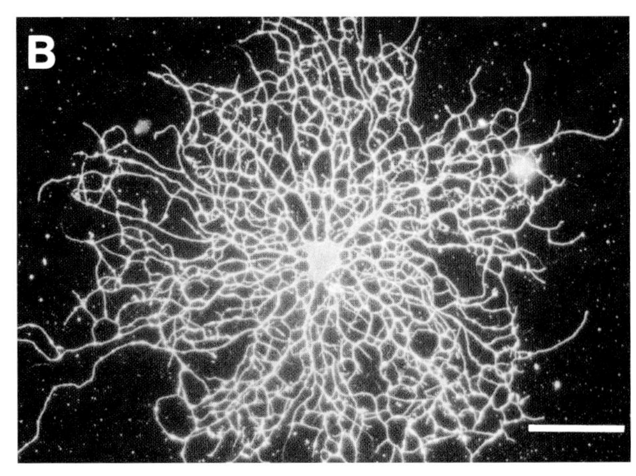

Figure 9: Oligodendrocytes stained in vitro with fluorescence-conjugated secondary antibodies. **(A)** A developing oligodendrocyte after primary antibody staining with mAb O4. **(B)** A morphologically more mature oligodendrocyte after primary antibody staining with anti-GalC. Note the complex arborization of fine branched cell processes, the small round nucleus, and the scant amount of cytoplasm. (original magnifications: rhodamine optics × 40 [A]; fluorescein optics × 40 [B]; scale bars = 50 μm)

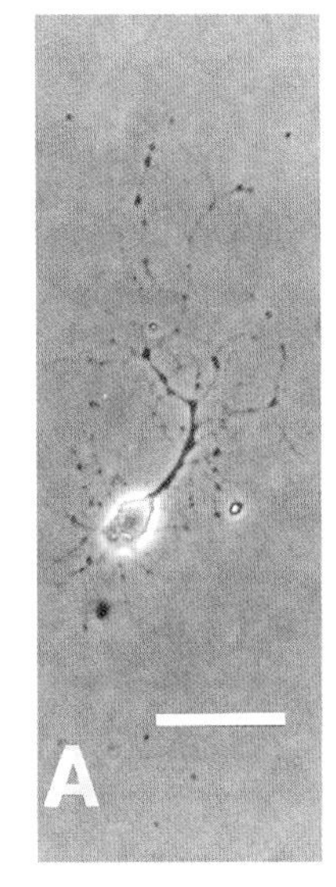

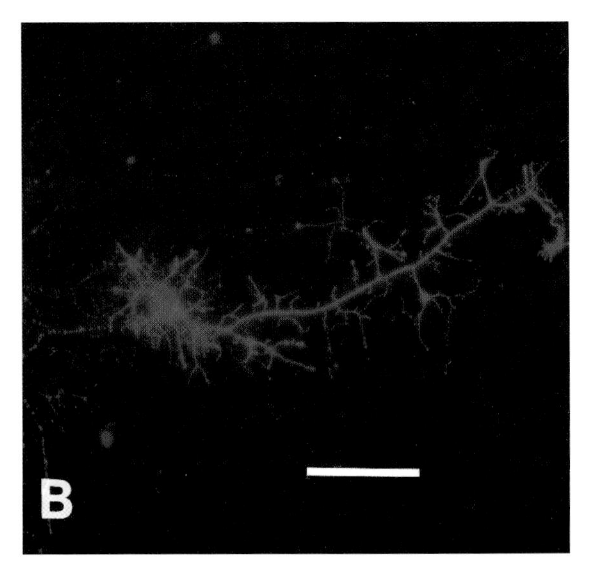

Figure 10: Adult O-2A progenitor cells in vitro. **A)** A live adult O-2A progenitor cell viewed with inverted phase-contrast microscopy. **B)** An adult O-2A progenitor cell stained with mAb A2B5 followed by a fluorescein-conjugated secondary antibody viewed with fluorescence microscopy using fluorescein optics. Note the multiple fine cell processes as well as the single large, prominent process leading to the "unipolar" designation of this cell type. Compare this morphology with the bipolar morphology of the perinatal O-2A progenitor cells in Figure 7. (Photomicrographs courtesy of Guus Wolswijk.) (original magnification × 30 [A], × 40 [B]; scale bars = 50 μm)

fate,[98] while T1As do not. The voltage-gated and neurotransmitter-gated ion channel status of adult O-2A progenitor cells has yet to be determined.

Using ^{1}H NMR spectra to analyze cell metabolites in vitro (Table 1 and Figure 3), one can distinguish perinatal O-2A progenitor cells from oligodendrocytes and T1As by the presence of a high concentration of N-acetyl-aspartate (NAA), and from neurons by the almost complete absence of β-hydroxybutyrate.[298,299] Oligodendrocytes could be distinguished from T1As by their high concentration of glycine (also present in perinatal O-2A progenitor cells) and their low ratio of choline-containing compounds to amino acids.[298]

While both T1A and O-2A lineage cells appear to express the neural cell adhesion molecule (N-CAM) in vitro,[205] mature oligodendrocytes can be distinguished from less mature O-2A lineage cells by both the type of N-CAM expressed and the percentage of cells that continue to express N-CAM. As perinatal O-2A progenitor cells differentiate into oligodendrocytes, they progress from expressing the embryonic form of the N-CAM (perinatal O-2A progenitor cell) to expressing predominantly adult N-CAM (immature oligodendrocyte), then to expressing exclusively the adult form of N-CAM (mature oligodendrocyte).[295] In addition, while all perinatal O-2A progenitor cells appear to express N-CAM, the percentage of cells that continue to express N-CAM progressively declines as the cells differentiate into oligodendrocytes. Trotter and colleagues[295] noted that 80% of mAb $O4^{+}$, mAb $O1^{-}$ (an mAb that recognizes an epitope similar to GalC) cells expressed N-CAM, while only 54% to 87% of mAb $O1^{+}$ cells were N-CAM^{+}. Others have noted N-CAM expression in as few as 5% of mAb $O1^{+}$ cells.[139]

While all glial cell types express major histocompatibility (MHC) T1As, oligodendrocytes can be distinguished from other glial cell types by their inability to be induced to express MHC T2As in vitro. Gamma interferon can induce T1As, T2As, and both perinatal and adult O-2A progenitor cells to express MHC T2As (immune-associated antigens (IA)) in vitro, while oligodendrocytes appear to lose this ability with maturation.[48]

In addition to differences within in vitro morphology and subtle differences in antigenic phenotype, adult O-2A progenitor cells differ from their perinatal counterparts in several other characteristics. Adult O-2A progenitor cells (and oligodendrocytes as well) are susceptible to the lytic effects of complement in the absence of antibody in vitro while perinatal O-2A progenitor cells, T2As, and T1As are not.[325] Adult O-2A progenitor cells have a longer average cell cycle time (65 hours versus 18 hours) and both a slower migratory rate (4 μm/hr versus 21 μm/hr) and a slower differentiation rate than their perinatal counterparts.[320,322,323] Finally, while perinatal O-2A progenitor cells are precursor cells that tend to undergo symmetric cell division (giving rise to two cells of similar type and maturity), adult O-2A progenitor cells appear to resemble true stem cells in that they can undergo asymmetric cell division in vitro (reproducing another adult O-2A progenitor cell along with a cell destined to terminally differentiate).[321,324]

Radial Glia and Specialized Glia

Radial glial cells extend from the internal limiting membrane all the way to the external limiting membrane of the CNS. They emerge very early in development, prior to the formation of cortical astrocytes and prior to the earliest migratory wave of neurons,[97,253] and are the first glial cell type that can be identified by morphological criteria. They provide the structural scaffolding for all five zones of the thickening wall of the neural tube, and provide the "tracks" that serve as a guide for migrating neurons (and possibly migrating glial precursor cells) on their way from the ventricular and subventricular zones to the cortical plate.[238,239] Antigenically, radial glia are reported to be mAb $RC1^{+}$, mAb $RC2^{+}$, and mAb Rat-401^{+}.[75,123,194,195] In nonprimates, radial glial cells are $vimentin^{+}$ and $GFAP^{-}$,[217,253,306] while they appear to be $GFAP^{+}$ in primates.[159]

Ependymal cells, tanycytes, cerebellar Bergmann glial cells, and retinal Müller cells share many morphological, immunological, and biochemical features with radial glial cells.[24,75,83,254]

This observation has led some researchers to postulate that these cells may represent divergent forms of radial glia that persist into adulthood in mammals.[49]

Multipotential Neuroglial Precursor Cells

All CNS cells originally arise from neuroectoderm and thus T1A and O-2A lineage cells as well as neurons and other specialized glia must share a common origin at some point in development. Temple[288] has been able to isolate cells from embryonic day (E) 13.5 and E14.5 (the rat gestational period is 21 days) that are capable of producing both neurons and glial cells as demonstrated by clonal analysis. Kilpatrick and Bartlett[143] have isolated precursor cells from E10 mouse telencephalon and mesencephalon that could produce both neurons and astrocytes as demonstrated by clonal analysis. Reynolds et al[249,250] isolated precursor cells from E14 mouse striatum, which can proliferate in vitro and form both neurons and astrocytes. Using retroviral gene transfer techniques, several groups have reported detecting β-galactosidase activity in vivo in clones containing both neurons and glia, indicating a common cellular origin from the originally infected cell.[222,224,297,309,310,316] The distinguishing antigenic phenotype of these earlier multipotential precursor cells has not yet been worked out.

Progression and Control of Gliogenesis

Timing In Vitro vs. In Vivo

Primary cultures taken from rat optic nerves[1,164,210,231,315] or from whole brain[315] as early as E10 and grown under proper conditions antigenically progress on schedule in vitro, suggesting that glial differentiation proceeds independently of cell location and/or orientation from at least that point. Proper conditions for reconstituting in vivo cell developmental timing for O-2A lineage cells in vitro include growing cultures in less than 0.5% FCS,[1,164,231,236,315] and growing cells either in T1A-CM,[164,231,236,315] or in media supplemented by platelet-derived growth factor (PDGF).[162,210]

Type-1 Astrocyte Lineage

The T1A lineage is the only cell lineage that appears to arise from the original optic stalk.[278] T1A precursors are detectable in whole-brain cultures stained with mAb RAN-2 as early as E10,[1] the earliest stage that has been tested. Mature T1As are first detected in optic nerve between E16 and E17.[189,232] Mature T1As continue to divide for up to 1 week after expressing GFAP.[189,209] T1As are stimulated to proliferate by epidermal growth factor (EGF),[153,230] by PDGF,[30] by basic fibroblast growth factor (bFGF),[127,198,215,227,308] and to a lesser extent by acidic fibroblast growth factor (aFGF)[215,308] (Table 4). T1As continue to form in vivo until approximately postnatal day (P) 15, when adult numbers of T1As are present in the optic nerve.[189,276,277] T1As will form on schedule in vitro whether grown in FCS or in chemically defined media, suggesting that induction from environmental factors is not necessary for their terminal differentiation. However, it is not known whether a specific factor found in chemically defined media[42] is critical for their differentiation.

Oligodendrocyte-Type-2 Astrocyte Lineage

O-2A lineage cells are not indigenous to the optic stalk and appear to migrate into the optic stalk from an adjacent subventricular zone (possibly the preoptic recess overlying the optic chiasm).[278] A similar process of O-2A lineage cell migration has been found in the cerebellum and the forebrain.[67,104,113,225,251]

Perinatal O-2A Progenitor Cells

If perinatal O-2A progenitor cells are grown in isolated cell culture in the absence of mitogens, they will go on to differentiate prematurely into either oligodendrocytes or T2As, regardless of the time of removal from the optic nerve.[209,232,234,236] T1As and neurons are the

TABLE 4

Established Growth Factor Effects on Normal Glial Proliferation, Differentiation, and Survival, and Their Potential Role in Glioma Biology

Growth Factor	Normal Cell(s) Stimulated to Proliferate	Normal Cell(s) Stimulated to Differentiate	Normal Cell(s) Dependent on Factor for Survival	Potential Role as a Glioma Auto/ Paracrine Factor
TGF-α	Multipotential neuroglial precursor	—	—	+
TGF-β	?	?	?	+
EGF	Multipotential neuroglial precursor T1A	—	—	+
PDGF	T1A Perinatal O-2A progenitor Adult O-2A progenitor	—	Young oligodendrocyte Perinatal O-2A progenitor	+
bFGF	Multipotential neuroglial precursor T1A Perinatal O-2A progenitor Adult O-2A progenitor	—	—	+
aFGF	T1A	?	—	+
IGF-1	Perinatal O-2A progenitor	O-2A progenitor (oligodendrocyte)	Oligodendrocyte Perinatal O-2A progenitor	+
IGF-2	—	?	Oligodendrocyte	+
CNTF	—	O-2A progenitor	Oligodendrocyte	+
NT-3	Perinatal O-2A progenitor*	?	Oligodendrocyte	+
BDNF	?	?	?	+
NGF	?	?	?	+
LIF	?	?	Oligodendrocyte	?
IL-6	?	?	Oligodendrocyte	?

*Effect in combination with PDGF.

major cell types missing (neurons) or present in reduced numbers (T1As) in these isolated cultures, but present in vivo, that might promote further perinatal O-2A progenitor proliferation.

If perinatal O-2A progenitor cells are grown in co-culture with excess T1As, the cells do not prematurely differentiate but continue proliferating as perinatal O-2A progenitor cells.[4,209,231] Dissociated T1As are not as effective as a T1A monolayer in producing this effect.[231] Growing perinatal O-2A progenitor cells in T1A-CM has an effect equivalent to growing the cells in physical contact with T1As, suggesting that the mitogen is a soluble factor secreted by T1As.[4,209]

Accumulated data suggest that the physiologic mitogen produced by T1As is PDGF: 1) exogenous PDGF can replace T1A as a mitogen for perinatal O-2A progenitor cells;[26,131,210,233] 2) PDGF receptors have been identified on perinatal O-2A progenitor cells;[116] 3) PDGF has been shown to be present in extracts of embryonic rat optic nerve;[233] 4) PDGF has been identified in T1A-CM;[252] 5) the active molecule in T1A-CM and PDGF is the same size and molecular weight;[252] 6) PDGF messenger RNA has been isolated from T1As;[252] 7) anti-PDGF antibodies inhibit most of the mitogenic effect of T1A-CM;[210,233,234] and 8) perinatal O-2A progenitor cells express the same properties (e.g., morphology, antigenic phenotype, cell motility, and average cell-cycle time) in T1A-CM as in serum-free media supplemented with PDGF.[210,233] The mitogenic response of perinatal O-2A progenitor cells to PDGF can be increased by simultaneous treatment with insulin[26] or bFGF.[181]

Other growth factors tested as possible mitogens for perinatal O-2A progenitor cells but not found to be effective include: interleukin (IL)-1,

IL-2, IL-3, IL-4, IL-5, IL-6, gamma interferon, transforming growth factor (TGF)-α, TGF-β, EGF, glial maturation factor, and tri-iodothyronine.[28,131,210] Hunter and Bottenstein[131] reported that FGF alone was not mitogenic for perinatal O-2A progenitor cells. Bögler et al[38] noted that FGF alone was mitogenic for perinatal O-2A progenitor cells, but did not mimic T1A in terms of effect on perinatal O-2A progenitor cell motility or restoring the proper timing for in vivo differentiation.

It has been found that only 70% of the mitogenic activity of optic nerve extracts is eliminated by anti-PDGF antibodies, suggesting that factors other than PDGF from T1As may play a role in influencing perinatal O-2A progenitor cell proliferation and the timing of terminal differentiation.[233] There is some evidence to suggest that neurons may also make a contribution as a mitogenic stimulus for perinatal O-2A progenitor cells. Soluble factors produced by cultures of rat cerebral cortical neurons have been shown to be mitogenic for O-2A lineage precursor cells, even in the presence of anti-PDGF and anti-bFGF antibodies.[114] Soluble factors produced by the CNS neuronal cell line B104 (neuroblastoma cell line) also have been shown to be mitogenic for perinatal O-2A progenitor cells, even in the presence of anti-PDGF antibodies.[41,130,131] The factor is soluble, sensitive to both trypsin and treatment for 20 minutes at 100°C (suggesting that it is a protein), and is estimated to be 30 to 100 KD in size.[41] IL-2, EGF, TGF-β, and 0.5% FCS all inhibit B104 cell-CM action.[131]

Additional evidence that neurons may stimulate perinatal O-2A progenitor cell proliferation comes from studies that have shown that, in addition to T1As, neurons express and secrete PDGF.[114,262,329] In vivo studies in which the optic nerve was cut just behind the orbit or in which the eye was enucleated at birth (leading to neuronal axon degeneration) demonstrate a subsequent marked reduction in oligodendrocyte and T2A production in optic nerve without any change in T1A cell numbers, suggesting that perinatal O-2A progenitor cells may depend upon axons, or factors from axons, for normal development.[68,93] Another study, using tetrodotoxin to selectively eliminate optic nerve electrical activity in vivo, suggested that electrical activity of neurons may play a role in modulating the production and release of perinatal O-2A progenitor cell mitogens whatever their cellular source.[21] However, the fact that perinatal O-2A progenitor cells and oligodendrocytes still form in neuron-free cultures from rat optic nerve suggests that the growth-promoting effect of neurons is beneficial but not obligatory.[2,93] Thus, cell-cell interactions via diffusible factors from T1As, with or without neurons, are necessary in order to restore the normal timing of O-2A lineage differentiation.

Oligodendrocytes

In vivo, oligodendrocyte production begins in the optic nerve at P0 and continues for several weeks.[189,276,277] Unlike T1As which can continue to divide for up to 1 week after achieving antigenic maturity,[189,276,277] immature oligodendrocytes stop dividing at about the time they differentiate into GalC$^+$ oligodendrocytes.[231,234,276,277] If perinatal O-2A progenitor cells are grown in vitro in less than 0.5% FCS with either T1A-CM or PDGF-supplemented Bottenstein-Sato medium, they will differentiate at the appropriate time into oligodendrocytes rather than T2As.[1,26,67,113,155,156,181,231,234,236] The fact that an environmental stimulus does not appear to be necessary to induce oligodendrocyte differentiation has led some investigators to suggest that oligodendrocyte differentiation is the constitutive pathway for perinatal O-2A progenitor cells.[236,289] Clonal analysis of individual perinatal O-2A progenitor cells shows that all daughter cells of a clone differentiate into oligodendrocytes after the same number of divisions, but that the number of divisions varies from clone to clone.[231,233,289,324] This difference in the number of cell divisions required to reach unresponsiveness from clone to clone probably reflects the varying age or maturity of the "seed" perinatal O-2A progenitor cells, which are continuously being produced between P0 and P7.[289]

It has been proposed that the perinatal O-2A progenitor cell contains an internal "biological clock" that "counts" cell divisions. PDGF is necessary as an environmental stimulus to drive the "clock," and it is an acquired unresponsiveness to PDGF rather than decreased availability of

PDGF that determines when the cell will differentiate.[116,231] Excess PDGF will not alter the timing of oligodendrocyte differentiation once unresponsiveness is reached.[233] It does not appear to be the loss of PDGF receptors that causes unresponsiveness, since PDGF receptors are not lost until after oligodendrocyte maturation has been completed.[182] Recently, McKinnon and colleagues[183] suggested that TGF-β might play a role in inhibiting perinatal O-2A progenitor cell proliferation in the presence of PDGF since antibodies against TGF-β partially neutralize this inhibition in vitro. Interestingly, the TGF-β seems to be produced by the perinatal O-2A progenitor cells themselves.[183]

It appears that the perinatal O-2A progenitor cell "biological clock" can be overridden in vitro by the synergistic or cooperative effect of bFGF along with PDGF.[37,38,181,204,206,207] The simultaneous exposure of perinatal O-2A progenitor cells to both of these growth factors leads to continuous cell renewal without differentiation into oligodendrocytes. TGF-β is a less potent inhibitor of perinatal O-2A progenitor proliferation in the presence of bFGF, which suggests that bFGF may interfere with TGF-β signaling.[183] Perinatal O-2A progenitor cells have been grown continuously in culture for over 1 month using this strategy, without affecting their ability to subsequently differentiate in a normal fashion.[107] However, growing perinatal O-2A progenitor cells with both bFGF and PDGF for several weeks is associated with increased rapidity of differentiation into oligodendrocytes (cells undergo fewer cell divisions before differentiation) following removal of bFGF (2 days versus 5 days for 50% of cells to differentiate).[37] Recently, Barres and colleagues[22] have shown that neurotrophin (NT)-3 will also cooperate with PDGF to override the perinatal O-2A progenitor cell "biological clock" and promote continued progenitor cell renewal in vitro. They have also shown that antibodies to NT-3 will lead to decreased numbers of perinatal O-2A progenitor cells and oligodendrocytes in the optic nerve in vivo, which suggests that NT-3 may be a true physiological mediator. No one has yet tested whether antibodies to bFGF will have the same effect in vivo or whether NT-3 and bFGF may act through a common mechanism to interfere with the stop signal of the "biological clock."

While it is an attractive hypothesis to regard oligodendrocyte differentiation as merely constitutive for perinatal O-2A progenitor cells, there is some evidence that it may also be inducible (Table 4). The chemically defined, serum-free media used by most groups to study developmental glial biology contains 5 mg/ml insulin.[42] Insulin is known to lower intracellular cAMP levels,[318] and there is evidence to suggest that insulin and/or insulin-like growth factor 1 (IGF-1) may be mitogens, differentiation factors, and survival factors for the oligodendrocyte pathway. Insulin and IGF-1 (also known as somatomedin C) have both been shown to increase the number of oligodendrocytes from cultures of perinatal O-2A progenitor cells.[26,72,178,185,186] IGF-1 and IGF-2 messenger RNA has been demonstrated in rat brain and T1As.[14,255] IGF-1 receptors have been identified on perinatal O-2A progenitor cells and oligodendrocytes.[178,186] The effect of IGF-1 was most pronounced on immature oligodendrocytes, but perinatal O-2A progenitor cells were also induced to proliferate.[185] IGF-1 was effective at a low concentration, while insulin required a dose that secondarily saturates IGF-1 receptors, suggesting that IGF-1 may be the true physiological mediator.[178,186]

Oligodendrocyte differentiation involves three physiological (as opposed to antigenic) stages.[237] The first stage involves exiting from the cell cycle, which occurs while the oligodendrocyte is immature.[231,234] The second stage involves the synthesis of myelin components, and the third stage is the actual assembly of myelin and the maintenance of extended cell membranes. Cells in isolated culture only reach the second stage, since structural myelin is not produced in the absence of neurons.[237]

One of the first myelin components produced in the second stage is CNP, a myelin-associated enzyme. cAMP analogs have been shown to increase the specific activity of CNP in oligodendrocytes in cell culture,[184] and to accelerate oligodendrocyte differentiation from perinatal O-2A progenitor cells, but only 1 to 2 days before they would have done so anyway.[237] Thus, the sensitivity of perinatal O-2A progenitor cells to cAMP also seems to progress according to an endogenous schedule. Although cAMP analogs do not influence the number of perinatal O-2A progenitor cells that go on to become oligodendrocytes, they do accelerate the rate at which cells express CNP after they have entered their last S-phase. It has been shown that cAMP analogs inhibit perinatal O-2A progenitor proliferation,[237] which is consistent with speculation that IGF-1 may stimulate perinatal O-2A progenitor cell proliferation by lowering intracellular cAMP.

Two other factors that may promote the maturation of oligodendrocytes are ciliary neurotrophic factor (CNTF) and leukemia inhibitory factor (LIF) (Table 4). Mayer and colleagues,[179] using purified cultures of perinatal O-2A progenitor cells, showed that either factor would promote oligodendrocyte maturation compared with untreated controls, as determined by expression of myelin basic protein.

Oligodendrocytes, like neurons,[63,213] are normally overproduced during development in vivo and redundant cells subsequently undergo a process of programmed cell death (apoptosis).[326,327] Barres and colleagues[18] have provided evidence that about 50% of oligodendrocytes undergo apoptosis in the developing rat optic nerve. Apoptosis peaked between P4 and P10 and had ceased by P45. Oligodendrocyte apoptosis appears to be triggered by inadequate amounts of critical growth factors required for in vivo survival (Table 4). Factors that have been found to promote long-term oligodendrocyte survival in vitro include IGF-1, IGF-2, insulin (but only at concentrations that secondarily saturate IGF-1 receptors), CNTF, LIF, NT-3, and IL-6 (at very high doses).[18,23,168,179] PDGF also promotes early oligodendrocyte survival but, since oligodendrocytes go on to lose their PDGF receptors,[182] this response is short-lived.[18] Combinations of these growth factors appear to be more effective for maintaining the survival effect over the long term.[23]

Adult O-2A Progenitor Cells

Adult O-2A progenitor cells appear in the developing rat optic nerve as a distinct population of cells that coexist with perinatal O-2A progenitor cells until this latter population has disappeared from the nerve.[322] Adult O-2A progenitor cells can be isolated from the optic nerve as early as P7.[322] Cultures from adult optic nerves contain only adult O-2A progenitor cells.[320]

Mounting evidence suggests that adult O-2A progenitor cells are derived from a subset of perinatal O-2A progenitor cells.[321] Time-lapse cinemicroscopy of cultures of perinatal O-2A progenitor cells from P21 optic nerve grown in T1A-CM revealed that some of the subsequent perinatal O-2A progenitor cell progeny had the characteristics of adult O-2A progenitor cells (e.g., "unipolar" morphology, slowly dividing, and slowly migrating).[324] In addition, serial passage of P0 optic nerve cultures (which lack adult O-2A progenitor cells) onto monolayers of T1As is associated with the appearance of cells with the antigenic phenotype, morphology, and rate of division characteristic of adult O-2A progenitor cells.[324] Finally, in vitro clonal analysis studies have documented that a subset of colonies of perinatal O-2A progenitor cells go on to contain cells with some of the properties of adult O-2A progenitor cells.[72]

Since perinatal O-2A progenitor cells eventually disappear from the developing optic nerve, how are populations of adult O-2A progenitor cells maintained throughout life in the adult animal? The answer appears to lie in the distinction between "progenitor" (or "precursor") cells and true "stem" cells.[111,219] Adult O-2A progenitor cells (unlike perinatal O-2A progenitor cells) possess true stem cell properties, including a long cell-cycle time,[320,323,324] and the ability to undergo asymmetric division and differentiation.[321,324] Like stem cells in other organs, adult O-2A progenitor cells can support their own replenishment as well as that of the oligodendrocyte population throughout life. Thus, the label "adult O-2A progenitor cells" is somewhat of a misnomer and a more accurate term for these cells would probably be "adult O-2A stem cells."

Known mitogens for adult O-2A progenitor cells include PDGF[323] and bFGF.[319] In fact, when applied together, both factors act synergistically and have the ability to convert adult O-2A progenitor cells in vitro into cells with the characteristics of perinatal O-2A progenitor cells (e.g., bipolar morphology, rapid cell-cycle time and migration rate, and an mAb $O4^-$, $vimentin^+$ phenotype).[319] It has been proposed that this growth factor cooperation may provide a mechanism to rapidly amplify the in vivo O-2A progenitor population in adults in the setting of CNS injury or demyelination in order to facilitate repair mechanisms.[321]

Type-2 Astrocytes

FCS will induce nearly 100% of perinatal O-2A progenitor cells to permanently express GFAP within 3 days after exposure in vitro.[5,26,67,155,156,158,160,211,230,234,236,289] Rat serum has a similar effect, horse serum has little or no effect, and calf serum (nonfetal) has an intermediate effect.[158,234] The active factor(s) in FCS migrates at 500 kD by gel filtration, is nondialyzable, is inactivated by boiling for 10 minutes, precipitates in 60% (v/v) saturated $(NH_4)_2SO_4$, is trypsin-sensitive, and is present in dilipidated and fibronectin-free FCS.[158,234] The factor in FCS works without coating the culture plates with poly-L-lysine, works despite disruption of actin filaments with cytochalasin D, and is not mimicked by increases in cAMP, cyclic guanosine monophosphate (cGMP), or pH changes.[234] The effect is reversible for 1 to 2 days but then becomes fixed. Both perinatal O-2A progenitor cells and immature oligodendrocytes (mAb $O4^+$,$GalC^-$) can be induced to differentiate into T2As, but $GalC^+$ oligodendrocytes cannot.[4,155,163]

Extracts made from optic nerve can induce T2A differentiation from perinatal O-2A progenitor cells, and this factor is 50 times more concentrated in extracts of optic nerve that the correct age for purported in vivo T2A differentiation than in extracts from younger optic nerve.[129] This factor is inactivated by heating to 96°C for 10 minutes or by trypsin digestion, which suggests that it is a protein.[129,163] Extracts made from rat brain contain a similar protein.[163] The observation that mechanical damage to T1As in vitro leads to release of a similar inducing factor into the medium suggests that the source of this protein might be T1As.[163]

The possibility that the T2A inducer protein made by T1As and found in optic nerve extracts might be CNTF is suggested by several supporting pieces of data. First, exogenous CNTF is as effective as CNS tissue extract at the same concentration in inducing T2A differentiation. Second, CNTF and the inducing factor in optic nerve extract have the same relative molecular weight. Third, optic nerve extract supports the survival of ciliary ganglion cells in vitro just as CNTF does.[128,129,163]

While CNTF may be the inducer protein present in CNS tissue extract, neither CNTF nor tissue extract is equivalent in effect to FCS. CNTF and/or tissue extract only induce T2A differentiation transiently in cell culture, while FCS does so permanently. T2As induced by CNTF and/or tissue extract eventually lose GFAP expression and go on to differentiate into oligodendrocytes if they are cultured in less than 0.5% FCS. CNTF and/or tissue extract only induce 15% to 45% of perinatal O-2A progenitor cells to differentiate into T2As, while FCS induces close to 100%. Other investigators have called into question the in vitro T2A-inducing ability of CNTF. Mayer and colleagues,[179] who did not see any induction of T2As when purified cultures of perinatal O-2A progenitor cells were exposed to CNTF alone, suggested that the T2A induction in response to CNTF seen by Lillien et al[128,162,163] may have been due to the presence of inductive factors from other cell types in less homogeneous cultures.

Lillien and colleagues[163] also noted that an extracellular matrix (ECM)-associated molecule left behind on culture dishes after the cultured cells were removed with ammonia and Triton X-100 led to stable T2A differentiation, and its effect was additive with CNTF for T2A induction. The ECM-associated molecule is extractable with 2N NaCl and has been shown to be present in the optic nerve at the time of purported T2A differentiation in vivo. ECM-associated molecules from cultures of T1As or macrophages were not as effective as those from cultures of meningeal or endothelial cells, suggesting that the ECM-associated molecule may not be of glial origin. These findings have been confirmed by others using ECM molecules derived from cultured endothelial cells.[179] The fact that CNTF enhances the ability of the ECM-derived molecule to induce T2A differentiation and also enhances the differentiation of oligodendrocytes from perinatal O-2A progenitor cells in the absence of the ECM-derived molecule suggests that CNTF is a pleiotrophic modulator (Table 4) that is capable of enhancing the process of differentiation *per se*, while the actual path of differentiation promoted is dependent on the presence of other factors.[179]

Cell density in culture has also been shown to influence whether perinatal O-2A progenitor cells differentiate into oligodendrocytes or T2As. High cell density favors oligodendrocytic differentiation, while low cell density favors astrocytic differentiation.[3,103,129,154] Levi and colleagues[154] have suggested that perinatal O-2A progenitor cells produce a high-molecular-weight (>30 kD), nonmitogenic autocrine factor when grown in high density that promotes oligodendrocyte differentiation. The exact role of cell-cell contact as opposed to cell-cell interactions via diffusible mediators in O-2A lineage differentiation determination has yet to be completely elucidated.

The In Vivo Type-2 Astrocyte Controversy

While the distinctions between T1As and T2As seem clear, reproducible, and verifiable in vitro, a great deal of controversy has arisen over confirming the actual presence of T2As in vivo.[94,204,273-275] The evidence for the in vivo existence of T2As is based primarily on antibody staining of suspensions of freshly dissociated cells from both rat optic nerve and rat brain demonstrating the presence of mAb A2B5$^+$, GFAP$^+$ cells beginning at P7 to P10.[189,315] Supporting evidence came from studies demonstrating that CNTF, one of the factors purported to induce T2A formation in vitro, also occurred in optic nerve during this same time period,[162,163] as well as from tissue section stains purporting to identify mAb A2B5$^+$, GFAP$^+$ cells in rat optic nerve.[189,190]

Doubts about the presence of T2As in vivo began when a combined [^{3}H]-thymidine autoradiographic and immunocytochemical study using thin-section electron microscopy in the rat optic nerve failed to identify a second wave of astrocytic proliferation following oligodendrocyte proliferation to correspond with T2A proliferation.[273-275] Re-examination of the cell suspension data revealed that the proportion of mAb A2B5$^+$, GFAP$^+$ cells was unexpectedly small and that this proportion did not increase with increasing age of the animal.[94] It was possible that the mAb A2B5$^+$, GFAP$^+$ cells did not represent a stable, but a transient phenotype for cells that might later still become oligodendrocytes.[128,162-164] Tissue section staining for mAb A2B5 was also called into question when it was noted that in vivo astrocytic mAb A2B5 staining was often intracellular rather than surface staining.[189,190]

Even if T2As are found to exist in vivo, it is unlikely that the original anatomic and functional distinctions between T1As and T2As remain valid. T2As were postulated to perform an axonal conduction role, occupying the interior of the optic nerve and the cerebral white matter, and contributing to the structures surrounding nodes of Ranvier.[84,85,190,191] T1As were thought to perform a more structural role, occupying gray matter and the periphery of the optic nerve and contributing to the formation of the blood-brain barrier, glial scar, and the glial limiting membrane.[130,135,188,191] More recently, in vivo intracellular dye injection studies[47] as well as thin-section electron microscopy studies[285] of rat optic nerve have shown that some astrocytes associated with either the pial surface or blood vessels also make contact with nodes of Ranvier. Furthermore, while the astrocytic processes associated with nodes of Ranvier have been labeled with the markers HNK-1, NSP-4 and J1 (erroneously purported to be T2A markers), none has been labeled with mAb A2B5.[84,85]

While it seems clear that both perinatal and adult O-2A progenitor cells retain the ability to form astrocytes given the right cellular microenvironment, current evidence for the presence of T2As under normal conditions in vivo remains weak. Either the number of T2As present in vivo is quite small, or we do not yet have sufficient tools to identify and distinguish these cells.

Radial Glia

In nonmammalian species, radial glia represent a permanent telencephalic cell population.[145] In mammalian species they are a transient cell population in the telencephalon, disappearing after the end of neuronal migration.[238,266] It now seems clear that most mammalian telencephalic radial glial cells transform into mature astrocytes with the same antigenic phenotype as T1As.[306] As these radial glial cells become GFAP+, they lose reactivity to mAb RC1 (and presumably to mAb RC2 and mAb Rat-401).[65]

Since most radial glia have been studied only in vivo, it has been difficult to investigate the biological signals that control radial glial formation, or their transition to cortical astrocytes in mammalian telencephalon. However, the fact that their transition temporally coincides with the cessation of neuronal migration as well as the arrival of cortical astrocytes in the cortical plate would suggest that signals from one or both of these cell types are likely to be involved. The biological signals surrounding the formation and persistence of specialized glial cells (ependymal cells, tanycytes, cerebellar Bergmann glial cells, and retinal Müller cells) are unknown.

Multipotential Neuroglial Precursor Cells

Little is known about the progression and control of maturation of multipotential neuroglial precursor cells. However, it appears that EGF, TGF-α, and bFGF, are all mitogens for these cells in vitro[202,249,250,306] (Table 4).

Subventricular Zone Heterogeneity and Precursor Migration

The description in 1935 of interkinetic nuclear migration by Sauer[263] was thought to have resolved the controversy between those who agreed with His[122] (that the ventricular and subventricular zone was composed of more than one type of neuroglial precursor cell) and those who agreed with Schaper[265] (that the ventricular and subventricular zone was composed of a homogeneous population of precursor cells), in favor of the latter group. The different "layers" of precursor cells simply reflected the different position of nuclei in cells in differing stages of the mitotic cycle. However, it now seems clear that His and his followers were actually closer to the truth, but for different reasons.

Ventricular and Subventricular Zone Composition

While at some very early point in development the ventricular and subventricular zone cells might be totipotent and could therefore be considered a homogeneous population, this population appears to rapidly become segregated into multipotent neuroglial precursors, neuronal precursors, and glial precursors.

Many telencephalic neuronal precursors proliferate in the subventricular zone and migrate only along radial glia to reach the cortical plate once they are postmitotic. A prominent exception involves cerebellar neuronal precursor cells, which migrate along radial glia to reach the external granular layer while they are still proliferating precursor cells. The external granular layer of the cerebellum acts as a "secondary subventricular zone" where neuronal precursor cells continue to proliferate and then migrate inward to the appropriate cortical layer once they are postmitotic.

Morshead and colleagues[200] have recently presented data suggesting that the EGF-responsive multipotential neuroglial precursor cells isolated from both E14 and adult murine brain were all derived from the ventricular and subventricular zones. Their group demonstrated that EGF-responsive "neurospheres" would be produced only when CNS dissections for primary culture included the ventricular and subventricular zones,[200] and that a new "neurosphere specific" monoclonal antibody (mAb 10B5) mainly labeled patches of cells lining the lateral ventricles.[317] These findings suggest (but do not prove) that these cells do not migrate until they become more restricted in their potential differentiation fate.

Perinatal O-2A progenitor cells (which are still proliferative while migrating, and probably continue to proliferate for a while once they reach their destination) can be identified from primary cultures of optic nerve taken as early as E16.[190,278] In vitro cultures of selected optic nerve segments revealed that perinatal O-2A progenitor cells first appeared at the brain end of the optic nerve at about E16 and reached the orbit end of the nerve by E21.[278] Time-lapse photography shows that T1As promote perinatal O-2A progenitor cell motility and this T1A effect can be mimicked by exogenously administered PDGF.[211,278] The entrance of perinatal O-2A progenitor cells into the chiasmal portion of the optic nerve also coincides with the arrival of axons at the chiasm.[170] A possible chemotactic and/or guiding role for perinatal O-2A progenitor cell migration by T1As and/or axons has been postulated.[278] Armstrong and colleagues[11] have shown that perinatal O-2A progenitor cells will migrate toward PDGF in vitro.

As previously stated, T1A precursors appear to arise from indigenous cells within the optic nerve.[278] If this finding holds true for the rest of the CNS (and it is not clear that it does), then it would appear that T1A precursors do not arise and migrate out from the subventricular zone but, like radial glial cells, are already present in the cell structure of the primative CNS mantle at the time that the subventricular zone forms.

It is now apparent that, although the cells of the ventricular and subventricular zones appear morphologically homogeneous, they are most likely a heterogeneous population of multipotential neuroglial precursors, neuronal precursors, and perinatal O-2A progenitor cells. Ventricular and subventricular zone heterogeneity does not exist just on a cellular level, but also appears to be operative on a regional level within both zones. For example, using retroviral gene transfer techniques, Luskin[172] has shown that the subventricular zone has specialized and highly localized regions that serve as sources for neuronal precursor cells. Similarly, perinatal O-2A progenitor cells do not arise from all parts of the ventricular (spinal cord) or subventricular (brain) zones, but appear to arise from very specific regions of these zones.

Warf and colleagues[311] were the first to make this discovery when they noticed that cells isolated from the dorsal half of spinal cords of E14 rats were not able to produce oligodendrocytes while those isolated from the ventral half were. Apparently, perinatal O-2A precursor cells in the spinal cord originate in the ventral half of the ventricular zone and then migrate into the dorsal half as well as out to the periphery of the spinal cord. These findings are in agreement with studies using in situ hybridization for PDGF-α receptor messenger RNA (expressed by perinatal O-2A progenitor cells),[226] and DM-20 messenger RNA (a splice-variant of the proteolipid protein, which is purported to be expressed by perinatal O-2A progenitor cells[169, 291] (B. Zalc, personal communication, January 1994). The in situ hybridization studies also suggest that perinatal O-2A progenitor cells arise from distinct regions of the subventricular zone of the brain.[226,291] The first pool of cells to express DM-20 is in the caudal rhombencephalon and the second pool is found in the lateral basal plate of the diencephalon.[291]

Mechanisms of Migration

The molecular mechanisms for CNS cellular migration have been best defined for neurons. Most research has focused upon cell-surface molecules that are involved in cell adhesion, including: calcium-dependent cadherins,[117] calcium-independent N-CAM,[290] neuroglial-CAM,[108] and L1,[165,246] cytotactin,[57] the adhesion molecule on glia,[9] astrotactin,[74] and the β_1-class integrins (cell-surface receptors for the ECM molecules, fibronectin, laminin, and type IV collagen).[46,126,161] Extracellular proteases have also been implicated.[197] Cell-cell adhesion can be either homotypic (between similar cell types) or heterotypic (between different types of cells). In vitro antibody perturbation studies have revealed that neuronal homotypic adhesion relies on members of the immunoglobulin superfamily (e.g., N-CAM, neuroglial-CAM, and L1), while heterotypic adhesion relies on astrotactin.[283] Since neurons migrate along radial glia and through the surrounding primitive ECM, it is not surprising that active neuronal migration has been found to depend more upon astrotactin and the β_1-class integrins than upon N-CAM or L1.[88,89,283]

The cellular and molecular mechanisms underlying perinatal O-2A progenitor cell migration in vivo are mostly unknown. It is not known whether perinatal O-2A progenitor cells simply migrate through the primitive ECM, or whether they migrate along "cellular rails" such as radial glia or even neuronal axons. Furthermore, while it is known that perinatal O-2A progenitor cells express N-CAM in vitro,[205,295] the status of expression of other known adhesion molecules is still under investigation. A major hindrance to piecing together the molecular mechanisms underlying O-2A progenitor migration has been the lack of a good in vitro model to study the process, as has been established for the study of neuronal migration.[73]

Confirmation of Nonprimate Mammalian Data in Humans

Studies of the process of normal glial differentiation have long been hampered by the limited availability of high-quality human fetal and even adult tissue samples, as well as political controversy surrounding the use of human fetal tissue in scientific experimentation. While rats are mammals, they are not primates, which raises the theoretical concern that data obtained from studying the rat system, or other nonprimate mammalian systems, will not necessarily apply to the human situation.

While theoretical concerns are difficult to dispel, there is no evidence of significant differences in the progression and control of gliogenesis between primates and nonprimates within the mammalian system. Indeed, what little human gliogenesis data are available would seem to be consistent with the schema outlined in this chapter. Kennedy and Fok-Seang[140] isolated mAb A2B5$^+$ perinatal O-2A progenitor-like cells from human optic nerve from human fetal tissue obtained from saline abortions. Aloisi et al[6] were able to isolate mAb O4$^+$, GalC$^-$ precursor cells in cultures taken from 7- to 8-week-old human embryos. Kim[144] confirmed the presence of transitional or bipotential glial cells in glial cultures of adult human corpus callosum obtained at autopsy. Armstrong et al[10] isolated an mAb O4$^+$, GalC$^-$ population of precursor cells in cultures as well as "tissue prints" of white matter taken from epileptic temporal lobe surgical specimens from adult humans. Whittemore et al[314] isolated mAb O4$^+$, mAb O1$^+$ precursor cells (which were bipotential in vitro) from adult spinal cord tissue freshly taken from organ donors. Finally, Wolswijk grew mAb O4$^+$, mAb O1$^-$ adult O-2A progenitor cells in short-term primary culture from adult human optic nerve taken from orbit enucleation specimens (G. Wolswijk, personal communication, December 1993).

Implications for Neuro-Oncology

Rapid proliferation, cellular migration or "invasion," and loss of contact inhibition are just some of the characteristics essential for malignancy that are normal cellular characteristics during the course of glial differentiation. Since the genes controlling normal cellular differentiation are still present in the genome of mature cells and since nature tends to conserve cellular processes, it is attractive to speculate whether oncogenesis involves the reactivation and loss of control of normal, or subtly altered, differentiation genes.

Growth Factors and the Autocrine Hypotheses

Growth factors provide a key link between cellular proliferation, cellular differentiation, cell survival, and oncogenesis. Table 4 summarizes our current knowledge of the established growth factor dependence of all four processes. Rapid and continued cellular division is normal during the proliferative phase of gliogenesis, while the absence of adequate amounts of certain growth factors can normally lead to cell death in even nonproliferative cells.

The autocrine hypothesis of oncology posits that the persistent and uncontrolled proliferation seen with malignant cells can result from abnormal autoproduction of a growth factor to which that cell normally responds, over-autoproduction of a growth factor to which that cell normally responds, overproduction of a receptor or production of an uncontrollable receptor to a growth factor, or a combination of these possibilities. Support for this hypothesis came when two oncogenes, *sis* and *int*-2, were found to encode the β chain of PDGF and an FGF-like factor, respectively, while the oncogenes *erb* B, *neu*, *ros*, and *trk* were found to encode the EGF receptor, an EGF-like receptor, an insulin-like receptor, and a neurotrophic factor receptor, respectively.

Consistent with this hypothesis are findings that human gliomas respond to many growth factors with known roles during normal gliogenesis (e.g., EGF, PDGF, IGF-1, nerve growth factor (NGF), aFGF, and bFGF).[81,319] Along with these mitogenic responses, human gliomas have been shown to actively express growth factors (e.g., EGF, bFGF, IGF-1, IGF-2, NGF, brain-derived neurotrophic factor (BDNF), NT-3, TGF-β, and TGF-α),[77,112,187,199,260,286,292] and several normal as well as rearranged growth factor receptors (e.g., EGF and PDGF receptors).[77,90,132]

While the effects of individual growth factors on gliomas have been studied, we have yet to explore the potential role of cooperative combinations of growth factors in glioma biology. Growth factor cooperation has been shown to play an important role in normal neuronal-glial development biology; examples being the synergistic effects of bFGF and PDGF in perpetuating the self-renewal of perinatal and adult O-2A progenitor cells,[37,38,181,204,206,207,319] the synergistic effects of NT-3 and PDGF in perpetuating the self-renewal of perinatal O-2A progenitor cells,[22] the cooperative effect of many different growth factors in promoting oligodendrocyte survival,[23] and the cooperative effect of FGF in making neuronal precursor cells competent to respond to NGF.[51,120]

Intracellular Second-Messenger Pathways

For growth factors (as well as other signaling molecules such as steroid hormones or vitamin derivatives) to effect cell proliferation, cell differentiation, and cell survival, they must ultimately cause gene transcription within the nucleus. Steroid hormones and vitamin derivatives (e.g., retinoic acid and vitamin D_3) are freely diffusible across the plasma membrane and interact with an intracellular receptor (all members of the "steroid receptor superfamily") which undergoes a conformational change allowing it to directly bind to DNA and effect gene transcription. Other signaling molecules (including growth factors) are not freely diffusible across lipid membranes and must achieve their effects through interaction with a cell membrane receptor. Intracellular second-messenger pathways provide the common pathway for many activated cell surface receptors to ultimately cause gene transcription. The specific details of the cascade of connections between cell-surface receptors and gene transcription have not yet been worked out for most second-messenger pathways; however, this is one of the most active areas of current research effort.[39]

A common second-messenger pathway begins with activation of a 7-pass (containing seven separate transmembrane hydrophobic regions) transmembrane receptor; this activates a gap (G) protein, which then activates adenylate cyclase to form cAMP. cAMP then activates A-kinase (a powerful serine/thryonine kinase) which in turn activates certain "effector proteins" which go on to affect cellular processes, including gene transcription, in specific ways that have yet to be determined. Most growth factors, however, appear to activate single-pass transmembrane receptors, which act through dimerization to form tyrosine kinases that autophosphorylate the receptor, thereby allowing it to bind to proteins that begin one or more of several second-messenger pathways.

One major pathway involves binding and subsequent activation of a G protein, which may be similar in function to the G protein associated with 7-pass transmembrane receptors. Insulin is one signaling molecule active in gliogenesis that is known to elevate cAMP levels.[318]

Another major pathway involves the activation of phospholipase C (PLC), which cleaves phosphatidyl-inositol-biphosphate (PIP_2) to form inositol triphosphate ($InsP_3$) and diacylglycerol. At this point the cascade branches. $InsP_3$ interacts with a receptor on the intracellular calcium sequestering compartment, which leads to calcium release into the cytosol. The calcium has at least two effects. It activates certain "effector proteins" by interacting with calmodulin, and it activates protein kinase C (PKC), which in turn goes on to activate certain "effector proteins" through phosphorylation. Diacylglycerol goes on to activate PKC by increasing its affinity for calcium, and it can be further cleaved to form arachidonic acid, which can then participate in the prostaglandin signaling pathway. The "effector proteins" (serine/thryonine kinases?) activated by calmodulin and/or PKC go on to affect cellular processes including gene transcription in ways that have yet to be determined.

A third major pathway (the *ras*/*raf*-1 pathway) is the best defined second-messenger pathway from membrane receptor to nuclear transcription factor. It involves binding and subsequent activation of a growth factor receptor-binding protein (GRB2)-mammalian son of sevenless (mSOS) complex;[53,110] this subsequently activates the *ras* protein (another G protein), which activates the *raf*-1 kinase (another serine/thryonine kinase), with or without help from a small number of other proteins.[196,301] The *raf*-1 kinase activates the rest of the mitogen-activated protein kinase cascade, ultimately leading to the phosphorylation and subsequent activation of the transcription factors such as *c-myc*.[269]

Not surprisingly, many other oncogenes have been found to encode proteins that interact with growth factor intracellular second-messenger pathways from the cell membrane to nuclear transcription factors. Some of these oncogenes such as *ras*, *raf*, *mos*, *abl*, and the *src* family encode cytosolic transducing proteins, while others such as *fos*, *jun*, *myc*, *erb* A, *myb*, *ets*, and *rel* encode transcription factors or parts of transcription factors. Continued research into the details of intracellular second-messenger pathways should provide insights that advance both developmental glial biology and glioma biology.

Improved Methods for the In Vitro Study of Glioma Biology

Most in vitro studies of glioma biology involve either chemically induced glioma cell lines from rats or low-passage human glioma cell lines from the primary culture of human gliomas. Ideally, one would like to apply the lineage analysis and antigenic phenotype data obtained from the study of glial developmental biology to these glioma cell lines. Unfortunately, while a few established lines do express GFAP, no glioma cell lines (either chemically induced or from primary culture) have been reported to be of O-2A lineage. In addition, most primary human glioma cell lines eventually lose their GFAP expression and go on to express mesenchymal antigens such as fibronectin (normally not expressed in gliomas) with serial passage under routine culture conditions. Attempts to stain standard formalin-fixed, paraffin-embedded human tumor specimens for differentiation ganglioside, sulfatide, and cerebroside antigens in order to perform cell lineage analysis have met with only limited success,[32,64,69] since these are very suboptimal fixation and embedding conditions for these antigens.

The major problem hindering the merger of in vitro developmental biology and glioma biology may in large part be due to the habit of growing the glioma cell lines in media containing animal serum (usually FCS). It was only with the establishment of serum-free culture conditions that human gliomas were finally shown to respond to growth factors.[218] Indeed, if human glioma specimens in vitro are treated like glial progenitor cells by growing them under serum-free conditions in astrocyte-CM (conditions more likely to mimic their in vivo setting, since serum proteins are not normally present in CNS extracellular fluid and since astrocytes are primarily responsible for maintaining extracellular fluid homeostasis in the CNS), then human glioma cell lines can be established that are of O-2A lineage. Noble and colleagues have used this strategy to isolate a new human glioma cell line (Hu-O-2A/Gb1) which has the same ^{1}H NMR spectrum as O 2A progenitor cells in vitro, responds to growth factors in vitro in a similar fashion as O-2A progenitor cells, expresses O-2A antigens, and can be manipulated in culture toward either oligodendrocytic or astrocytic end points (Figures 4 and 11) (M. Noble, et al, unpublished data). Continued application of this serum-free primary culture strategy should provide us with additional glioma cell lines for study that also behave more consistently with the principles discovered through the study of glial developmental biology.

In addition to performing glioma lineage analysis through the use of serum-free T1A-CM primary culture, it might be possible to perform lineage analysis on human gliomas in vivo through the application of ^{1}H NMR spectroscopy data.[298,299] Whether successful and accurate glioma lineage analysis will provide us with improved diagnostic and prognostic infor-

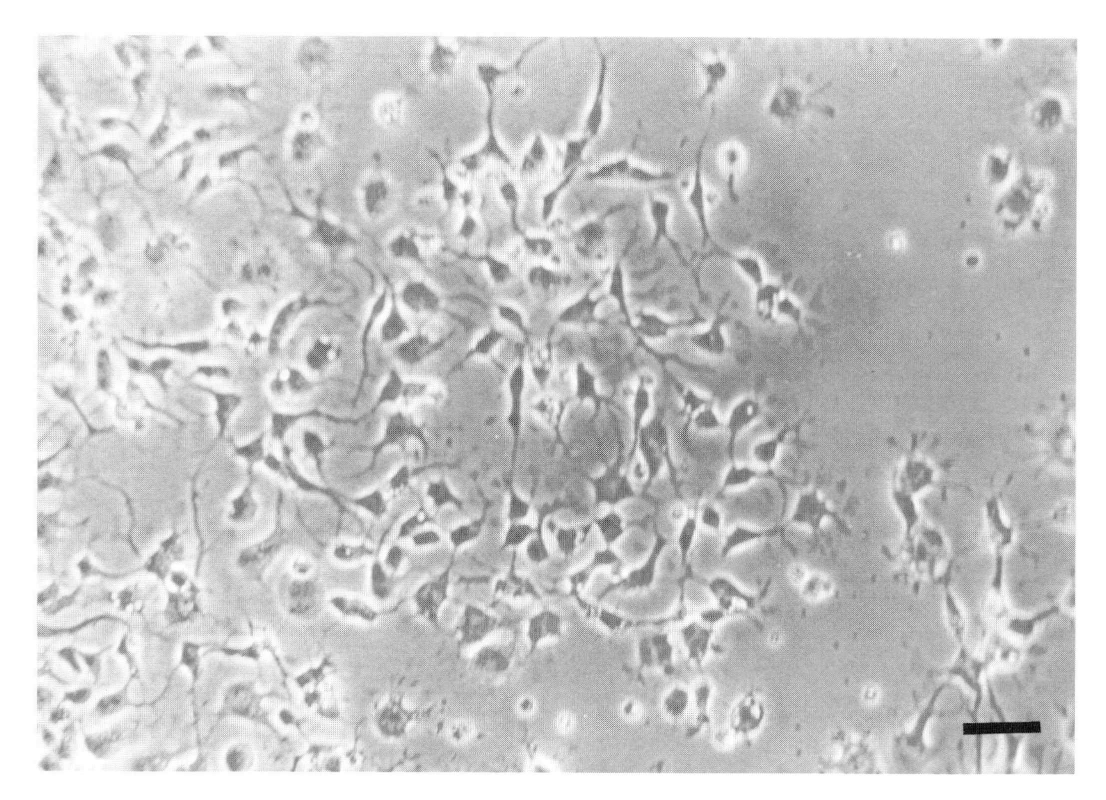

Figure 11: Inverted phase-contrast microscopic view of passage 15 of human glioblastoma cell line Hu-O-2A/Gb1 in vitro. Grown exclusively under serum-free conditions using T1A-conditioned medium,[209] Hu-O-2A/Gb1 is the first O-2A lineage human glioma line to be isolated. Possessing the same ^{1}H NMR spectrum as perinatal O-2A progenitor cells, expressing all O-2A antigens, responding to growth factors in a similar way as perinatal O-2A progenitor cells, and able to move toward either astrocytic or oligodendrocytic endpoints under various conditions, this new glioma cell line should serve as a powerful tool for applying developmental glial biology to glioma biology. The application of serum-free, astrocyte-conditioned medium to primary glioma culture should allow for the isolation of other similar cell lines in the future (cf Figure 4 which shows this same cell line grown in three-dimensional culture as a multicellular tumor spheroid). (original magnification × 20; scale bar = 50 μm)

mation compared with current histological classifications and whether it would provide a useful tool for choosing and predicting subsequent response to therapies remain to be determined.

Rat glioma cell lines are produced by transplacental chemical induction during periods of maximum glial progenitor proliferation. Most are induced by alkylating agents such as the nitrosoureas (usually ethylnitrosourea). These lines are attractive for studying glioma biology because they are from the same species that has been used for most of the studies of normal mammalian gliogenesis, and because they have remained relatively stable over long periods of time. Despite the fact that they are normally grown in serum-containing media, they can be weaned to serum-free conditions. Using these techniques, investigators have shown that the rat glioma lines C6, A2B5, F98, and 9L[27,147,150] bind mAb A2B5 but not mAb RAN-2 under serum-free conditions (M. Linskey and M. Gilbert, unpublished data), suggesting that these glioma cell lines may be of O-2A lineage. In the future, even better rat glioma cell lines for study can no doubt be obtained by immediately culturing chemically induced gliomas under serum-free conditions in astrocyte-CM, rather than waiting for later passages to make the switch.

Another area where developmental glial biology can assist the study of glioma biology is in providing three-dimensional in vitro substrates for studying glioma-brain interactions including CNS tumor invasion. Bjerkvig and colleagues[33,35] have developed a technique where three-dimensional fetal rat brain aggregates (FRBAs) can be created in vitro by dissociating E18 rat brain cells and allowing them to reaggregate under nonadherent agar-liquid media overlay conditions (Figure 4). Once mature (after 21 days), the resultant FRBAs are of homogeneous density and contain astrocytes, neurons, oligodendrocytes, neuropil, and myelinated axons. FRBAs provide a useful in vitro substrate for studying glioma invasion (Figure 4) and this in vitro model provides much more controlled conditions and requires fewer research animals than available in vivo glioma invasion models.[34,80,81,171]

New Directions for Glioma Therapy

Chromosomal loss of heterozygosity data based on chromosomal restriction polymorphisms would suggest that there are at least two possible routes to formation of a glioblastoma multiforme. Loss of heterozygosity on chromosomes 13, 17, and 22 has been observed in all three histological grades of glioma (astrocytoma, anaplastic astrocytoma, and glioblastoma multiforme).[78,91,95,133,248,302] Loss of heterozygosity on chromosome 9p has been observed in anaplastic astrocytoma and glioblastoma multiforme.[133,302] Loss of heterozygosity on chromosome 10 appears to occur exclusively with glioblastoma multiforme.[95,245,302,312] Thus, while it is possible for glioblastoma multiforme to arise directly from normal glia through an isolated alteration of chromosome 10, it can also arise from "low-grade" gliomas via a progressive stepwise series of acquired genetic alterations.

This loss of heterozygosity data is consistent with clinical data from the long-term follow-up of patients with "low-grade" gliomas. If subependymal giant cell astrocytomas, pilocytic astrocytomas, gangliogliomas, and pure oligodendrogliomas are removed from consideration, the median survival time for patients with "low-grade" gliomas is only 5.2 years (hardly that of a "benign" or "low-grade" neoplasm).[271] The most common cause of death for patients with these "low-grade" gliomas is transformation into a more malignant glioma.[152,201,216,280,304] A recent review demonstrated that by a median of 5 years after diagnosis, 28% of patients with "low-grade" gliomas exhibited transformation to a more malignant form.[304] If one waits until the point of symptomatic recurrence or death, 80% to 96% of "low-grade" gliomas will have transformed into a more malignant form.[201,280]

The question as to whether or not patients with these "low-grade" gliomas should be treated can thus be answered with an emphatic "yes!" The new question becomes, "can we come up with a form of treatment that is not worse than the natural history of the disease, and which is not itself known to induce malignancy?," since many patients with "low-grade" gliomas maintain an excellent quality of life without treatment, right up to the point of malignant transformation.

Differentiation Agents

One form of treatment that deserves closer scrutiny for potential use in patients with "low-grade" gliomas is the class of drugs known as "differentiation agents."[96,166] This term refers to a heterogeneous group of pharmacological agents that have been shown to induce malignant hematopoietic and solid tumor cell lines to recapitulate normal phenotypical, morphological, and biochemical stages of differentiation in vitro.[12,29,45,56,61,92,138,151,284] The three most studied and clinically applicable classes of differentiation agents are the vitamin derivatives (retinoic acid), the polar-apolar compounds (hexamethylene bisacetamide (HMBA) and dimethyl sulfoxide (DMSO)), and the short-chain fatty acids (sodium butyrate).

While the exact mechanisms of action of each of these agents is still being determined, the effects of all three classes appear to be mediated through one or both of two mechanisms that affect gene transcription. The first involves nonspecific effects on chromatin configuration through combinations of nucleosome disruption,[59,259,272] DNA hypomethylation,[54,55] hyperacetylation of histone proteins,[50,267] decreased binding of core histones,[167] and a general decrease in the number of non-histone nuclear proteins.[270] Why these nonspecific effects would act on genes that favor the differentiated state over the undifferentiated state is not clear, but may have something to do with the way that these different types of gene are packaged in chromatin.

The second mechanism appears to involve the induction or activation of specific transcription activators or transcription factors. Retinoic acid receptors (members of the "steroid receptor superfamily"), when bound to retinoic acid, are known to act as transcription activators by binding as heterodimers to specific DNA sequences.[71,136] Retinoic acid has been shown to induce homeobox (DNA-binding) genes in vitro.[44,60,151] HMBA alters the transcription rates of c-*myc*, c-*myb*, and c-*fos*,[175,176] while sodium butyrate has been shown to suppress the expression of c-*myc* [293] at the same time it induces the expression of c-*fos*.[287,293]

All three classes of differentiation agents have demonstrated promising morphological effects on rat glioma cell lines in vitro (Figure 12).[52,87,115,121,146,166] Recently, using both morphological and antigenic phenotype criteria under serum-free conditions, investigators have found that retinoic acid moves cell lines C6 and F98 toward astrocytic differentiation, sodium butyrate moves cell lines C6, 9L, and F98 toward oligodendrocytic differentiation, and HMBA moves cell lines C6 and A15A5 toward oligodendrocytic differentiation (M. Linskey and M. Gilbert, unpublished data). Retinoic acid has now entered clinical trials for use against neuroblastoma in vivo,[86] but none of these agents has yet been tried in vivo against gliomas.

The ideal role for differentiation agents in the treatment of "low-grade" gliomas would be as a low-toxicity chronic treatment agent (preferably oral), which would "stabilize" the chromatin of the neoplasm, inducing the cells to favor a more differentiated phenotype and hopefully preventing or significantly delaying malignant transformation. Their effects would most likely be tumor-static, rather than tumoricidal. However, since most patients with "low-grade" gliomas die from malignant transformation of their tumor, the delay or prevention of that transformation would make a significant contribution to the length and quality of their lives. Even if these three differentiation agents do not prove useful as therapeutic agents, one of the many newer related experimental agents may prove to be effective.[174,203,220,247]

Potential for Specifically Targeted Therapies

As progress continues to be made in the related fields of glial developmental biology and glioma biology, one can envision a day when therapies for any given glioma will be targeted to respond to the specific defect leading to oncogenesis present in that tumor, thereby maximizing the therapeutic index for treatment in each patient. An optimistic scenario might go something like this:

> In lieu of the need to reduce symptomatic mass effect through surgical debulking, a sample of the tumor, which is identified and localized through neuroimaging, is removed stereotactically. Instead of simply going to the pathology laboratory for histological diagnosis, a portion is also sent to the neuro-oncology laboratory. A portion of the neuro-oncology laboratory specimen is sectioned and stained with a battery of glial lineage markers as frozen tissue while another portion is cultured under both serum-containing and serum-free conditions in order to perform lineage analysis on the tumor. By means of polymerase chain reaction technology, the tumor genome in the final portion is screened against an ever-growing library of known genetic defects leading to glial oncogenesis. In this way, the specific genetic defects operative in that particular neoplasm are identified. If the problem is found to be loss or malfunction of a tumor suppressor gene, then the necessary gene is re-inserted into the neoplastic cells using gene therapy techniques. If the problem is defined as the presence of an oncogene, then the therapy would involve treatment with a pharmacological agent specifically tailored to interfere with the molecular mechanism of action of that oncogene without interfering with the cell processes of normal cells that do not contain the oncogene.

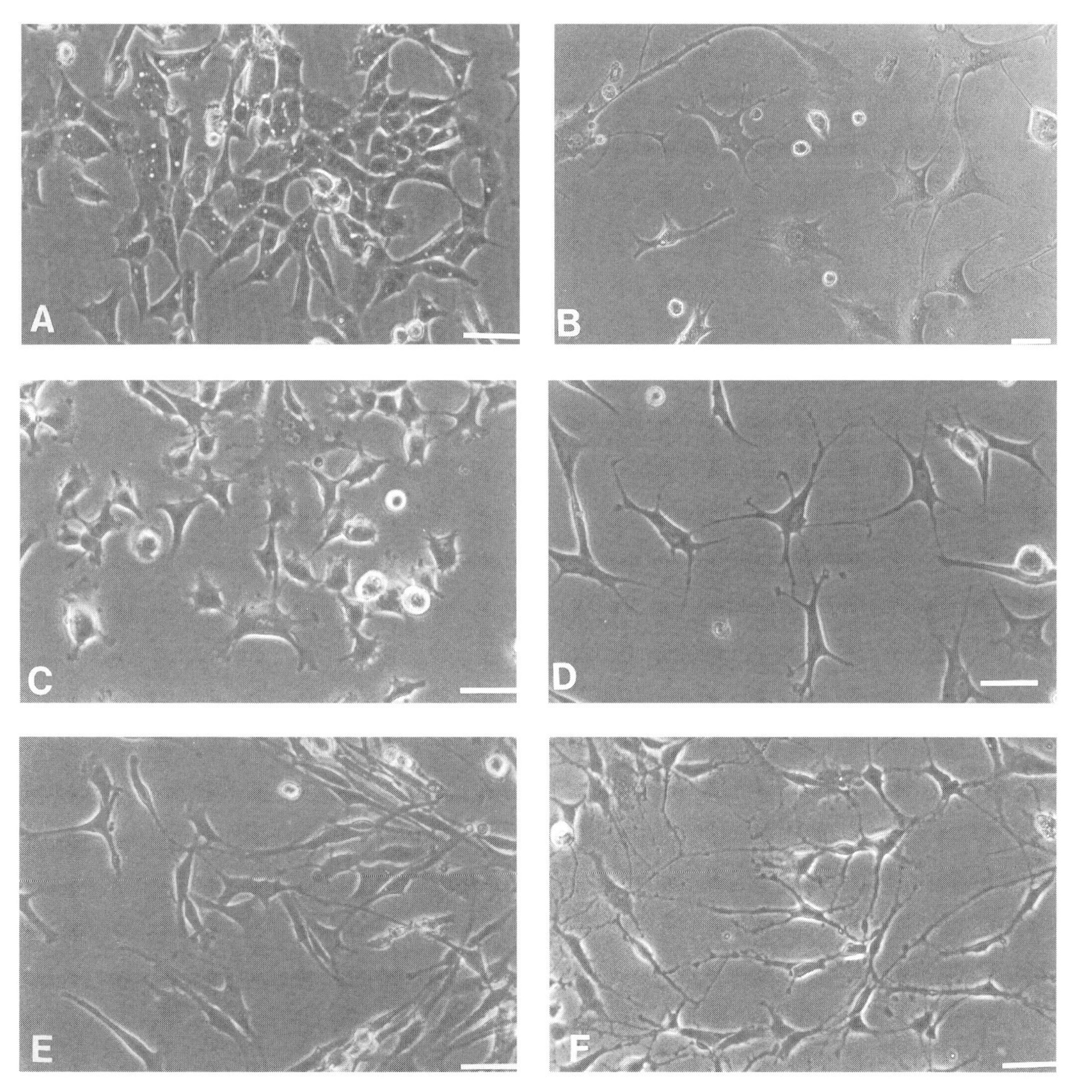

Figure 12: The effects of three differentiation agents on rat glioma cell line morphology in vitro under serum-free conditions. **A)** Control F98 glioma cells. **B)** F98 glioma cells after a 6-day exposure to 1 mM sodium butyrate in Bottenstein-Sato (B-S) medium.[42] Note the reduced cell density, the increased cell size (despite the reduced magnification), and the marked increase in cell process formation in these cells treated with sodium butyrate. **C)** Control F98 glioma cells. **D)** F98 glioma cells after a 6-day exposure to 10 mM hexamethylene bisacetamide (HMBA) in B-S medium. Note the reduced cell density, the increase in cell size, and the increase in the number, length, and complexity of the cell processes in the cells treated with HMBA. **E)** Control C6 glioma cells. **F)** C6 glioma cells after a 6-day exposure to 10^{-7} M all-trans retinoic acid in B-S medium. Note the decrease in cell density and the increase in cell process number, length, and complexity in the cells treated with retinoic acid. (original magnification × 30 [A, C-F], × 20 [B]; scale bars = 50 μm)

While this scenario seems to be a long way from practical reality, significant strides have already been made on all fronts necessary to bring it into being. At the same time that normal molecular mechanisms of cellular pathways and defects in those pathways leading to oncogenesis are being cataloged, normal human genome is being mapped through the human genome project and other related projects.[54] Additional researchers are simultaneously developing the biotechnology necessary to deliver genetic material to neoplastic glial cells in vivo.[7,177,212,240,241] Most current glioma genetic therapies are designed to selectively kill neoplastic cells; however, the same biotechnology should be adaptable to deliver genes designed to "fix" neoplastic cells rather than kill them. Still other researchers are simultaneously developing novel anticancer pharmaceutical agents designed to specifically interfere with oncogene molecular pathways. Within the last year, two separate groups have published results reportedly "curing" cancer cells (malignant due to the presence of the *ras* oncogene) in vitro using agents that specifically interfere with the attachment of the *ras* oncogene product to the cell membrane.[134,148] While still a long way from clinical reality, these new agents (or their improved successors) are the first of their kind and serve as examples of what might be possible in the future.

References

1. Abney ER, Bartlett PP, Raff MC: Astrocytes, ependymal cells, and oligodendrocytes develop on schedule in dissociated cell cultures of embryonic rat brain. **Dev Biol 83:**301-310, 1981
2. Abney ER, Williams BP, Raff MC: Tracing the development of oligodendrocytes from precursor cells using monoclonal antibodies, fluorescence-activated cell sorting, and cell culture. **Dev Biol 100:**166-171, 1983
3. Agresti C, Aloisi F, Levi G: Heterotypic and homotypic cellular interactions influencing the growth and differentiation of bipotential oligodendrocyte-type-2 astrocyte progenitors in culture. **Dev Biol 144:**16-29, 1991
4. Aloisi F, Agresti C, D'Urso D, et al: Differentiation of bipotential glial precursors into oligodendrocytes is promoted by interaction with type-1 astrocytes in cerebellar cultures. **Proc Natl Acad Sci USA 85:**6167-6171, 1988
5. Aloisi F, Agresti C, Levi G: Establishment, characterization, and evolution of cultures enriched in type-2 astrocytes. **J Neurosci Res 21:**188-198, 1988
6. Aloisi F, Giampaolo A, Russo G, et al: Developmental appearance, antigenic profile, and proliferation of glial cells of the human embryonic spinal cord: An immunocytochemical study using dissociated cultured cells. **Glia 5:**171-181, 1992
7. Anderson WF: Human gene therapy. **Science 256:**808-813, 1992
8. Antoniades HN, Scher CD, Stiles CD: Purification of human platelet-derived growth factor. **Proc Natl Acad Sci USA 76:**1809-1813, 1979
9. Antonicek H, Persohn E, Schachner M: Biochemical and functional characterization of a novel neuron-glia adhesion molecule that is involved in neuronal migration. **J Cell Biol 104:**1587-1595, 1987
10. Armstrong RC, Dorn HH, Kufta CV, et al: Pre-oligodendrocytes from adult human CNS. **J Neurosci 12:**1538-1547, 1992
11. Armstrong RC, Harvath L, Dubois-Dalcq ME: Type 1 astrocytes and oligodendrocyte-type 2 astrocyte glial progenitors migrate towards distinct molecules. **J Neurosci Res 27:**400-407, 1990
12. Augeron C, Laboisse CL: Emergence of permanently differentiated cell clones in a human colonic cancer cell line in culture after treatment with sodium butyrate. **Cancer Res 44:**3961-3969, 1984
13. Bailey P, Cushing H: **A Classification of the Tumors of the Glioma Group on a Histogenetic Basis with a Correlated Study of Prognosis.** Philadelphia: JB Lippincott, 1926
14. Ballotti R, Nielson FC, Pringle N, et al: Insulin-like growth factor-I in cultured rat astrocytes: expression of the gene, and receptor tyrosine kinase. **EMBO J 6:**3633-3639, 1987
15. Barres BA, Chun LL, Corey DP: Glial and neuronal forms of the voltage-dependent sodium channel: characteristics and cell-type distribution. **Neuron 2:**1375-1388, 1989
16. Barres BA, Chun LL, Corey DP: Ion channel expression by white matter glia. I. Type 2 astrocytes and oligodendrocytes. **Glia 1:**10-30, 1988
17. Barres BA, Chun LL, Corey DP: Ion channels in vertebrate glia. **Annu Rev Neurosci 13:**441-474, 1990
18. Barres BA, Hart IK, Coles HSR, et al: Cell death and control of cell survival in the oligodendrocyte lineage. **Cell 70:**31-46, 1992
19. Barres BA, Koroshetz WJ, Chun LL, et al: Ion channel expression by white matter glia: the type-1 astrocyte. **Neuron 5:** 527-544, 1990
20. Barres BA, Koroschetz WJ, Swartz KJ, et al: Ion channel expression by white matter glia: the O-2A glial progenitor cell. **Neuron 4:**507-524, 1990
21. Barres BA, Raff MC: Proliferation of oligodendrocyte precursor cells depends on electrical activity in axons. **Nature 361:**258-260, 1993 (Letter)
22. Barres BA, Raff MC, Gaese F, et al: A crucial role for neurotrophin-3 in oligodendrocyte development. **Nature 367:**371-375, 1994
23. Barres BA, Schmid R, Sendnter M, et al: Multiple extracellular signals are required for long-term oligodendrocyte survival. **Development 118:** 283-295, 1993
24. Bartlett PP, Noble MD, Pruss RM, et al: Rat neural antigen-2 (Ran-2): a cell surface antigen on astrocytes, ependymal cells, Müller cells and leptomeninges defined by a monoclonal antibody. **Brain Res 204:**339-351, 1981
25. Bartlett WP, Li XS, Williams M: Expression of IGF-1 mRNA in the murine subventricular zone during postnatal development. **Brain Res Mol Brain Res 12:**285-291, 1992
26. Behar T, McMorris FA, Novotny EA, et al: Growth and differentiation properties of O-2A progenitors purified from rat cerebral hemispheres. **J Neurosci Res 21:**168-180, 1988
27. Benda P, Lightbody J, Sato G, et al: Differentiated rat glial cell strain in tissue culture. **Science 161:** 370-371, 1968
28. Benveniste EN, Whitaker JN, Gibbs DA, et al:

Human B cell growth factor enhances proliferation and glial fibrillary acidic protein gene expression in rat astrocytes. **Int Immunol 1:**219-228, 1989
29. Berg RW, McBurney MW: Cell density and cell cycle effects on retinoic acid-induced embryonal carcinoma cell differentiation. **Dev Biol 138:**123-135, 1990
30. Besnard F, Perrand F, Sensenbrenner M, et al: Platelet-derived growth factor is a mitogen for glial but not for neuronal rat brain cells *in vitro*. **Neurosci Lett 73:**287-292, 1987
31. Bignami A, Eng LF, Dahl D, et al: Localization of the glial fibrillary acidic protein in astrocytes by immunofluorescence. **Brain Res 43:**429-435, 1972
32. Bishop M, de la Monte SM: Dual lineage of astrocytomas. **Am J Pathol 135:**517-527, 1989
33. Bjerkvig R: Reaggregation of fetal rat brain cells in a stationary culture system. II: Ultrastructural characterization. **In Vitro 22:**193-200, 1986
34. Bjerkvig R, Laerum OD, Mella O: Glioma cell interactions with fetal rat brain aggregates *in vitro* and with brain tissue *in vivo*. **Cancer Res 46:**4071-4079, 1986
35. Bjerkvig R, Steinsvag SK, Laerum OD: Reaggregation of fetal rat brain cells in a stationary culture system. I: Methodology and cell identification. **In Vitro 22:**180-192, 1986
36. Black JA, Sontheimer H, Minturn JE, et al: The expression of sodium channels in astrocytes *in situ* and *in vitro*. **Prog Brain Res 94:**89-107, 1992
37. Bögler O, Noble M: Studies relating differentiation to a mechanism that measures time in O-2A progenitor cells. **Ann NY Acad Sci 633:**505-507, 1991
38. Bögler O, Wren D, Barnett S, et al: Cooperation between two growth factors promotes extended self-renewal and inhibits differentiation of oligodendrocyte-type-2 astrocyte (O-2A) progenitor cells. **Proc Natl Acad Sci USA 87:**6368-6372, 1990
39. Boguski MS, McCormick F: Proteins regulating Ras and its relatives. **Nature 366:**643-654, 1993
40. Bormann J, Kettenmann H: Patch-clamp study of γ-aminobutyric acid receptor Cl^- channels in cultured astrocytes. **Proc Natl Acad Sci USA 85:**9336-9340, 1988
41. Bottenstein JE, Hunter SF, Seidel M: CNS neuronal cell line-derived factors regulate gliogenesis in neonatal rat brain cultures. **J Neurosci Res 20:** 291-303, 1988
42. Bottenstein JE, Sato GH: Growth of a rat neuroblastoma cell line in serum-free supplemented medium. **Proc Natl Acad Sci USA 76:**514-517, 1979
43. Boulder Committee: Embryonic vertebrate central nervous system: revised terminology. **Anat Rec 166:**257-262, 1970
44. Breier G, Búcan M, Francke U, et al: Sequential expression of murine homeo box genes during F9 EC cell differentiation. **EMBO J 5:**2209-2215, 1986
45. Breitman TR, Selonick SE, Collins SJ. Induction of differentiation of the human promyelocytic leukemia cell line (HL-60) by retinoic acid. **Proc Natl Acad Sci USA 77:**2936-2940, 1980
46. Buck CA, Horwitz AF: Integrin, a transmembrane glycoprotein complex mediating cell substratum adhesion. **J Cell Sci 8 (suppl):**231-250, 1987
47. Butt AM, Ransom BR: Visualization of oligodendrocytes and astrocytes in the intact rat optic nerve by intracellular injection of lucifer yellow and horseradish peroxidase. **Glia 2:**470-475, 1989
48. Calder VL, Wolswijk G, Noble M: The differentiation of O-2A progenitor cells into oligodendrocytes is associated with a loss of inducibility of Ia antigens. **Eur J Immunol 18:**1195-1201, 1988
49. Cameron RS, Rakic P: Glial cell lineage in the cerebral cortex: a review and synthesis. **Glia 4:** 124-137,1991
50. Candido EPM, Reeves R, Davie JR: Sodium butyrate inhibits histone deacetylation in cultured cells. **Cell 14:**105-113, 1978
51. Cattaneo E, McKay R: Proliferation and differentiation of neuronal stem cells regulated by nerve growth factor. **Nature 347:**762-765, 1990
52. Chapman SK: Antitumor effects of vitamin A and inhibitors of ornithine decarboxylase in cultured neuroblastoma and glioma cells. **Life Sci 26:** 1359-1366, 1980
53. Chardin P, Camonis JH, Gale NW, et al: Human Sos1: a guanine nucleotide exchange factor for Ras that binds to GRB2. **Science 260:**1338-1343, 1993
54. Christman JK, Price P, Pedrinan L, et al: Correlation between hypomethylation of DNA and expression of globin genes in Friend erythroleukemia cells. **Eur J Biochem 81:**63-61, 1977
55. Christman JK, Weich N, Schoenbrun B, et al: Hypomethylation of DNA during differentiation of Friend erythroleukemia cells. **J Cell Biol 86:** 366-370, 1980
56. Chung YS, Song IS, Erickson RH, et al: Effect of growth and sodium butyrate on brush border membrane-associated hydrolases in human colorectal cancer cell lines. **Cancer Res 45:**2976-2982, 1985
57. Chuong CM, Crossin KL, Edelman GM: Sequential expression and differential function of multiple adhesion molecules during the formation of cerebellar cortical layers. **J Cell Biol 104:**331-342, 1987
58. Cohen D, Chumakov I, Weissenbach J: A first generation physical map of the human genome. **Nature 366:**698-701, 1993 (Letter)
59. Cohen RB, Sheffery M: Nucleosome disruption precedes transcription and is largely limited to the transcribed domain of globin genes in murine erythroleukemia cells. **J Mol Biol 182:**109-129, 1985
60. Colberg-Poley AM, Voss SD, Chowdhury K, et al: Clustered homeo boxes are differentially expressed during murine development. **Cell 43:**39-45, 1985
61. Collins SJ, Bodner A, Ting R, et al: Induction of morphological and functional differentiation of human promyelocytic leukemia cells (HL-60) by compounds which induce differentiation of murine leukemia cells. **Int J Cancer 25:**213-218, 1980
62. Corvalan V, Cole R, de Vellis J, et al: Neuronal modulation of calcium channel activity in cultured rat astrocytes. **Proc Natl Acad Sci USA 87:**4345-4348, 1990
63. Cowan WM, Fawcett JW, O'Leary DDM, et al:

Regressive events in neurogenesis. **Science 225:**1258-1265, 1984
64. Cudkowicz M, De la Monte SM: Histogenesis and cell lineage analysis of medulloblastomas. **J Neurol Sci 94:**221-229, 1989
65. Culican SM, Baumrind NL, Yamamoto M, et al: Cortical radial glia: identification in tissue culture and evidence for their transformation to astrocytes. **J Neurosci 10:**684-692, 1990
66. Cull-Candy SG, Mathie A, Symonds CJ, et al: Distribution of quisqualate and kainate receptors in rat type-2 astrocytes and their progenitor cells in culture. **J Physiol (Lond) 418:**195p, 1989
67. Curtis R, Cohen J, Fok-Seang J, et al: Development of macroglial cells in rat cerebellum. I. Use of antibodies to follow early *in vivo* development and migration of oligodendrocytes. **J Neurocytol 17:** 43-54, 1988
68. David S, Miller RH, Patel R, et al: Effects of neonatal transection on glial cell development in the rat optic nerve: evidence that the oligodendrocyte-type 2 astrocyte cell lineage depends on axons for its survival. **J Neurocytol 13:**961-974, 1984
69. de la Monte SM: Uniform lineage of oligodendrogliomas. **Am J Pathol 135:**529-540, 1989
70. del Rio Hortega P: Estudios sobre la neuroglia: La glia de ecasas radiciones (oligodendroglia). **Bol Soc Espan Hist Nat** 1921
71. De Luca LM: Retinoids and their receptors in differentiation, embryogenesis, and neoplasia. **FASEB J 5:**2924-2933, 1991
72. Dubois-Dalcq M: Characterization of a slowly proliferative cell along the oligodendrocyte differentiation pathway. **EMBO J 6:**9:2587-2595, 1987
73. Edmondson JC, Hatten ME: Glial-guided granule neuron migration *in vitro*: a high-resolution time-lapse video microscopic study. **J Neurosci 7:**1928-1934, 1987
74. Edmondson JC, Liem RKH, Kuster JE, et al: Astrotactin: a novel neuronal cell surface antigen that mediates neuron astroglial interactions in cerebellar microcultures. **J Cell Biol 106:**505-517, 1988
75. Edwards MA, Yamamoto M, Caviness VS Jr: Organization of radial glia and related cells in the developing murine CNS. An analysis based upon a new monoclonal antibody marker. **Neuroscience 36:**121-144, 1990
76. Eisenbarth GS, Walsh FS, Nirenberg M: Monoclonal antibody to a plasma membrane antigen of neurons. **Proc Natl Acad Sci USA 76:**4913-4917, 1979
77. Ekstrand AJ, James CD, Cavanee WK, et al: Genes for epidermal growth factor receptor, transforming growth factor a, and epidermal growth factor and their expression in human gliomas *in vivo*. **Cancer Res 51:**2164-2172, 1991
78. El-Azouzi M, Chung RY, Farmer GE, et al: Loss of distinct regions of the short arm of chromosome 17 associated with tumorigenesis of human astrocytomas. **Proc Natl Acad Sci USA 86:**7186-7190, 1989
79. Eng LF, Vanderhaeghen JJ, Bignami A, et al: An acidic protein isolated from fibrous astrocytes. **Brain Res 28:**351-354, 1971
80. Engebraaten O, Bjerkvig R, Lund-Johansen M, et al: Interaction between human brain tumor biopsies and fetal rat brain tissue *in vitro*. **Acta Neuropathol 81:**130-140, 1990
81. Engebraaten O, Bjerkvig R, Pedersen PH, et al: Effects of EGF, bFGF, NGF, and PDGF(bb) on cell proliferative, migratory and invasive capacities of human brain-tumor biopsies *in vitro*. **Int J Cancer 53:**209-214, 1993
82. Farinelli SE, Nicklas WJ: Glutamate metabolism in rat cortical astrocyte cultures. **J Neurochem 58:**1905-1915, 1992
83. Fedoroff S, Vernadakis A (eds): **Astrocytes: Development, Morphology, and Regional Specialization of Astrocytes. Vol 1.** New York: Academic Press, 1986
84. ffrench-Constant C, Miller RH, Kruse J, et al: Molecular specialization of astrocyte processes at nodes of Ranvier in rat optic nerve. **J Cell Biol 102:**844-852, 1986
85. ffrench-Constant C, Raff MC: The oligodendrocyte-type-2 astrocyte cell lineage is specialized for myelination. **Nature 323:**335-338, 1986
86. Finklestein JZ, Krailo MD, Lenarsky C, et al: 13-cis-retinoic acid (NSC 122758) in the treatment of children with metastatic neuroblastoma unresponsive to conventional chemotherapy: report from the Childrens Cancer Study Group. **Med Pediatr Oncol 20:**307-311, 1992
87. Fischer I, Nolan CE, Shea TB: Effects of retinoic acid on expression of the transformed phenotype in C6 glioma cells. **Life Sci 41:**463-470, 1987
88. Fishell G, Hatten ME: Astrotactin provides a receptor system for CNS neuronal migration. **Development 113:**755-765, 1991
89. Fishman RB, Hatten ME: Multiple receptor systems promote CNS neural migration. **J Neurosci 13:**3485-3495, 1993
90. Fleming TP, Saxena A, Clark WC, et al: Amplification and/or overexpression of platelet-derived growth factor receptors and epidermal growth factor receptor in human glial tumors. **Cancer Res 52:**4550-4553, 1992
91. Frankel RH, Bayona W, Koslow M, et al: p53 Mutations in human gliomas: comparison of loss of heterozygosity with mutation frequency. **Cancer Res 52:**1427-1433, 1992
92. Friend C, Scher W, Holland JG, et al: Hemoglobin synthesis in murine virus-induced leukemic cells *in vitro*: stimulation of erythroid differentiation by dimethy sulfoxide. **Proc Natl Acad Sci USA 68:** 378-382, 1971
93. Fulcrand J, Privat A: Neuroglial reactions secondary to Wallerian degeneration in the optic nerve of the postnatal rat: ultrastructural and quantitative study. **J Comp Neurol 176:**189-224, 1977
94. Fulton BP, Burne JF, Raff MC: Glial cells in the rat optic nerve: The search for the type-2 astrocyte. **Ann NY Acad Sci 633:**27-34, 1991
95. Fults D, Brockmeyer D, Tullous MW, et al: p53 Mutation and loss of heterozygosity on chromosomes 17 and 10 during human astrocytoma progression. **Cancer Res 52:**674-679, 1992
96. Gabrilove JL: Differentiation factors. **Semin Oncol**

13:228-233, 1986

97. Gadisseux JF, Evrard P, Misson JP, et al: Dynamic structure of the radial glial fiber system of the developing murine cerebral wall: An immunocytochemical analysis. **Brain Res Dev Brain Res 50:**55-67, 1989
98. Gallo V, Bertolotto A, Levi G: The proteoglycan chondroitin sulfate is present in a subpopulation of cultured astrocytes and in their precursors. **Dev Biol 123:**282-285, 1987
99. Gallo V, Giovannini C, Suergiu R, et al: Expression of excitatory amino acid receptors by cerebellar cells of the type-2 astrocyte cell lineage. **J Neurochem 52:**1:1-9, 1989
100. Gallo V, Suergiu R, Levi G: Kainic acid stimulates GABA release from a subpopulation of cerebellar astrocytes. **Eur J Pharmacol 133:**319-322, 1986
101. Gard AL, Pfeiffer SE: Oligodendrocyte progenitors isolated directly from developing telencephalon at a specific phenotypic stage: myelinogenic potential in a defined environment. **Development 106:**119-132, 1989
102. Gard AL, Pfeiffer SE: Two proliferative stages of the oligodendrocyte lineage (A2B5+O4- and O4+ GalC-) under different mitogenic control. **Neuron 5:**615-625, 1990
103. Goldman JE, Geier S, Hirano M: Differentiation of astrocytes and oligodendrocytes from germinal matrix cells in primary culture. **J Neurosci 6:** 52-60, 1986
104. Goldman JE, Hirano M, Yu RK, et al: GD3 ganglioside is a glycolipid characteristic of immature neuroectodermal cells. **J Neuroimmunol 7:**179-192, 1984
105. Goldman JE, Vaysse PJ: Tracing glial cell lineages in the mammalian forebrain. **Glia 4:**149-156, 1991
106. Gospodarowicz D, Bialecki H, Greenberg G: Purification of the fibroblast growth factor activity from bovine brain. **J Biol Chem 253:**3736-3743, 1978
107. Groves AK, Barnett SC, Franklin RJM, et al: Repair of demyelinated lesions by transplantation of purified O-2A progenitor cells. **Nature 362:**453-455, 1993
108. Grumet M, Edelman GM: Heterotypic binding between neuronal membrane vesicles and glial cells is mediated by a specific cell adhesion molecule. **J Cell Biol 98:**1746-1756, 1984
109. Guentert-Lauber B, Honegger P: Responsiveness of astrocytes in serum-free aggregate cultures to epidermal growth factor: dependence on the cell cycle and the epidermal growth factor concentration. **Dev Neurosci 7:**286-295, 1985
110. Gulbins E, Coggeshall KM, Baier G, et al: Tyrosine kinase-stimulated guanine nucleotide exchange activity of Vav in T cell activation. **Science 260:** 822-825, 1993
111. Hall PE, Watt FM: Stem cells: the generation and maintenance of cellular diversity. **Development 106:**619-633, 1989
112. Hamel W, Westphal M, Szönyi E, et al: Neurotrophin gene expression by cell lines derived from human gliomas. **J Neurosci Res 34:**147-157, 1993
113. Hardy R, Reynolds R: Proliferation and differentiation potential of rat forebrain oligodendroglial progenitors both *in vitro* and *in vivo*. **Development 111:**1061-1080, 1991
114. Hardy R, Reynolds R: Rat cerebral cortical neurons in primary culture release a mitogen specific for early (G_{D3}^+/$O4^-$) oligodendrocyte progenitors. **J Neurosci Res 34:**589-600, 1993
115. Hargreaves AJ, Yusta B, Avila J, et al: Sodium butyrate induces major morphological changes in C6 glioma cells that are correlated with increased synthesis of a spectrin-like protein. **Brain Res Dev Brain Res 45:**291-295, 1989
116. Hart IK, Richardson WD, Heldin CH, et al: PDGF receptors on cells of the oligodendrocyte-type-2 astrocyte (O-2A) cell lineage. **Development 105:**595-603, 1989
117. Hatta K, Okada TS, Takeichi M: A monoclonal antibody disrupting calcium-dependent cell-cell adhesion of brain tissue: possible role of its target antigen in animal pattern formation. **Proc Natl Acad Sci USA 82:**2789-2793, 1985
118. Hatten ME: Neuronal inhibition of astroglial cell proliferation is membrane mediated. **J Cell Biol 104:**1353-1360, 1987
119. Hatten ME: Neuronal regulation of astroglial morphology and proliferation *in vitro*. **J Cell Biol 100:**384-396, 1985
120. Heuer JG, von Bartheld CS, Kinoshita Y, et al: Alternating phases of FGF receptor and NGF receptor expression in developing chicken nervous system. **Neuron 5:**283-296, 1990
121. Higashida H, Miki N, Ito M, et al: Cytotoxic action of retinoidal butenolides on mouse neuroblastoma and rat glioma cells. **Int J Cancer 33:**677-681, 1984
122. His W: Die Neuroblatsen und deren Entstehung im embryonalen Mark. Abhandl. **Math Phys Kl Konigl Sachs Ges Wiss 26:**313-372, 1889
123. Hockfield S, McKay RDG: Identification of major cell classes in the developing mammalian nervous system. **J Neurosci 5:**3310-3328, 1985
124. Honegger P, Lenoir P, Favrod P: Growth and differentiation of aggregating fetal brain cells in a serum-free defined medium. **Nature 282:**305-307, 1979
125. Hoppe D, Kettenmann H: Carrier-mediated Cl^- transport in cultured mouse oligodendrocytes. **J Neurosci Res 23:**467-475, 1989
126. Horwitz A, Duggan K, Greggs R, et al: The cell substrate attachment (CSAT) antigen has properties of a receptor for laminin and fibronectin. **J Cell Biol 101:**2134-2144, 1985
127. Huff KR, Schreier W: Fibroblast growth factor inhibits epidermal growth factor-induced responses in rat astrocytes. **Glia 3:**193-204, 1990
128. Hughes SM, Lillien LE, Raff MC, et al: Ciliary neurotrophic factor induces type-2 astrocyte differentiation in culture. **Nature 335:**70-73, 1988.
129. Hughes SM, Raff MC: An inducer protein may control the timing of fate switching in a bipotential glial progenitor cell in rat optic nerve. **Development 101:**157-167, 1987
130. Hunter SF, Bottenstein JE: Bipotential glial progenitors are targets of neuronal cell line-derived growth factors. **Brain Res Dev Brain Res** 49:33-49, 1989
131. Hunter SF, Bottenstein JE: Growth factor responses

of enriched bipotential glial progenitors. **Brain Res Dev Brain Res 54**:235-248, 1990
132. Hurtt MR, Moossy J, Donovan-Peluso M, et al: Amplification of epidermal growth factor receptor gene in gliomas: histopathology and prognosis. **J Neuropathol Exp Neurol 51**:84-90, 1992
133. James CD, Carlbom E, Dumanski JP, et al: Clonal genomic alterations in glioma malignancy stages. **Cancer Res 48**:5546-5551, 1988
134. James GL, Goldstein JL, Brown MS, et al: Benzodiazepine peptidomimetics: potent inhibitors of ras farnesylation in animal cells. **Science 260**: 1937-1942, 1993
135. Janzer RC, Raff MC: Astrocytes induce blood-brain barrier properties in endothelial cells. **Nature 325**:253-257, 1987
136. Jetten AM: Multi-stage program of differentiation in human epidermal keratinocytes: regulation by retinoids. **J Invest Dermatol 95 (suppl)**:44S-46S, 1990
137. Johnstone SR, Levi G, Wilkin GP, et al: Subpopulations of rat cerebellar astrocytes in primary culture: morphology, cell surface antigens and [3H]GABA transport. **Brain Res 389**:63-75, 1986
138. Joshi SS, Sinangil F, Sharp JG, et al: Effects of differentiation inducing chemicals on *in vivo* malignancy and NK susceptibility of metastatic lymphoma cells. **Cancer Detect Prev 11**:405-417, 1988
139. Keilhauer G, Faissner A, Schachner M: Differential inhibition of neurone-neurone, neurone-astrocyte and astrocyte-astrocyte adhesion by L1, L2, and N-CAM antibodies. **Nature 316**:728-730, 1985
140. Kennedy PGE, Fok-Seang J: Studies on the development, antigenic phenotype and function of human glial cells in tissue culture. **Brain 109**:1261-1277, 1986
141. Kettenmann H, Blankenfeld GV, Trotter J: Physiological properties of oligodendrocytes during development. **Ann NY Acad Sci 633**:64-77, 1991
142. Kettenmann H, Okland RK, Lux HD, et al: Single potassium channel currents in cultured mouse oligodendrocytes. **Neurosci Lett 32**:41-46, 1982
143. Kilpatrick TJ, Bartlett PF: Cloning and growth of multipotential neural precursors: requirements for proliferation and differentiation. **Neuron 10**: 255-265, 1993
144. Kim SU: Antigenic expression by glial cells grown in culture. **J Neuroimmunol 8**:255-282, 1985
145. King JS: A comparative investigation of neuroglia in representative vertebrates: A silver carbonate study. **J Morphol 119**:435-466, 1966
146. Ko LW, Koestner A: Morphologic and morphometric analyses of butyrate-induced alterations of rat glioma cells *in vitro*. **J Natl Cancer Inst 65**:1017-1027, 1980
147. Koestner A, Swenberg JA, Wechsler W: Transplacental production with ethylnitrosourea of neoplasms of the nervous system in Sprague-Dawley rats. **Am J Pathol 63**:37-56, 1971
148. Kohl NE, Mosser SD, deSolms SJ, et al: Selective inhibition of *ras*-dependent transformation by a farnesyltransferase inhibitor. **Science 260**:1934-1937, 1993
149. Kozak LP, Eppig JJ, Dahl D, et al: Ultrastructural and immunohistological characterization of a cell culture model for the study of neuronal-glial interactions. **Dev Biol 59**:206-227, 1977
150. Lantos PL, Roscoe JP, Skidmore CJ: Studies on the morphology and tumorigenicity of experimental brain tumours in tissue culture. **Br J Exp Pathol 57**:95-104, 1976
151. LaRosa GJ, Gudas LJ: Early retinoic acid-induced F9 teratocarcinoma stem cell gene *ERA*-1: alternate splicing creates transcripts for a homeobox-containing protein and one lacking the homeobox. **Mol Cell Biol 8**:3906-3917, 1988
152. Laws ER Jr, Taylor WF, Clifton MB, et al: Neurosurgical managment of low-grade astrocytoma of the cerebral hemispheres. **J Neurosurg 61**:665-673, 1984
153. Leutz A, Schachner M: Epidermal growth factor stimulates DNA-synthesis of astrocytes in primary cerebellar cultures. **Cell Tissue Res 220**:393-404, 1981
154. Levi G, Agresti C, D'Urso D, et al: Is the oligodendroglial differentiation of bipotential oligodendrocyte-type 2 astrocyte progenitors promoted by autocrine factors? **Neurosci Lett 128**:37-41, 1991
155. Levi G, Aloisi F, Wilkin GP: Differentiation in cerebellar bipotential glial precursors into oligodendrocytes in primary culture: developmental profile of surface antigens and mitotic activity. **J Neurosci Res 18**:407-417, 1987
156. Levi G, Gallo V, Ciotti MT: Bipotential precursors of putative fibrous astrocytes and oligodendrocytes in rat cerebellar cultures express distinct surface features and "neuron-like" γ-aminobutyric acid transport. **Proc Natl Acad Sci USA 83**:1504-1508, 1986
157. Levi G, Wilkin GP, Ciotti MT, et al: Enrichment of differentiated stellate astrocytes in cerebellar interneuron cultures as studied by GFAP immunofluorescence and autoradiographic uptake patterns with [^{3}H] D-aspartate and [3H]GABA. **Brain Res 312**:227-241, 1983
158. Levison SW, McCarthy KD: Characterization and partial purification of AIM: a plasma protein that induces rat cerebral type 2 astroglia from bipotential glial progenitors. **J Neurochem 57**:782-794, 1991
159. Levitt P, Cooper ML, Rakic P: Coexistence of neuronal and glial precursor cells in the cerebral ventricular zone of the fetal monkey: an ultrastructural immunoperoxidase analysis. **J Neurosci 1**:27-39, 1981
160. Liepelt U, Kindler-Röhrborn A, Lennartz K, et al: Differentiation potential of a monoclonal antibody-defined neural progenitor cell population isolated from prenatal rat brain by fluorescence-activated cell sorting. **Brain Res Dev Brain Res 51**:267-278, 1990
161. Liesi P: Extracellular matrix and neuronal movement. **Experientia 46**:900-907, 1990
162. Lillien LE, Raff MC: Analysis of the cell-cell interactions that control type-2 astrocyte development *in vitro*. **Neuron 4**:525-534, 1990
163. Lillien LE, Sendtner M, Raff MC: Extracellular matrix-associated molecules collaborate with ciliary neurotrophic factor to induce type-2 astrocyte development. **J Cell Biol 111**:635-644, 1990

164. Lillien LE, Sendtner M, Rohrer H, et al: Type-2 astrocyte development in rat brain cultures is initiated by a CNTF-like protein produced by type-1 astrocytes. **Neuron 1**:485-494, 1988
165. Lindner J, Rathjen FG, Schachner M: L1 mono- and polyclonal antibodies modify cell migration in early postnatal mouse cerebellum. **Nature 305**:427-430, 1983
166. Linskey ME, Gilbert MR: Glial differentiation: a review with implications for new directions in neuro-oncology. **Neurosurgery 36**:1-22, 1995
167. Long BH, Huang CY, Pogo AO: Isolation and characterization of the nuclear matrix in Friend erythroleukemia cells: chromatin and hnRNA interactions with the nuclear matrix. **Cell 18**:1079-1090, 1979
168. Louis JC, Magal E, Takayama S, et al: CNTF protection of oligodendrocytes against natural and tumor necrosis factor-induced death. **Science 259**:689-692, 1993
169. Lubetzki C, Goujet-Zalc C, Gansmüller A, et al: Morphological, biochemical, and functional characterization of bulk isolated glial progenitor cells. **J Neurochem 56**:671-680, 1991
170. Lund RD, Bunt AH: Prenatal development of central optic pathways in albino rats. **J Comp Neurol 165**:247-264, 1976
171. Lund-Johansen M, Bjerkvig R, Humphrey PA, et al: Effect of epidermal growth factor on glioma cell growth, migration, and invasion *in vitro*. **Cancer Res 50**:6039-6044, 1990
172. Luskin MB: Restricted proliferation and migration of postnatally generated neurons derived from the forebrain subventricular zone. **Neuron 11**:173-189, 1993
173. MacVicar BA: Voltage-dependent calcium channels in glial cells. **Science 226**:1345-1347, 1984
174. Marks PA, Breslow R, Rifkind RA, et al: Polar/apolar chemical inducers of differentiation of transformed cells: strategies to improve therapeutic potential. **Proc Natl Acad Sci USA 86**:6358-6362, 1989
175. Marks PA, Ramsay R, Sheffery M, et al: Changes in gene expression during hexamethylene bisacetamide induced erythroleukemia differentiation, in Stamatoyannopoulos G, Wienhuis A (eds): **Developmental Control of Globin Gene Expression**. New York: Alan R Liss, 1987, pp 253-268
176. Marks PA, Sheffery M, Rifkind RA: Induction of transformed cells to terminal differentiation and the modulation of gene expression. **Cancer Res 47**:659-666, 1987
177. Martuza RL, Malick A, Markert JM, et al: Experimental therapy of human glioma by means of a genetically engineered virus mutant. **Science 252**:854-856, 1991
178. Masters BA, Werner H, Roberts CT Jr, et al: Insulin-like growth factor I (IGF-I) receptors and IGF-I action in oligodendrocytes from rat brains. **Regul Pept 33**:117-131, 1991
179. Mayer M, Bhakoo K, Noble M: Ciliary neurotrophic factor and leukemia inhibitory factor promote the generation, maturation, and survival of oligodendrocytes *in vitro*. **Development 120**:143-153, 1994
180. McKay RD: The origins of cellular diversity in the mammalian central nervous system. **Cell 58**: 815-821, 1989
181. McKinnon RD, Matsui T, Aranda M, et al: A role for fibroblast growth factor in oligodendrocyte development. **Ann NY Acad Sci 638**:378-386, 1991
182. McKinnon RD, Matsui T, Dubois-Dalcq M, et al: FGF modulates the PDGF-driven pathway of oligodendrocyte development. **Neuron 5**:603-614, 1990
183. McKinnon RD, Piras G, Ida JA Jr, et al: A role for TGF-β in oligodendrocyte differentiation. **J Cell Biol 121**:1397-1407, 1993
184. McMorris FA: Cyclic AMP induction of the myelin enzyme 2',3'-cyclic nucleotide 3'-phosphohydrolase in rat oligodendrocytes. **J Neurochem 41**:2:506-515, 1983
185. McMorris FA, Dubois Dalcq M: Insulin-like growth factor I promotes cell proliferation and oligodendroglial commitment in rat glial progenitor cells developing *in vitro*. **J Neurosci Res 21**:199-209, 1988
186. McMorris FA, Smith TM, DeSalvo S, et al: Insulin-like growth factor I/somatomedin C: a potent inducer of oligodendrocyte development. **Proc Natl Acad Sci USA 83**:822-826, 1986
187. Melino G, Stephanou A, Annicchiarico-Petruzzelli M, et al: IGF-II mRNA expression in LI human glioblastoma cell line parallels cell growth. **Neurosci Lett 144**:25-28, 1992
188. Miller RH, Abney ER, David S, et al: Is reactive gliosis a property of a distinct subpopulation of astrocytes? **J Neurosci 6**:22-29, 1986
189. Miller RH, David S, Patel R, et al: A quantitative immunohistochemical study of macroglial cell development in the rat optic nerve: *in vivo* evidence for two distinct astrocyte lineages. **Dev Biol 111**:35-41, 1985
190. Miller RH, Fulton BP, Raff MC: A novel type of astrocyte contributes to the structure of nodes of Ranvier in rat optic nerve. **Eur J Neurosci 1**: 172-180, 1989
191. Miller RH, Raff MC: Fibrous and protoplasmic astrocytes are biochemically and developmentally distinct. **J Neurosci 4**:585-592, 1984
192. Minturn JE, Black JA, Angelides KJ, et al: Sodium channel expression detected with antibody 7493 in A2B5-positive and A2B5-negative astrocytes from rat optic nerve in vitro. **Glia 3**:358-367, 1990
193. Minturn JE, Sontheimer H, Black JA, et al: Membrane-associated sodium channels and cytoplasmic precursors in glial cells. Immunocytochemical, electrophysiological, and pharmacological studies. **Ann NY Acad Sci** 633:255-271, 1991
194. Misson JP, Edwards MA, Yamamoto M, et al: Identification of radial glial cells within the developing murine central nervous system: studies based upon a new immunohistochemical marker. **Brain Res Dev Brain Res 44**:95-108, 1988
195. Misson JP, Edwards MA, Yamamoto M, et al: Mitotic cycling of radial glial cells of the fetal murine cerebral wall: A combined autoradiographic and immunohistochemical study. **Brain Res Dev 466**:183-190, 1988
196. Moodie SA, Willumsen BM, Weber MJ, et al: Com-

plexes of Ras-GTP with Raf-1 and mitogen-activated protein kinase. **Science 260:**1658-1661, 1993
197. Moonen G, Grau-Wagemans MP, Selak I: Plasminogen activator-plasmin system and neuronal migration. **Nature 298:**753-755, 1982
198. Morrison RS, deVellis J: Growth of purified astrocytes in a chemically defined medium. **Proc Natl Acad Sci USA 78:**7205-7209, 1981
199. Morrison RS, Giordano S, Yamaguchi F, et al: Basic fibroblast growth factor expression is required for clonogenic growth of human glioma cells. **J Neurosci Res 34:**502-509, 1993
200. Morshead C, Reynolds B, Weiss S, et al: Neural stem cells are located in the subependymal region of the adult mammalian forebrain. **Soc Neurosci Abstr 19:**870, 1993
201. Müller W, Afra D, Schroder R: Supratentorial recurrences of gliomas: Morphological studies with relation to time intervals with astrocytomas. **Acta Neurochir 37:**75-91, 1977
202. Murphy M, Drago J, Bartlett PF: Fibroblast growth factor stimulates the proliferation and differentiation of neural precursor cells *in vitro*. **J Neurosci Res 25:**463-475, 1990
203. Nastruzzi C, Simoni D, Manfredini S, et al: New synthetic retinoids: Effects on proliferation and differentiation. **Anticancer Res 9:**1377-1384, 1989
204. Noble M: Points of controversy in the O-2A lineage: clocks and type-2 astrocytes. **Glia 4:**157-164, 1991
205. Noble M, Albrechtsen M, Moller C, et al: Glial cells express N-CAM/D2-CAM-like polypeptides *in vitro*. **Nature 316:**725-728, 1985
206. Noble M, Ataliotis P, Barnett SC, et al: Development, regeneration, and neoplasia of glial cells in the central nervous system. **Ann NY Acad Sci 633:**35-47, 1991
207. Noble M, Barnett SC, Bögler O, et al: Control of division and differentiation in oligodendrocyte-type-2 astrocyte progenitor cells. **Ciba Found Symp 150:**227-249, 1990
208. Noble M, Fok-Seang J, Cohen J: Glia are a unique substrate for the *in vitro* growth of central nervous system neurons. **J Neurosci 4:**1892-1903, 1984
209. Noble M, Murray K: Purified astrocytes promote the *in vitro* division of a bipotential glial progenitor cell. **EMBO J 3:**2243-2247, 1984
210. Noble M, Murray K, Stroobant P, et al: Platelet-derived growth factor promotes division and motility and inhibits premature differentiation of the oligodendrocyte/type-2 astrocyte progenitor cell. **Nature 333:**560-562, 1988 (Letter)
211. Norton WT, Farooq M: Astrocytes cultured from mature brain derive from glial precursor cells. **J Neurosci 9:**769-775, 1989
212. Oldfield EH, Ram Z, Culver KW, et al: Gene therapy for the treatment of brain tumors using intra-tumoral transduction with the thymidine kinase gene and intravenous ganciclovir. **Hum Gene Ther 4:** 39-69, 1993
213. Oppenheim RW: Cell death during development of the nervous system. **Annu Rev Neurosci 14:** 453-501, 1991
214. Osborn M, Debus E, Weber K: Monoclonal antibodies specific to vimentin. **Eur J Cell Biol 34:** 137-143, 1984
215. Pettmann B, Weibel M, Sensenbrenner M, et al: Purification of two astroglial growth factors from bovine brain. **FEBS Lett 189:**102-108, 1985
216. Piepmeier JM: Observations on the current treatment of low-grade astrocytic tumors of the cerebral hemispheres. **J Neurosurg 67:**177-181, 1987
217. Pixley SK, de Vellis J: Transition between immature radial glia and mature astrocytes studied with a monoclonal antibody to vimentin. **Brain Res 317:**201-209, 1984
218. Pollack IF, Randall MS, Kristofik MP, et al: Response of low-passage human malignant gliomas *in vitro* to stimulation and selective inhibition of growth factor-mediated pathways. **J Neurosurg 75:**284-293, 1991
219. Potten CS, Loeffler M: Stem cells: attributes, cycles, spirals, pitfalls and uncertainties. Lessons for and from the crypt. **Development 110:**1001-1020, 1990
220. Pouillart P, Cerutti I, Ronco G, et al: Butyric monosaccharide ester-induced cell differentiation and anti-tumor activity in mice. Importance of their prolonged biological effect for clinical applications in cancer therapy. **Int J Cancer 49:**89-95, 1991
221. Price J: Retroviruses and the study of cell lineage. **Development 101:**409-419, 1987
222. Price J, Thurlow L: Cell lineage in the rat cerebral cortex: a study using retroviral-mediated gene transfer. **Development 104:**473-482, 1988
223. Price J, Turner D, Cepko C: Lineage analysis in the vertebrate nervous system by retrovirus-mediated gene transfer. **Proc Natl Acad Sci USA 84:** 156-160, 1987
224. Price J, Williams B, Grove E: Cell lineage in the cerebral cortex. **Development (Suppl 2):**23-28, 1991
225. Pringle NP, Mudhar HS, Collarini EJ, et al: PDGF receptors in the rat CNS: during late neurogenesis, PDGF alpha-receptor expression appears to be restricted to glial cells of the oligodendrocyte lineage. **Development 115:**535-551, 1992
226. Pringle NP, Richardson WD: A singularity of PDGF alpha-peceptor expression in the dorsoventral axis of the neural tube may define the origin of the oligodendrocyte lineage. **Development 117:** 525-533, 1993
227. Pruss RM, Bartlett PF, Gavrilovic J, et al: Mitogens for glial cells: a comparison of the response of cultured astrocytes, oligodendrocytes, and Schwann cells. **Brain Res 229:**19-35, 1982
228. Pukel CS, Lloyd KO, Travassos LR, et al: G_{D3}, a prominent ganglioside of human melanoma. Detection and characterization by mouse monoclonal antibody. **J Exp Med 155:**1133-1147, 1982
229. Raff MC: Glial cell diversification in the rat optic nerve. **Science 243:**1450-1455, 1989
230. Raff MC, Abney ER, Cohen J, et al: Two types of astrocytes in cultures of developing rat white matter: differences in morphology, surface gangliosides, and growth characteristics. **J Neurosci 3:**1289-1300, 1983
231. Raff MC, Abney ER, Fok-Seang J: Reconstitution of a developmental clock *in vitro*: a critical role for as-

trocytes in the timing of oligodendrocyte differentiation. **Cell 42**:61-69, 1985

232. Raff MC, Abney ER, Miller RH: Two glial cell lineages diverge prenatally in rat optic nerve. **Dev Biol 106**:53-60, 1984
233. Raff MC, Lillien LE, Richardson WD, et al: Platelet-derived growth factor from astrocytes drives the clock that times oligodendrocyte development in culture. **Nature 333**:562-565, 1988
234. Raff MC, Miller RH, Noble M: A glial progenitor cell that develops *in vitro* into an astrocyte or an oligodendrocyte depending on culture medium. **Nature 303**:390-396, 1983
235. Raff MC, Mirsky R, Fields KL: Galactocerebroside is a specific cell-surface antigenic marker for oligodendrocytes in culture. **Nature 274**:813-816, 1978
236. Raff MC, Williams BP, Miller RH: The *in vitro* differentiation of a bipotential glial progenitor cell. **EMBO J 3**:1857-1864, 1984
237. Raible DW, McMorris FA: Cyclic AMP regulates the rate of differentiation of oligodendrocytes without changing the lineage commitment of their progenitors. **Dev Biol 133**:437-446, 1989
238. Rakic P: Mode of cell migration to the superficial layers of fetal monkey neocortex. **J Comp Neurol 145**:61-84, 1972
239. Rakic P: Specification of cerebral cortical areas. **Science 241**:170-176, 1988
240. Ram Z, Culver KW, Walbridge S, et al: *In situ* retroviral-mediated gene transfer for the treatment of brain tumors in rats. **Cancer Res** 53:83-88, 1993
241. Ram Z, Culver KW, Walbridge S, et al: Toxicity studies of retroviral-mediated gene transfer for the treatment of brain tumors. **J Neurosurg** 79:400-407, 1993
242. Ramon y Cajal S: **Histologie du systeme nerveux de L' homme et des vertebres. Vols I-II.** Paris: Maloine, 1955
243. Ranscht B, Clapshaw PA, Price J, et al: Development of oligodendrocytes and Schwann cells studied with a monoclonal antibody against galactocerebroside. **Proc Natl Acad Sci USA 79**:2709-2713, 1982
244. Ransom BR, Kettenmann H: Electrical coupling, without dye coupling, between mammalian astrocytes and oligodendrocytes in cell culture. **Glia** 3:258-266, 1990
245. Rasheed BK, Fuller GN, Friedman AH, et al: Loss of heterozygosity for 10q loci in human gliomas. **Genes Chromosom Cancer** 5:75-82,1992
246. Rathjen FG, Schachner M: Immunocytological and biochemical characterization of a new neuronal cell surface component (L1 antigen) which is involved in cell adhesion. **EMBO J 3**:1-10, 1984
247. Rephaeli A, Rabizadeh E, Aviram A, et al: Derivatives of butyric acid as potential anti-neoplastic agents. **Int J Cancer** 49:66-72, 1991
248. Rey JA, Bello MJ, Jiménez-Lara AM, et al: Loss of heterozygosity for distal markers on 22q in human gliomas. **Int J Cancer 51**:703-706, 1992
249. Reynolds BA, Tetzlaff W, Weiss S: A multipotent EGF-responsive striatal embryonic progenitor cell produces neurons and astrocytes. **J Neurosci** 12:4565-4574, 1992
250. Reynolds BA, Weiss S: Generation of neurons and astrocytes from isolated cells of the adult mammalian central nervous system. **Science 255**: 1707-1710, 1992
251. Reynolds R, Wilkin GP: Development of macroglial cells in rat cerebellum. II. An *in situ* immunohistochemical study of oligodendroglial lineage from precursor to mature myelinating cell. **Development 102**:409-425, 1988
252. Richardson WD, Pringle N, Mosley MJ, et al: A role for platelet-derived growth factor in normal gliogenesis in the central nervous system. **Cell 53**: 309-319, 1988
253. Rickmann M, Amaral DG, Cowan WM: Organization of radial glial cells during the developmentof the rat dentate gyrus. **J Comp Neurol** 264:449-479, 1987
254. Robinson SR, Dreher Z: Müller cells in adult rabbit retinae: morphology, distribution and implications for function and development. **J Comp Neurol 292**:178-192, 1990
255. Rotwein P, Burgess SK, Milbrandt JD, et al: Differential expression of insulin-like growth factor genes in rat central nervous system. **Proc Natl Acad Sci USA 85**:265-269, 1988
256. Russell DS, Rubinstein LJ: **Pathology of Tumours of the Nervous System, 5th ed.** Baltimore, Md: Williams & Wilkins, 1989
257. Saiki RK, Gelfand DH, Stoffel S, et al: Primer-directed enzymatic amplification of DNA with a thermostable DNA polymerase. **Science 239**: 487-491, 1988
258. Saiki RK, Scharf S, Faloona F, et al: Enzymatic amplification of b-globin genomic sequences and restriction site analysis for diagnosis of sickle cell anemia. **Science 230**:1350-1354, 1985
259. Salditt-Georgieff M, Sheffery M, Krauter K, et al: Induced transcription of the mouse b-globin transcription unit erythroleukemia cells. Time course of induction and of changes in chromatin structure. **J Mol Biol 172**:437-450, 1984
260. Sandberg-Nordqvist AC, Stahlbom PA, Reinecke M, et al: Characterization of insulin-like growth factor 1 in human primary brain tumors. **Cancer Res 53**:2475-2478, 1993
261. Sanes JR, Rubenstein JLR, Nicolas JF: Use of a recombinant retrovirus to study post-implantation cell lineage in mouse embryos. **EMBO J 5**:3133-3142, 1986
262. Sasahara M, Fries JW, Raines EW, et al: PDGF B-chain in neurons of the central nervous system, posterior pituitary, and in a transgenic model. **Cell 64**:217-227, 1991
263. Sauer FC: The cellular structure of the neural tube. **J Comp Neurol 63**:13-23, 1935
264. Savage CR Jr, Inagami T, Cohen S: The primary structure of epidermal growth factor. **J Biol Chem 247**:7612-7621, 1972
265. Schaper A: The earliest differentiation in the central nervous system of vertebrates. **Science 5**:430-431, 1897
266. Schmechel DE, Rakic P: A Golgi study of radial glial cells in developing monkey telencephalon: morpho-

genesis and transformation into astrocytes. **Anat Embryol 156:**115-152, 1979

267. Sealy L, Chalkley R: The effect of sodium butyrate on histone modification. **Cell 14:**115-121, 1978
268. Seeds NW, Haffke SC: Cell junctions and ultrastructural development of reaggregated mouse brain cultures. **Dev Neurosci 1:**69-79, 1978
269. Seth A, Gonzalez FA, Guptas S, et al: Signal transduction within the nucleus by mitogen-activated protein kinase. **J Biol Chem 267:**24796-24804, 1992
270. Seyedin SM, Pehrson JR, Cole RD: Loss of chromosomal high mobility group proteins HMG1 and HMG2 when mouse neuroblastoma and Friend erythroleukemia cells become committed to differentiation. **Proc Natl Acad Sci USA 78:**5988-5992, 1981
271. Shaw EG, Scheithauer BW, Gilbertson DT, et al: Postoperative radiotherapy of supratentorial low-grade gliomas. **Int J Radiat Oncol Biol Phys 16:** 663-668, 1989
272. Sheffery M, Marks PA, Rifkind RA: Gene expression in murine erythroleukemia cells: transcriptional control and chromatin structure of the a_1-globin gene. **J Mol Biol 172:**417-436, 1984
273. Skoff RP: Gliogenesis in rat optic nerve: astrocytes are generated in a single wave before oligodendrocytes. **Dev Biol 139:**149-168, 1990
274. Skoff RP, Knapp PE: Division of astroblasts and oligodendroblasts in postnatal rat brain: evidence for separate astrocyte and oligodendrocyte lineages. **Glia 4:**165-174, 1991
275. Skoff RP, Knapp PE: Lineage and differentiation of oligodendrocytes in the brain. **Ann NY Acad Sci 633:**48-55, 1991
276. Skoff RP, Price DL, Stocks A: Electron microscopic autoradiographic studies of gliogenesis in rat optic nerve. I. Cell proliferation. **J Comp Neurol 169:** 291-312, 1976
277. Skoff RP, Price DL, Stocks A: Electron microscopic autoradiographic studies of gliogenesis in rat optic nerve. II. Time of origin. **J Comp Neurol 169:** 313-333, 1976
278. Small RK, Riddle P, Noble M: Evidence for migration of oligodendrocyte-type-2 astrocyte progenitor cells into the developing rat optic nerve. **Nature 328:**155-157, 1987 (Letter)
279. Sobue G, Pleasure D: Astroglial proliferation and phenotype are modulated by neuronal plasma membrane. **Brain Res 324:**175-179, 1984
280. Soffietti R, Chiò A, Giordana MT, et al: Prognostic factors in well-differentiated cerebral astrocytomas in the adult. **Neurosurgery 24:**686-692, 1989
281. Sommer I, Schachner M: Monoclonal antibodies (O1 to O4) to oligodendrocyte cell surfaces: An immunocytological study in the central nervous system. **Dev Biol 83:**311-327, 1981
282. Sontheimer H, Trotter J, Schachner M, et al: Channel expression correlates with differentiation stage during the development of oligodendrocytes from their precursor cells in culture. **Neuron 2:**1135-1145, 1989
283. Stitt TN, Hatten ME: Antibodies that recognize astrotactin block granule neuron binding to astroglia. **Neuron 5:**639-649, 1990
284. Strickland S, Mahdavi V: The induction of differentiation in teratocarcinoma stem cells by retinoic acid. **Cell 15:**393-403, 1980
285. Súarez I, Raff MC: Subpial and perivascular astrocytes associated with nodes of Ranvier in the rat optic nerve. **J Neurocytol 18:**577-582, 1989
286. Tada T, Yabu K, Kobayashi S: Detection of active form of transforming growth factor-beta in cerebrospinal fluid of patients with glioma. **Jpn J Cancer Res 84:**544-548, 1993
287. Tang SJ, Ko LW, Lee YH, et al: Induction of *fos* and *sis* proto-oncogenes and genes of the extracellular matrix proteins during butyrate induced glioma differentiation. **Biochim Biophys Acta 1048:**59-65, 1990
288. Temple S: Division and differentiation of isolated CNS blast cells in microculture. **Nature 340:** 471-473, 1989
289. Temple S, Raff MC: Clonal analysis of oligodendrocyte development in culture: evidence for a developmental clock that counts cell divisions. **Cell 44:** 773-779, 1986
290. Thiery JP, Brackenbury R, Rutishauser U, et al: Adhesion among neural cells of the chick embryo. II. Purification and characterization of a cell adhesion molecule from neural retina. **J Biol Chem 252:** 6841-6845, 1977
291. Timsit SG, Bally-Cuif L, Colman DR, et al: DM-20 mRNA is expressed during the embryonic development of the nervous system of the mouse. **J Neurochem 58:**1172-1175, 1992
292. Torp SH, Helseth E, Dalen A, et al: Epidermal growth factor receptor expression in human gliomas. **Cancer Immunol Immunother 33:**61-64, 1991
293. Toscani A, Soprano DR, Soprano KJ: Molecular analysis of sodium butyrate-induced growth arrest. **Oncogene Res 3:**223-238, 1988
294. Trapp BD, Honegger P, Richelson E, et al: Morphological differentiation of mechanically dissociated fetal rat brain in aggregating cell cultures. **Brain Res 160:**235-252, 1980
295. Trotter J, Bitter-Suermann D, Schachner M: Differentiation-regulated loss of the polysialylated embryonic form and expression of the different polypeptides of the neural cell adhesion molecule by cultured oligodendrocytes and myelin. **J Neurosci Res 22:**369-383, 1989
296. Trotter J, Schachner M: Cells positive for the O4 surface antigen isolated by cell sorting are able to differentiate into astrocytes or oligodendrocytes. **Brain Res Dev Brain Res 46:**115-122, 1989
297. Turner DL, Cepko CL: A common progenitor for neurons and glia persists in rat retina late in development. **Nature 328:**131-136, 1987
298. Urenjak J, Williams SR, Gadian DG, et al: Proton nuclear magnetic resonance spectroscopy unambiguously identifies different neural cell types. **J Neurosci 13:**981-989, 1993
299. Urenjak J, Williams SR, Gadian DG, et al: Specific expression of N-acetylaspartate in neurons, oligodendrocyte-type-2 astrocyte progenitors, and im-

mature oligodendrocytes *in vitro*. **J Neurochem 59**:55-61, 1992
300. Usowicz MM, Gallo V, Cull-Candy SG: Multiple conductance channels in type-2 cerebellar astrocytes activated by excitatory amino acids. **Nature 339**:380-383, 1989
301. Van Aelst L, Barr M, Marcus S, et al: Complex formation between RAS and RAF and other protein kinases. **Proc Natl Acad Sci USA 90**:6213-6217, 1993
302. Verkhratsky AN, Trotter J, Kettenmann H: Cultured glial precursor cells from mouse cortex express two types of calcium currents. **Neurosci Lett 112**: 194-198, 1990
303. Vertosick FT Jr, Selker RG, Arena VC: Survival of patients with well-differentiated astrocytomas diagnosed in the era of computed tomography. **Neurosurgery 28**:496-501, 1991
304. Vescovi AL, Reynolds BA, Fraser DD, et al: bFGF regulates the proliferative fate of unipotent (neuronal) and bipotent (neuronal/astroglial) EGF-generated CNS progenitor cells. **Neuron 11**:951-966, 1993
305. Venter DJ, Thomas DGT: Multiple sequential molecular abnormalities in the evolution of human gliomas. **Br J Cancer 63**:753-757, 1991
306. Voigt T: Development of glial cells in the cerebral wall of ferrets: Direct tracing of their transformation from radial glia into astrocytes. **J Comp Neurol 289**:74-88, 1989
307. von Blankenfeld GJ, Trotter J, Kettenmann H: Expression of a distinct $GABA_A$ receptor subtype in the oligodendrocyte lineage and its developmental regulation. **Eur J Neurosci 3**:310-316, 1991
308. Walicke PA, Baird A: Neurotrophic effects of basic and acidic fibroblast growth factors are not mediated through glial cells. **Brain Res 468**:71-79, 1988
309. Walsh C, Cepko CL: Clonally related cortical cells show several migration patterns. **Science 241**:1342-1345, 1988
310. Walsh C, Cepko CL: Widespread dispersion of neuronal clones accross functional regions of the cerebral cortex. **Science 255**:434-440, 1992
311. Warf BC, Fok-Seang J, Miller RH: Evidence for the ventral origin of oligodendrocyte precursors in the rat spinal cord. **J Neurosci 11**:2477-2488, 1991
312. Watanabe K, Nagai M, Wakai S, et al: Loss of constitutional heterozygosity in chromosome 10 in human glioblastoma. **Acta Neuropathol 80**: 251-254, 1990
313. Watanabe T, Raff MC: Retinal astrocytes are immigrants from the optic nerve. **Nature 332**:834-837, 1988
314. Whittemore SR, Sanson HR, Wood PM: Concurrent isolation and characterization of oligodendrocytes, microglia, and astrocytes from adult human spinal cord. **Int J Dev Neurosci 11**:755-764, 1993
315. Williams BP, Abney ER, Raff MC: Macroglial cell development in embryonic rat brain: studies using monoclonal antibodies, fluorescence activated cell sorting, and cell culture. **Dev Biol 112**:126-134, 1985
316. Williams BP, Read J, Price J: The generation of neurons and oligodendrocytes from a common precursor cell. **Neuron 7**:685-693, 1991
317. Williams JS, Weiss S, Hawkes R: A nuclear antigen of EGF-responsive stem cell progeny in vitro is highly expressed in vivo by cells of the ventricular wall. **Soc Neurosci Abstr 19**:870, 1993
318. Willingham MC: Cyclic AMP and cell behavior in cultured cells. **Int Rev Cytol 44**:319-363, 1976
319. Wolswijk G, Noble M: Cooperation between PDGF and FGF converts slowly dividing $O\text{-}2A^{adult}$ progenitor cells to rapidly dividing cells with characteristics of $O\text{-}2A^{perinatal}$ progenitor cells. **J Cell Biol 118**: 889-900, 1992
320. Wolswijk G, Noble M: Identification of an adult-specific glial progenitor cell. **Development 105**: 387-400, 1989
321. Wolswijk G, Noble M: In vitro studies on the development and maintenance of the oligodendrocyte - type-2 astrocyte (O-2A) lineage in the adult central nervous system, in Kettenmann H, Ransom BR (eds): **Neuro-Glial Cells.** Oxford University Press (In press)
322. Wolswijk G, Riddle PN, Noble M: Coexistence of perinatal and adult forms of a glial progenitor cell during development of the rat optic nerve. **Development 109**:691-698, 1990
323. Wolswijk G, Riddle PN, Noble M: Platelet-derived growth factor is mitogenic for $O\text{-}2A^{adult}$ progenitor cells. **Glia 4**:495-503, 1991
324. Wren D, Wolswijk G, Noble M: *In vitro* analysis of the origin and maintainance of $O\text{-}2A^{adult}$ progenitor cells. **J Cell Biol 116**:167-176, 1992
325. Wren DR, Noble M: Oligodendrocytes and oligodendrocyte/type-2 astrocyte progenitor cells of adult rats are specifically susceptible to the lytic effects of complement in absence of antibody. **Proc Natl Acad Sci USA 86**:9025-9029, 1989
326. Wyllie AH, Kerr JFR, Currie AR: Cell death: the significance of apoptosis. **Int Rev Cytol 68**:251-307, 1980
327. Wyllie AH, Morris RG, Smith AL, et al: Chromatin cleavage in apoptosis: association with condensed chromatin morphology and dependence on macromolecular synthesis. **J Pathol 142**:67-77, 1984
328. Wyllie DJA, Mathie A, Symonds CJ, et al: Activation of glutamate receptors and glutamate uptake in identified macroglial cells in rat cerebellar cultures. **J Physiol (Lond) 432**:235-258, 1991
329. Yeh HJ, Ruit KG, Wang YX, et al: PDGF A-chain gene is expressed by mammalian neurons during development and in maturity. **Cell 64**:209-216, 1991

CHAPTER 3

THE PATHOLOGY OF BENIGN CEREBRAL ASTROCYTOMAS

MICHAEL L. RODRIGUEZ, MBBS, FRCPA, AND PARAKRAMA CHANDRASOMA, MD

For the pathologist, the concept of classifying a tumor as a benign astrocytoma is difficult to grasp, since many of the morphological features used to define malignancy outside the central nervous system (CNS) are not applicable within it. In general, these defining features include differentiation and anaplasia, growth rate, local invasion, and metastasis.[43] While benign tumors outside the CNS are, by definition, well differentiated and closely resemble their tissue of origin, this may not be true within the brain. For example, both pilocytic astrocytomas and subependymal giant cell astrocytomas are considered to be benign, but neither is composed of cells resembling normal components of the mature nervous system. In contrast, local invasion by astrocytomas into surrounding brain tissue is universal, and metastatic spread is exceedingly rare and has a negligible effect on survival.

Conceptually, it becomes a little easier to understand benign and malignant astrocytomas if malignancy is defined biologically or clinically rather than histologically. A benign astrocytoma has a long clinical course and is not fatal to the patient, while a malignant astrocytoma has a short clinical course and is fatal. This definition introduces several new parameters that contribute to malignant behavior. First, since the CNS is structurally inhomogeneous, the effects of a tumor are dependent on its anatomical location. For example, a tumor involving vital structures, such as the brain stem, or located in a therapeutically inaccessible site will behave in a less benign fashion than a histologically similar tumor involving the frontal pole. Second, tumors behave as expanding space-occupying lesions within the brain so that even the most "benign" slow-growing astrocytoma may eventually cause fatal mass effects. A consequence of this definition is that malignancy is not solely dependent on the intrinsic biological properties of a tumor and hence, in some cases, the reliability of histological findings to predict prognosis is limited. As well as the location, the growth characteristics of an astrocytoma are important for defining its malignant behavior. These characteristics include growth rate and the ability to infiltrate brain.

ASTROCYTOMA GRADING SYSTEMS

Numerous grading systems, based on histological criteria, have been proposed to distinguish astrocytomas that behave favorably ("benignly") from those that behave aggressively ("malignantly"). Although histological grading is undoubtedly important, it should be remembered that it reflects only one aspect of the complex interrelationship between tumor and host which determines behavior (benign or malig-

TABLE 1

WHO Histological Typing of CNS Tumors

1	Tumors of Neuroepithelial Tissue	
1.1	Astrocytic tumors	
1.1.1	Astrocytoma	
1.1.1.1	Variants:	Fibrillary
1.1.1.2		Protoplasmic
1.1.1.3		Gemistocytic
1.1.2	Anaplastic (malignant) astrocytoma	
1.1.3	Glioblastoma	
1.1.3.1	Variants:	Giant cell glioblastoma
1.1.3.2		Gliosarcoma
1.1.4	Pilocytic astrocytoma	
1.1.5	Pleomorphic xanthoastrocytoma	
1.1.6	Subependymal giant cell astrocytoma (Tuberous sclerosis)	

*From reference 113.

nant) and prognosis. Several of the more commonly used grading systems have been reviewed in a recent monograph in this series,[32] to which the reader is referred for further information. Since that monograph appeared, the World Health Organization (WHO) has published a new edition of *Histological Typing of Tumors of the Central Nervous System*[113] includes a revised classification and grading system for astrocytic tumors (Table 1). In this classification, a clear distinction is made between diffusely infiltrating astrocytic neoplasms and the less common, more circumscribed pilocytic astrocytoma (PA), pleomorphic xanthoastrocytoma, and subependymal giant cell astrocytoma.[114] The infiltrating tumors—astrocytoma, anaplastic astrocytoma, and glioblastoma multiforme—seem to form a biological continuum in terms of both histological appearance and behavior that is paralleled by sequential genetic events. There is also a tendency for diffuse astrocytomas to become more malignant with time, a phenomenon rarely seen with the more circumscribed astrocytic tumors.

Until relatively recently, apart from counting mitotic figures, the measurement of proliferative activity to assess tumor growth was difficult and not widely practiced, requiring either the administration of potentially mutagenic bromodeoxyuridine to patients preoperatively or manipulation of fresh tumor tissue after excision. The use of immunohistochemical means to detect nuclear antigens such as proliferating cell nuclear antigen or Ki-67, which are regulated during the cell cycle, now allows proliferative activity to be measured easily in both current and archival material. The use of these techniques to predict tumor behavior is discussed by Hinton in Chapter 8 in this monograph.

The new WHO grading system for astrocytic tumors is essentially three-tiered and is largely based on the histological criteria used in the St. Anne/Mayo classification system (Table 2).[45] WHO grading is based on the presence or absence of only four well-defined features: atypia, mitotic figures, endothelial proliferation, and necrosis. One feature (usually atypia) is present in grade II, two (usually atypia and mitotic figures) are present in grade III, and three or four features are present in grade IV tumors. The original St. Anne/Mayo system also included as

TABLE 2

Comparison of the WHO and St. Anne/Mayo Grading Systems for Astrocytomas*

WHO		St. Anne/Mayo	
Grade	Designation	Astrocytoma Grade	Histological Criteria
I	Pilocytic astrocytoma		
II	Astrocyoma (low-grade)	1	No criteria
		2	One criterion, usually nuclear atypia
III	Anaplastic astrocytoma	3	Two criteria, usually nuclear atypia & mitotic activity
IV	Glioblastoma multiforme	4	Three criteria, usually nuclear atypia, mitoses, endothelial proliferation, & or necrosis

*WHO data modified from reference 117; St. Anne/Mayo data modified from reference 48.

grade 1, tumors that showed none of the four features. However such tumors are exceptionally rare (0.7% of "ordinary," i.e., nonpilocytic astrocytomas[45]) and are not included in the new WHO system. One major advantage of this grading system, which is not shared by many other systems, is that the criteria for grading are binary and objective. This simplicity fosters both intra- and interobserver reproducibility, the lack of which has been a major stumbling block of several previous grading systems. Most importantly, this grading scheme correlates with prognosis.[45]

Grade I in the new WHO classification (as in the previous WHO system[236]) includes pilocytic astrocytomas and subependymal giant cell astrocytomas. In some ways this is unfortunate, as it may give the (unintentional) impression that the same grading criteria are used for grades I through IV and that, biologically, grade I tumors are similar to grade II to IV tumors. However, whereas the differences between grade II and grade III tumors are quantitative, those between grades I and II are not. In addition, the St. Anne/Mayo system is applicable only to diffuse or fibrillary astrocytomas, showing no correlation between grade and survival time when applied to pilocytic tumors.[45,53,79,224]

The literature dealing with benign gliomas is profuse and somewhat confusing. The term "benign glioma" has been used in several ways: to include both grade I and grade II astrocytomas (with or without identifying the actual grading system employed); as a synonym for cystic or cerebellar astrocytomas; to include both circumscribed and diffuse tumors; or without being defined. It is not surprising that conclusions drawn from these studies are often inconsistent. For the purposes of this review, we have included under the rubric of benign cerebral astrocytomas tumors classified as WHO grade I astrocytoma (pilocytic and subependymal giant cell), as well as pleomorphic xanthoastrocytoma, desmoplastic cerebral astrocytoma of infancy, and gliofibroma. We have chosen not to include diffuse astrocytomas (WHO grade II) within this group, as we believe that they are best classified as low-grade malignant neoplasms at the less aggressive end of a spectrum that encompasses anaplastic astrocytoma and glioblastoma multiforme. We have also confined our discussion to cerebral astrocytomas and have therefore not included a detailed discussion of PAs involving either the cerebellum and brain stem or the optic nerves and chiasm.

Pilocytic Astrocytoma

Clinical Features

PAs are typically slow-growing tumors that usually occur in children and young adults. Although the majority are found in the cerebellum, any level of the neuraxis may be involved. Common extracerebellar sites include the anterior optic pathways and the region around the hypothalamus and third ventricle. Rare examples have been described in the pineal gland.[48] Most tumors are sporadic, although tumors of the anterior optic structures and around the third ventricle may be associated with neurofibromatosis type I (NF1). Optic nerve gliomas, nearly all PAs, are found in 4% to 36% of patients with NF1.[8,12,20,78,122,125,146] The wide variation in incidence probably reflects differences in the age and race of the populations studied, the use of different neuroradiological techniques, and increased screening of asymptomatic individuals. Optic nerve gliomas appear to be very rare in Japanese patients with NF1 (reported incidence <2%).[112,202,232] Conversely, about 22% of patients with optic nerve gliomas will be found to have NF1,[52] with the reported incidence ranging from 10% to 70%.[122]

In the cerebral hemispheres, PAs are relatively uncommon, representing 3% of gliomas.[152] They are more frequent in the cerebral hemispheres of children, where they account for between 37%[80] and 56%[138] of astrocytomas. Two-thirds to three-quarters of PAs are diagnosed in patients under 20 years of age, with the median age at diagnosis being 14 to 15 years.[1,49,152] Cerebellar PAs tend to be diagnosed earlier, at a median age of 9 years.[169] This may reflect either a significant difference between the biological behavior of supra- and infratentorial PAs or the limited capacity of the posterior fossa to accommodate an enlarging space-occupying lesion. The median age at diagnosis for adults with cerebral PAs (22 years[62]) is significantly less than that for the more common diffuse astrocytoma (34 years[63]). The majority (60% to 80%) of cerebral hemisphere PAs are located in the temporal or temporoparietal region.[1,138,152,155,178] Although the brain is not a homogeneous organ, it appears that many of the radiological features, the gross and microscopic pathology, and the biological behavior of supratentorial PAs are similar to those of the more common cerebellar examples.[152,169]

Cerebral PAs present (depending on their location) with signs of cortical irritation, increased intracranial pressure, or a focal deficit. Although most patients have symptoms for less than 3 years prior to diagnosis,[1] some may be symptomatic for many years and preoperative symptoms for more than 50 years have been reported in cases of cerebellar PA.[110]

Neuroimaging Features

Radiologically, PAs have a characteristic although not pathognomonic appearance. They are round to oval, sharply demarcated, and smoothly marginated.[121] These features distinguish them from the more common diffuse astrocytomas in the cerebral hemispheres. They are usually cystic, the cyst being either unilocular (frequently with a mural nodule) or multilocular. Occasionally, and especially when they arise in the anterior optic pathways, PAs may be lobular and solid. Associated edema is rare. In nearly all cases, both computed tomography (CT)[121] and magnetic resonance imaging (MRI)[56] studies demonstrate marked tumor enhancement following intravenous administration of contrast material. Tumor enhancement indicates disruption of the blood-brain barrier and electron microscopy has demonstrated fenestration of endothelial cells and open intercellular tight junctions in PAs, which may facilitate extravascular leakage of contrast material.[173] In most astrocytomas, enhancement is associated with a high-grade tumor; however, in PAs this feature correlates with neither grade nor prognosis. In tumors presenting as mural nodules within cysts, usually only the nodule enhances.[151] In these cases, tumor is confined to the nodule microscopically and the cyst wall shows only reactive gliosis.[209] Contrast enhancement in the cyst wall is associated with neoplastic cell permeation. Rarely, cyst wall enhancement is seen in the absence of tumor. This may be related to inflammation associated with intracystic hemorrhage.[209] In one series, angiography showed an avascular mass in 48%, tumor hypervascularity in 31%, or was normal in 21%.[53]

Glucose utilization studies using fluorine-18 fluorodeoxyglucose positron emission tomography (FDG PET) have been used to assess the metabolic activity of PAs. Glucose utilization is similar to that observed in anaplastic astrocytomas and significantly higher than that reported in nonpilocytic low-grade astrocytomas.[57] The areas of high glucose utilization closely correspond to areas of contrast enhancement seen on MRI. This may reflect increased metabolic activity in hyperplastic vascular endothelial cells rather than in tumor astrocytes since, in some PAs, vascular endothelium expresses proliferation markers.[34,86] It has been suggested that the FDG PET findings may reflect increased expression of the glucose transporter GT1 on tumor endothelium.[56]

Pathological Findings

Cerebral PAs usually appear grossly circumscribed and may be described at operation as encapsulated with a distinct tumor margin (eight of 18 cases) or as having diffuse infiltrative margins (10 of 18 cases).[40] They may be cystic or solid, with the frequency of macroscopic cysts varying from 14%[53] to 43%.[40] Cystic tumors appear to be commoner in the cerebellum where only 20% of PAs are predominantly solid.[44,171] The cysts usually contain xanthochromic fluid, which is protein-rich and coagulates after aspiration. Following hemorrhage, the fluid may be brown. The mural nodule in cystic tumors is often reddish brown and may present as plaque or a multinodular mass.[152] While grossly circumscribed, all PAs show variable parenchymal infiltration microscopically. In one series of supratentorial PAs, microscopic infiltration was minor in 29%, moderate in 55%, and widespread in 16%.[53] This infiltration is usually much less than that encountered in fibrillary astrocytomas, allowing

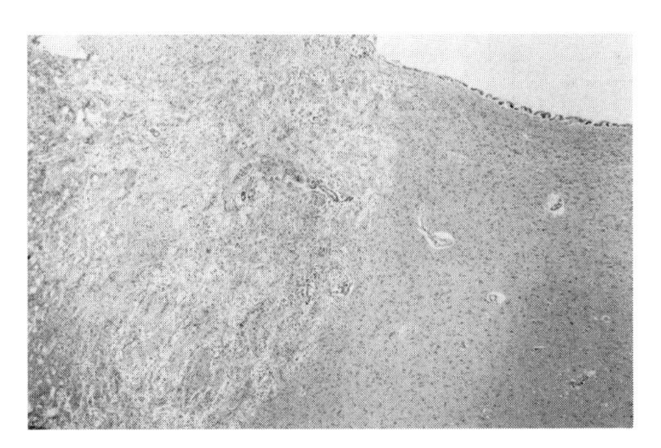

Figure 1: Photomicrograph of a pilocytic astrocytoma in the wall of the third ventricle. The tumor appears well circumscribed, distinguishing pilocytic astrocytoma from the more diffusely infiltrating fibrillary astrocytoma. (hematoxylin-eosin, original magnification × 50)

gross total excision of tumors in favorable locations (Figure 1). Local leptomeningeal extension is common[33,167,171] but is not associated with a poor prognosis.[228]

Microscopically, Russell and Rubinstein[171] distinguished two variants of PA: adult and juvenile. In the less common adult type, the histology is more uniform and the tumor consists of closely packed interwoven fascicles of relatively broad fibrillated bipolar cells with a classical pilocytic appearance that can be best appreciated on smears (Figure 2A). The nuclei are elongated and bland and the cytoplasm forms two extremely fine hair-like polar processes. The fascicles are not particularly related to blood vessels. In some areas, a few randomly oriented stellate and gemistocytic cells are encountered but microcysts are rare or absent. Variable calcification is present (Figure 2B), predominantly in capillary walls.[167] Although grossly discrete, in the adult type of PA there is microscopic infiltration into the surrounding brain, which is usually more pronounced than in the juvenile examples.[33] PAs also tend to occur in older patients and are more likely to undergo anaplastic change.[171]

The juvenile variant is more common and contains two histological patterns. The first (pilocytic pattern) is similar to the adult variant although the cells tend to be thinner and often form a longitudinal sheath around blood vessels (Figure 3A).[171] The second (microcystic pattern) consists of regions of less cohesive stellate astrocytes with microscopic cysts and spongiform areas containing eosinophilic proteinaceous material (Figure 3B to D). The microcysts may fuse to form macrocysts. The two patterns vary in proportion and are seen together in 43% of cases; in one study the microcystic pattern predominated in 31% and the pilocytic ("adult") pattern predominated in 26% (Figure 3E).[53]

Foci of oligodendroglial cells are occasionally found in cerebellar PAs[33] and are associated with local leptomeningeal infiltration and a favorable prognosis.[228] Since areas of PA may be found in mixed gliomas and have been associated with oligodendroglioma,[192] the diagnosis of PA should be made with caution when only a small amount of tissue is available, especially if

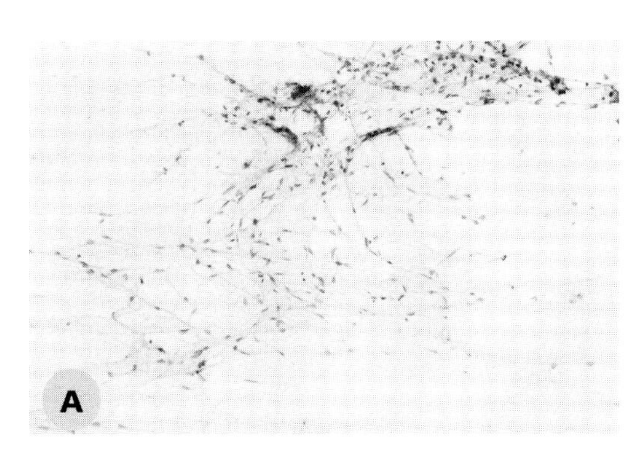

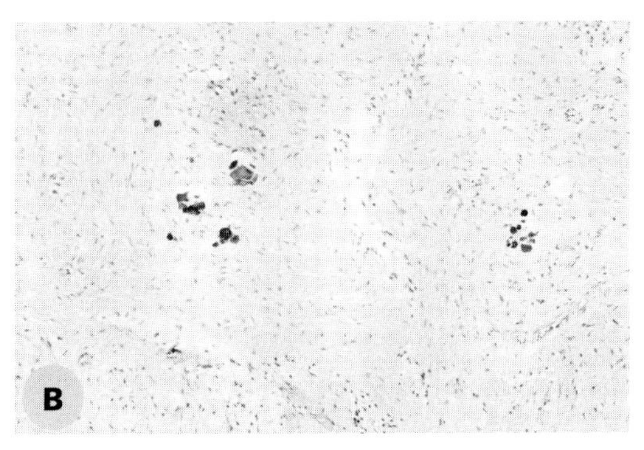

Figure 2: Photomicrographs showing pilocytic astrocytomas in adults. **A)** Smear preparation revealing bland astocytic nuclei with fine hair-like bipolar processes. **B)** Focal calcification can be seen. (hematoxylin-eosin, original magnification × 125)

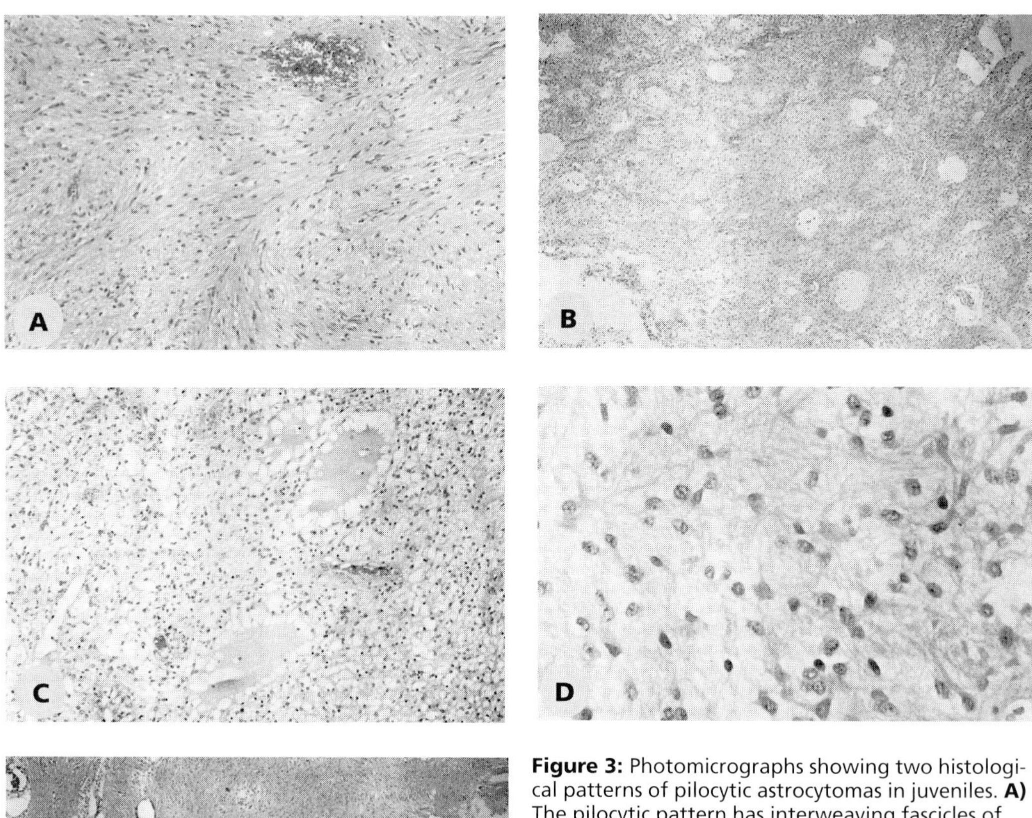

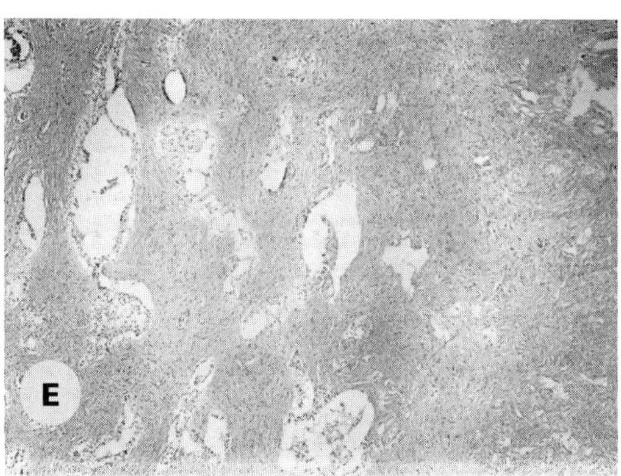

Figure 3: Photomicrographs showing two histological patterns of pilocytic astrocytomas in juveniles. **A)** The pilocytic pattern has interweaving fascicles of thin, elongated spindle cells. This is predominant in the "adult" variant and is found admixed with microcystic areas in the more common "juvenile" variant. (**B** to **E**) The microcystic pattern. **B)** A predominantly microcystic pattern is demonstrated. **C)** Microcystic area containing pale eosinophilic proteinaceous material can be seen. **D)** Example of plump protoplasmic and stellate astrocytes commonly found in microcystic areas. **E)** Small scattered microcystic areas are seen in a predominantly spindle-cell tumor. The proportion of microcystic and pilocytic patterns may vary widely. (hematoxylin-eosin, original magnification × 125 [A and C], × 50 [B and E], × 500 [D])

the clinical or radiological features are atypical.

Although cytological atypia with nuclear hyperchromasia and enlargement, multinucleation, and giant cell formation may be seen in infratentorial PAs, they are believed to be degenerative and are not associated with an adverse prognosis (Figure 4).[171] These changes are more common in supratentorial PA, being observed in 94% of cases, and were mild in 49%, moderate in 43%, and marked in 4%.[53] Mitotic figures are usually infrequent but in one series were found occasionally in 35% of cases, readily in 6%, and commonly in 2%.[53] Necrosis is usually absent.[53] Vascular proliferation and endothelial hyperplasia with the formation of glomeruloid capillaries is relatively common and may be marked in up to 14% of supratentorial PAs (Figure 5).[53] While this feature has ominous prognostic significance in non-PAs, and is usually associated with high-grade tumors, in the context of PAs there is no association with a poor prognosis. It is, however, the morphological basis of the marked enhancement noted on CT or MRI. Some PAs contain focal areas with

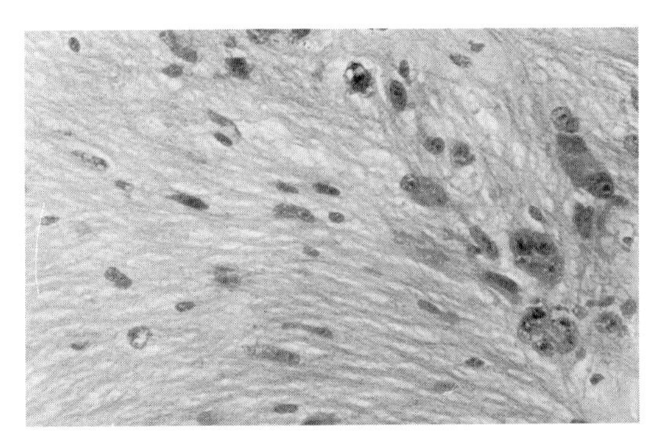

Figure 4: Pilocytic astrocytoma with atypia. Marked cytological pleomorphism with prominent nucleoli and multinucleated cells can be seen. (hematoxylin-eosin, original magnification × 500)

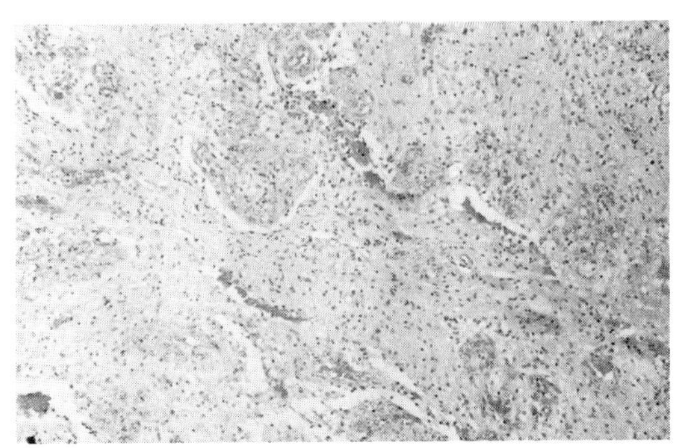

Figure 5: Pilocytic astrocytoma showing focal vascular and endothelial proliferation. This correlates with enhancement seen on CT scans. (hematoxylin-eosin, original magnification × 125)

abundant vascular channels, which mimic an arteriovenous malformation.[1,53] In one report, vascular proliferation was more common in supratentorial (12%) than in cerebellar (5%) tumors.[127] Frequently, these vessels are ectatic and hyalinized (Figure 6) rather than forming well-defined arteries and veins, and may show evidence of prior thrombosis with luminal obliteration or recanalization.[127] Perivascular hemosiderin may be evident and fatal hemorrhage has been described.[128]

Rosenthal fibers are a characteristic although not diagnostic feature of PAs (Figure 7). They appear as opaque, brightly eosinophilic rod-shaped, corkscrew, or beaded hyaline structures within the neuropil that stain blue with Luxol fast blue, purple with phosphotungstic acid hematoxylin (PTAH), and bright red with Masson's trichrome stains. They are present in variable numbers and are most often found in compact spindle-cell areas rather than in the microcystic areas. They may be absent in up to 24% of supratentorial PAs.[53] Ultrastructurally, Rosenthal fibers are irregularly shaped intracytoplasmic collections of granular or amorphous electron-dense material, surrounded by numerous bundles of 10-nm intermediate filaments.[81] On immunohistochemical examination they are either diffusely[70] or peripherally[94] positive for αB-crystallin, and positive for ubiquitin.[130] On light microscopy, they are negative for glial fibrillary acidic protein (GFAP), although

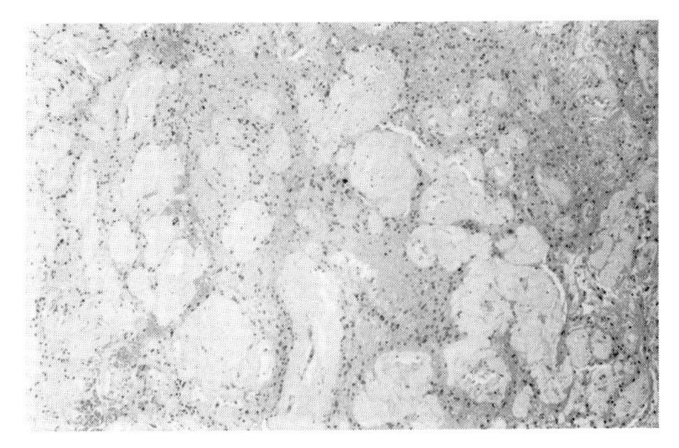

Figure 6: Pilocytic astrocytoma with numerous hyalinized thick-walled blood vessels. In some tumors, these vessels may be more numerous and mimic a vascular malformation. (hematoxylin-eosin, original magnification × 125)

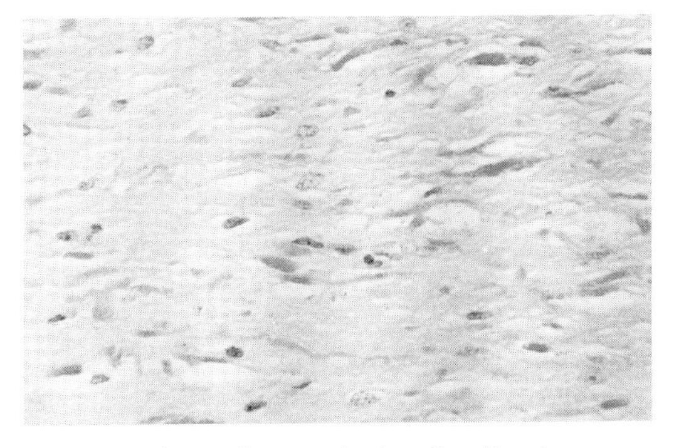

Figure 7: Photomicrograph of a pilocytic astrocytoma showing irregular, somewhat beaded Rosenthal fibers. These vary in number and stain intensely with eosin. (hematoxylin-eosin, original magnification × 500)

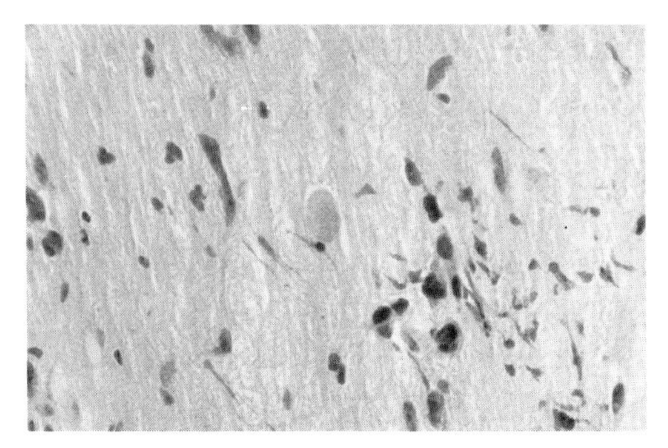

Figure 8: Eosinophilic granular bodies in a pilocytic astrocytoma. These are usually found in the microcystic areas of the tumor and, unlike Rosenthal fibers, are not immunoreactive for αB-crystallin (hematoxylin-eosin, original magnification × 500)

strong immunoreactivity at the periphery of the fiber may be seen.[97,219] Immunoelectron microscopy confirms the diffuse αB-crystallin immunoreactivity[211] and demonstrates some GFAP immunoreactivity within the central electron-dense matrix.[50]

Granular eosinophilic bodies are round hyaline bodies frequently seen in microcystic areas (Figure 8) and, like Rosenthal fibers, they may be absent in up to 26% of PAs.[53] Many correspond to aggregates of autophagocytic vacuoles[171] and are immunoreactive for α-1-antitrypsin and α-1-antichymotrypsin[54] but not for GFAP.[189] Some represent small Rosenthal fibers. The cells in PAs are immunoreactive for GFAP,[18,33] αB-crystallin,[94] and vimentin.[18,177] The fibrillary processes of the pilocytic cells are strongly positive, while the more protoplasmic cells in the microcystic areas are negative or only weakly stained. PAs also express other intermediate filament proteins, including various cytokeratin subunits and neurofilament proteins.[18] Bodey and colleagues[18] suggest that this may reflect a normal pattern of developmentally regulated expression of different intermediate filament proteins. Alternatively, in some cases, it may represent the detection of shared epitopes by monoclonal antibodies.

Cytogenetic Studies

Proliferation indices have been measured in a limited number of PAs using bromodeoxyuridine (66 cases)[66,86,92,139] or antibodies to nuclear antigens such as Ki-67 (23 cases)[34,49,68,185,214,235] or proliferating cell nuclear antigen (PCNA) (four cases).[15] For both bromodeoxyuridine and Ki-67, the mean labeling index is <1%, although indices between 0% and 5.6% for Ki-67[214] and up to 7.9% for bromodeoxyuridine have been described.[66] The mean PCNA labeling index for PAs (5.03 ± 3.20) was not significantly different from that for either fibrillary astrocytomas (4.80 ± 2.85) or gemistocytic astrocytomas (4.51 ± 1.35). However, only four cases were examined and it is unclear whether only tumor nuclei were counted or whether immunoreactive inflammatory cell and endothelial nuclei were included.[15] The bromodeoxyuridine index tends to be higher in younger patients, males, and cerebellar rather than hypothalamic tumors.[92] The labeling index does not appear to correlate with prognosis; however, only a few cases have been examined and the follow-up period is frequently short. The identification of occasional tumors with a high labeling index must be reconciled with the observation that PAs grow extremely slowly and, in cystic examples, this increase in size may be due to expansion of the cyst rather than growth of solid tumor. The apparent discrepancy between proliferation indices and behavior could be explained by a concomitant increase in the rate of cell loss by apoptosis. It has been suggested that the tumor growth rate decreases when patients reach the age of about 20 years.[92]

Cytogenetic analysis has been performed on a small number of PAs with variable results. Normal karyotypes with or without small numbers of double minute forms (20 cases),[98,100,163,165,205,212] complex clonal and nonclonal chromosomal abnormalities with or without marker chromosomes (seven cases),[73,98,164] and numerical aberrations without significant structural changes (six cases)[100,165,205,212] have been described but no common pattern has emerged. Of the cases with complex clonal abnormalities, two were recurrent tumors that had been treated with radiotherapy.[163] Since mitoses are rare in these tumors, primary short-term culture is usually required to obtain adequate numbers of cells in metaphase for karyotyping. PAs are very slow growing and it is likely that the majority of tumor cells are in a noncycling pool. Short-term culture may select rare abnormal karyotypes associated with an in vitro proliferative advantage, which will bias the final karyotype. In some cases, karyotypes may reflect proliferating endothelial or inflammatory cells rather than astrocytes.

Unlike karyotype analysis, flow cytometry performed on fresh tissue or following histological processing reflects deoxyribonucleic acid (DNA) content in vivo. While this eliminates the problem of in vitro selection, tissue heterogeneity remains, so that the DNA content of endothelial cells, fibroblasts, inflammatory cells, and non-neoplastic brain within the specimen will be included in the final result. In one series,[79] DNA flow cytometry analysis of cerebellar PAs classified 70% as diploid, 19% as aneuploid, and 11% as tetraploid (79 cases). In a similar series, the mean percentage of cells in S phase was 3.19% (72 cases).[211] Of 34 supratentorial PAs, 53% were diploid, 32% aneuploid, 12% aneuploid-polyploid, and 3% tetraploid.[53] For both supra- and infratentorial PAs, ploidy did not appear to influence survival.[53,80]

Limited molecular genetic data are available for PAs. It has been suggested that, in some cases, deletion of a tumor suppressor gene on the long arm of chromosome 17 may be associated with PA,[221] and loss of alleles from chromosome 11p has been described in one tumor.[164] Molecular analysis has shown no loss of genetic material from chromosomes 19[222] or 10,[230] or (in 15 cases) from multiple chromosomes.[96,163] Neither p53 protein expression[99] nor mutations in the p53 tumor suppressor gene,[147] located on the short arm of chromosome 17, have been detected in PAs, even though similar mutations are found in up to one-third of other low-grade astrocytomas.[59,149,220]

Prognosis

The prognosis for both adults[62] and children with cerebral PA is good, with 5- and 10- year survival rates of 85% and 79%, respectively. Patients surviving 27 years have been described.[58] Corresponding 5- and 10-year survival rates for cerebellar PAs are similar (85% and 81%, respectively).[79] Survival is largely dependent on the accessibility and degree of resection of the tumor.[53,138,155] The relative circumscription of the tumor with a predominantly expansile mode of growth often permits complete surgical resection of accessible lesions. Following gross total or radical subtotal resection of supratentorial PAs, the 5- and 10-year survival rate is 100%. This decreases to 95% and 84%, respectively, following subtotal removal and to only 44% following biopsy alone.[183] Some series describe a more favorable prognosis for cerebellar astrocytomas in childhood (25-year survival rate 94%).[70] This may reflect more complete resection at this site. Most studies show radiotherapy to be of no benefit,[11] although its role following incomplete resection is controversial, with some reports suggesting a small advantage.[183] Some also suggest a better prognosis for the microcystic variant than for predominantly pilocytic tumors in the cerebellum;[45,223] however, the number of cases is small and in one study patients were followed only for 2 years.[223]

A few PAs recur or behave aggressively, with extensive leptomeningeal dissemination[10,39,116,136,139] or in rare cases extracranial spread.[27] In most instances, it has proved difficult to identify atypical features in these tumors, either radiologically[195] or histologically.[11] Recurrence may be early, usually in the first few years following surgery, or delayed for more than 20 years.[16] Cases in which recurrence developed 36[149] or 48 years[233] after surgery have been described. Usually, the recurrent neoplasm shows the same benign histology as the original tumor[9,116,139,145] although, in some cases, bizarre atypical giant cells are seen, possibly related to prior radiotherapy.[233] In contrast, diffuse low-grade astrocytomas tend to recur earlier and to transform into higher-grade lesions. In some cases of PA, recurrence is associated with reaccumulation of cystic fluid rather than with growth of solid tumor.[152]

Rare cases of anaplastic transformation occurring many years after initial surgical treatment of cerebellar PAs have been described.[5,16,30,35,51,115,180,201,210,215] In all but four cases,[16,180,210] the initial surgery was followed by radiotherapy. At the present time, the role of radiotherapy in this transformation is unclear. It may provide a "second hit" to induce anaplastic transformation in residual tumor, it may initiate neoplastic transformation of residual benign astrocytes within the radiation field, or it may have no direct effect, with anaplasia being a rare manifestation of tumor progression, unrelated to radiotherapy. Unfortunately, in some reports describing tumor recurrence or malignant change, the initial pathology is not described in sufficient detail to unequivocally diagnose a PA or to exclude a diffuse, low-grade astrocytoma with or without pilocytic features.[181,182] The long symptom-free period between the initial diagnosis and an anaplastic recurrence suggests that incomplete sampling of a glioma containing areas of high-grade tumor *ab initio* is unlikely.

PAs may exhibit unusual growth characteristics. They may recur many years after gross total resection, may apparently stop growing following partial excision,[11,29,102] or may show evidence of increased proliferation and aneuploidy with no apparent worsening of prognosis. It has been suggested that some PAs evolve into simple non-neoplastic cerebellar cysts.[186] There is evidence, based on serial neuroimaging studies, that the growth rate of optic nerve PAs decreases with time.[7]

Attempts have been made to identify clinical or pathological features that correlate with prognosis. Since the natural history of PA is usually one of slow growth over decades, this requires prolonged follow-up. Unfortunately, some studies do not address homogeneous clinicopathological entities but refer to "benign astrocytomas" or "cerebellar astrocytomas" without distinguishing pilocytic from nonpilocytic lesions. In addition, most reports are confined to cerebellar tumors. While supra- and infratentorial PAs have many features in common and appear to behave similarly, we are not aware of a published study directly comparing these two entities, so the accuracy of extrapolating results from one site to the other may be questionable. Multivariate analysis of cerebellar PA cases has identified three variables associated with improved survival (good neurological function at diagnosis, the presence of microcysts, and gross total resection) and with improved disease-free survival (good neurological function at diagnosis, young patient age, and gross total resection).[79] The presence of necrosis, mitotic figures, and atypia did not affect prognosis. Preliminary data presented by Tomlinson and colleagues[210] compared the histological features of malignancy in typical (72 cases), atypical (six cases), and malignant (four cases) cerebellar PA. Associated with a malignant histology were a high mitotic index (2 to 5 mitoses/high-power field(hpf)), an elevated percentage of cells in S phase (5% to 11%), and aneuploidy or polyploidy. Atypical tumors had a mildly elevated mitotic rate (1 to 3 mitoses/hpf), had 2% to 6% of cells in S phase, and were diploid (five cases) or polyploid (one case); typical tumors were predominantly diploid (73%) with a mean (± standard deviation) of 3.19% ± 2.1% of cells in S phase. It was noted that endothelial proliferation was not a prognostic indicator. It is unclear from the published abstract whether these findings correlated with clinical behavior. Forsyth et al[53] examined 24 clinical, pathological, and therapeutic variables in supratentorial PAs and found that only the extent of surgical resection was strongly associated with survival time and that the presence of atypia, mitoses, necrosis, vascular proliferation, calcification, or cyst formation was not significant. Due to the paucity of examples with each feature, multivariate analysis could not be performed. It has been suggested that "appreciable" mitotic activity,[169] tumor necrosis, or infiltrative growth may identify tumors with a worse prognosis.[62] Although individual examples of recurrent PA may appear more atypical than the original tumor with increased cellularity and vascularity, endothelial proliferation, increased nuclear irregularity, and mitotic figures,[16] these features do not predict recurrence.

PAs must be distinguished from low-grade fibrillary astrocytomas that appear focally pilocytic. This may be seen when isomorphic structures such as the corpus callosum, internal capsule, or cerebral peduncles are infiltrated by tumor. In these situations, astrocytoma cells are constrained by the pre-existing microenvironment and appear elongated and thin with bipolar nuclei and thin, parallel fibrillar processes. However, other microscopic features of PA such as granular bodies, Rosenthal fibers, and microcysts are absent. This distinction is important because low-grade fibrillary astrocytomas are diffusely infiltrating, poorly demarcated neoplasms that cannot be resected in toto, have a tendency to transform into more aggressive tumors, and are ultimately fatal.[120] The prognosis is considerably worse for low-grade astrocytoma and oligoastrocytoma (5- and 10-year survival rates of 51% and 23%, respectively) than for supratentorial PA (5- and 10-year survival rates, 85% and 79%, respectively).[183] While many studies have associated diffuse cerebellar astrocytoma with a poor prognosis[69,171] (a 38% 25-year survival rate versus 94% for juvenile PA), others have found no difference in prognosis between "diffuse" and "discrete (juvenile pilocytic)" cerebellar astrocytomas.[152,154,155,201] In the cerebellum there appears to be considerable histological overlap, with both "diffuse" and "discrete" patterns being found in the same tumor.[33,91,154] Hayostek et al[79] also described a subgroup of cerebellar PA, which they designated "diffuse pilocytic astrocytoma," with a predominantly infiltrative growth pattern and at least focal areas of microcystic or compact PA. The presence of this subtype was not an independent prognostic factor for overall or disease-free survival.

Based purely on the morphological similarities between certain normal structures in the mature or developing brain and the cells in PAs, it has been suggested that these tumors are derived from the radial glia found during normal fetal development, from Bergmann astrocytes in the cerebellum,[171] or from subependymal astrocytes.[152,234] The latter is supported by the frequent close proximity of these tumors to the ventricular walls.[138,152,155,178]

Pleomorphic Xanthoastrocytoma

Pleomorphic xanthoastrocytoma (PXA) is an uncommon tumor that was first delineated as a separate clinicopathological entity by Kepes and colleagues[109] in 1979. Since then, fewer than 100 examples have been described, in varying detail.* The clinical and pathological characteristics of PXA have been recently reviewed.[104]

This tumor is most frequently encountered in children and young adults, mainly during the second decade of life, although it has been reported in three older patients aged 46,[153] 62,[131] and 66 years.[82] Clinically, 75% of patients present with seizures,[10] often of several years' duration. Less frequent presentations include a focal deficit or evidence of increased intracranial pressure.

Neuroimaging Features

Imaging studies demonstrate a superficially located, usually temporoparietal brain mass with distinct borders, frequently involving the leptomeninges. The dura is involved only exceptionally and bone erosion of the skull is rare.[231] Nearly all reported PXAs have been supratentorial. A cerebellar PXA was seen in consultation[124] and only a single example of a thoracic cord tumor has been described.[82] An associated cyst is very common and some tumors present as a mural nodule within a cyst. There may be calcification and the mass is usually avascular on carotid artery angiograms,[71,109,227] although in one case partial blood supply from the external carotid artery was demonstrated.[231] On CT scans, contrast enhancement is usual.[107,117] On MRI studies, most tumors are isointense with gray matter on T1-weighted images and mildly hyperintense on T2-weighted images; all tumors enhance following the administration of contrast material.[168,209]

Pathological Findings

Macroscopically, PXAs are firm and frequently well defined although nonencapsulated, with a variegated appearance. The cut surface is frequently gray-white or yellowish with one or more cysts and occasional areas of hemorrhage but no gross evidence of necrosis.

Microscopically, the tumor is moderately cellular and includes spindle cells and pleomorphic mono- and multinucleated giant cells (Figure 9A). The spindle cells form parallel and interlacing bundles which may appear storiform. In some areas, the cells appear cytologically bland. The leptomeninges are usually massively involved and tumor extends into the underlying brain by either direct invasion or within perivascular Virchow-Robin spaces.

*References 4,10,17,26,71,72,74,82,83,87,88,93,101, 107,117,118,125,126,131,148,153,156,168,174,175,196, 197,206,207,225,227,231,234

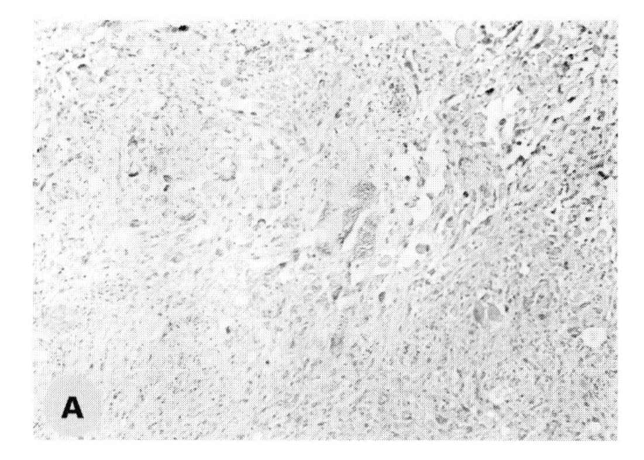

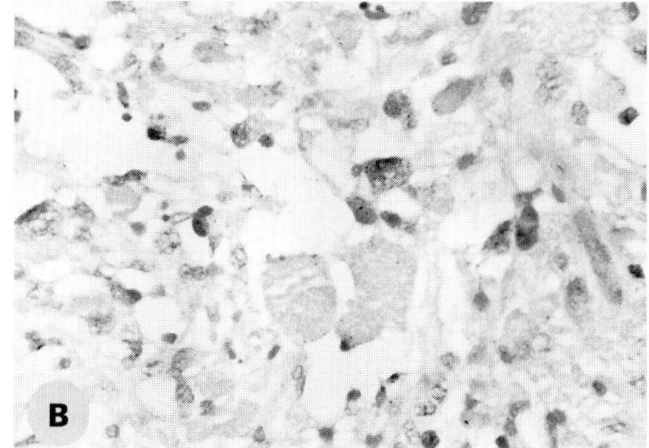

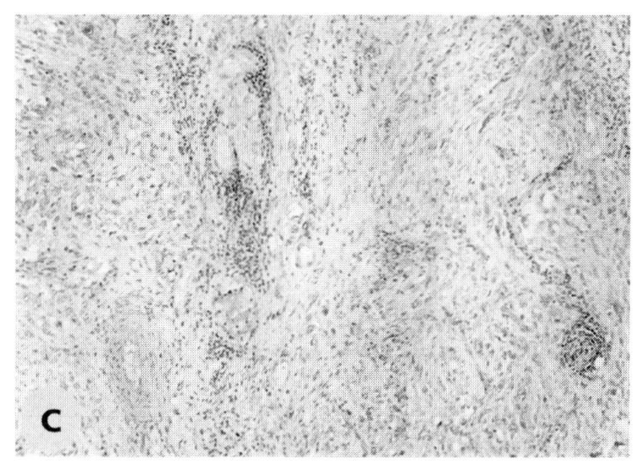

Figure 9: Photomicrographs of pleomorphic xanthoastrocytomas. **A)** Example of marked pleomorphism with multinucleated tumor giant cells. Mitotic figures are rare in these tumors and necrosis is absent. **B)** Numerous PAS-positive cytoplasmic inclusions are seen within the tumor cells. Note also the nuclear pleomorphism. **C)** Focal perivascular aggregates of lymphoid cells are present. (hematoxylin-PAS, original magnification × 125 [A and C]; × 500 [B])

Many cells contain lipid droplets that are birefringent under polarized light. These droplets may distend the cell body and displace the nucleus and other cytoplasmic constituents peripherally so that the cell does not resemble a typical astrocyte. However, other tumor cells are more recognizably astrocytic with fibrillary processes and eosinophilic cytoplasm. Occasional periodic acid-Schiff (PAS)-positive intracytoplasmic hyaline droplets are seen (Figure 9B).

Characteristically, PXA is rich in reticulin fibers. Although reticulin fibers are commonly seen in other types of gliomas that infiltrate the leptomeninges, where they represent a desmoplastic response to tumor invasion, in PXA, reticulin is noted between individual spindle cells and surrounds single and small groups of giant cells, both in the leptomeninges and within the brain substance. Reticulin is more commonly observed surrounding groups of cells in deeper areas of brain invasion. Scattered single and aggregates of lymphocytes and plasma cells are frequently found throughout these tumors (Figure 9C)[109,117,126,227] and, rarely, lymphoid follicles with germinal centers have been described.[109] Mitotic figures are absent or inconspicuous and necrosis is absent.

The astrocytic lineage of the tumor cells is supported by finding GFAP in both the obviously astrocytic cells and the xanthomatous cells in PXA. In the lipid-laden cells, GFAP immunoreactivity is displaced peripherally by the central lipid droplets and is present within cell processes and beneath the plasma membrane. Cells are also strongly immunoreactive for S100 protein[72,93] and vimentin,[117] and stain positively for the macrophage/histiocytic markers α-1-antitrypsin and α-1-antichymotrypsin.[117] They are occasionally positive for lysozyme[93] and some cells coexpress the macrophage marker CD68 and GFAP.[234] Cytokeratin expression has been detected in both the pleomorphic and spindle cells of PXA,[84] and rare cells immunoreactive for neurofilament proteins have been described in one case.[84] Cytokeratin expression has been described in astrocytomas in both adults[45] and children.[18]

Electron microscopy[83,87,109,119,225] complements the light microscopic and immunohistochemical findings. Tumor cells contain abundant 10-nm intermediate filaments, which are displaced peripherally by lipid droplets. Prominent basal lamina material surrounds individual and small groups of cells. Some hemidesmosomes and punctate attachments between tumor cells are also seen.

The superficial location and the presence of prominent reticulin has led to the hypothesis that PXAs are derived from subpial astrocytes,[109] which are superficial and are known to form both basement membrane[162] and hemidesmosomes.[161]

Although one does not normally think of astrocytes as generating fibrous tissue, both normal and neoplastic astrocytes can produce basement membrane components and collagen. Basement membrane has been demonstrated by electron microscopy on normal subpial astrocytes,[162] in cultured mouse embryo spinal cord astrocytes,[119] and in astrocytoma cell lines.[188] Laminin, a component of basement membrane, is expressed by astrocytoma cell lines in vitro[3] and by astrocytes in vivo following brain injury.[123] Other astrocytoma cell lines synthesize type IV collagen,[3,157] tenascin,[134] and extracellular matrix components.[135]

Cytogenetic Studies

Several features suggest that PXAs are slow-growing neoplasms. Clinical symptoms may be present for several years before diagnosis (15 years in one case[83]), mitotic figures are rare, necrosis is absent, and the peritumoral brain may be gliotic and contain Rosenthal fibers.[93,101] Proliferation potential has been assessed in several PXAs. Using silver stains for nucleolar organizer region-associated proteins (Ag-NORs), Sawada et al[174] found that the average number of Ag-NORs per nucleus in PXA (2.34) was less than in glioblastoma (3.27) and similar to that in low-grade astrocytoma (2.57). Immunostaining for the proliferation-associated nuclear antigen Ki-67 revealed a proliferation index of <1% in one case,[198] and an S-phase fraction of <0.25% was found in another tumor by DNA cytofluorometric analysis.[87] In the latter case, the mode cellular DNA content was diploid and a few polyploid nuclei were identified.

Karyotype analysis has been reported for one PXA. In short-term culture, 75% of the cells had a normal karyotype while 25% showed consistent numerical and structural changes.[175] The tumor recurred 1 year after surgical excision (without radiotherapy or chemotherapy or morphological evidence of transformation into a higher-grade tumor) and the karyotype contained chromosomal telomere fusions and ring chromosomes suggesting tumor progression .[176]

Prognosis

Optimal management of PXA remains controversial, although primary surgical resection with later surgery for residual or recurrent tumor has been advocated. The role of radiotherapy is uncertain,[227] and survival for 18 years has been reported following surgical treatment alone.[153]

The prognosis for patients with typical PXA is favorable, with almost 50% of patients alive with a mean follow-up of 7.4 years after diagnosis.[227] Some patients remain symptom-free for many years (in one case 17 years[109]). However, it is difficult to predict the clinical course following diagnosis. While originally described as a low-grade tumor that behaves more favorably than its morphology would imply, several examples of aggressive PXA with local recurrence or subarachnoid dissemination have been reported.[4,83,93,107,225,227] In these cases, transition to a more malignant anaplastic astrocytoma or glioblastoma was documented, either at the time of the original diagnosis, with subsequent recurrence, or at autopsy. In some cases a high-grade tumor developed many years after the diagnosis of PXA.[227]

The reasons for the relatively good prognosis of PXA are unknown, but possible contributing factors include the superficial location and relative circumscription of the tumor allowing gross total removal, the paucity of mitotic figures, the low labeling index, and the presence of lymphocytic infiltrates. Some studies have shown that, for both low-grade[226] and malignant[25,152] gliomas, lymphocytic infiltration correlates with prolonged survival.

Differential Diagnosis

Because PXA has a relatively good prognosis, it is important to distinguish it from true mesenchymal lesions involving the leptomeninges and from more malignant astrocytic neoplasms that are heavily lipidized. Prior to recognition as a distinct entity, PXA was frequently (mis)diagnosed as a mesenchymal lesion (such as fibroxanthoma, leptomeningeal xanthosarcoma,[105] or monstrocellular sarcoma[64]) based on leptomeningeal attachment, spindle-cell morphology (often with storiform areas), the presence of xanthoma cells, and obvious pericellular reticulin. However, the presence of recognizable astrocytes within the lesion and GFAP immunoreactivity in both xanthomatous and spindle cells distinguishes PXA from these mesenchymal lesions. True meningeal sarcomas are GFAP- and S100 protein-negative, are frequently immunoreactive for macrophage and leukocyte markers, and show other features of malignancy (including foci of necrosis and a high mitotic index).[72]

The presence of marked pleomorphism and tumor giant cells may suggest a glioblastoma. However, the young age of most patients, the paucity of mitotic figures, and the absence of necrosis or significant endothelial proliferation distinguish PXA from glioblastoma.

Other astrocytic neoplasms may contain lipid-rich cells, usually near areas of coagulative necrosis. However, the lipidized cells in PXA are distributed throughout the tumor, and necrosis is absent. Several examples of malignant gliomas containing heavily lipidized tumor cells have been described. Unlike PXA, these tumors occur in older individuals, are deeply situated in the cerebral hemispheres, and show obvious features of malignancy with a widely infiltrative growth pattern, areas of necrosis, and numerous, often atypical mitotic figures.[67,106,172] In one case examined by electron microscopy, no pericellular basal lamina was identified.[67] As in PXA, these tumors show heavily lipidized cells in non-necrotic areas. Occasionally, a heavily lipidized malignant astrocytoma may be cystic, superficially located, and occur in adolescents.[72] The importance of adhering to specific histological criteria when diagnosing PXA has been stressed. Specifically, the diagnosis of PXA should not be made in the presence of necrosis[103,109] even if other features are consistent with PXA.[64]

The origin of the lipid within astrocytes is unclear. While some may be derived from phagocytosis by cells surrounding foci of necrosis, fatty change may also reflect disordered metabolism within injured cells.[199] This seems to be a more plausible explanation for lipid accumulation in cells away from areas of necrosis, which may also be seen in areas of white matter injury following anoxia or radiation-induced damage.[106]

As is true of most pathological entities, with increasing experience atypical and unusual variants of PXA have been described. These variants include: tumors with "epithelioid" characteristics in which reticulin and basal lamina material surround nests of tumor cells rather than individual cells;[93] tumors with sparse reticulin;[101] with sparse lipid;[33] or tumors with numerous blood vessels ("angiomatous" variant).[198] Tumors have been reported in unusual locations including the suprasellar region, the floor of the middle cranial fossa,[196] the thalamus (without apparent meningeal contact),[117] the cerebellum,[124] and the thoracic spinal cord.[82] PXA has been described as a component of gangliogliomas,[60,124] in association with a classic PA[101,109] or "ordinary" fibrillary astrocytoma,[101] and in a patient with neurofibromatosis.[148] Several examples of tumors that appear to mimic PXA have also been described. Maleki and colleagues[132] reported as an atypical xanthoastrocytoma a tumor with some features of PXA including diagnosis when the patient was 15 years of age, superficial temporoparietal location with massive leptomeningeal involvement, relative circumscription and a cystic component, the presence of lipidized astrocytes, basement membrane material and hemidesmosomes on electron microscopy, and absent mitotic figures. However, the lipidized tumor cells were mainly surrounding necrotic foci and reticulin radiated from slightly hyperplastic blood vessels rather than being predominantly pericellular. In addition, atypical ganglion cells were scattered throughout the tumor. Despite the favorable prognosis in this case, with no evidence of recurrence at 12 months, the tumor does not appear to fulfill the diagnostic criteria for PXA. (For a discussion of the possible significance of neuronal differentiation in PXA, see the section on "Desmoplastic Cerebral Astrocytoma of Infancy," below.)

Subependymal Giant Cell Astrocytoma

Clinical Features

Subependymal giant cell astrocytomas (SGCAs) are rare benign tumors which in most but not all cases are associated with tuberous sclerosis (TS). Approximately 5% of people with TS develop SGCAs. The wide variation in the published incidence of SGCA in TS (1.7% to 26%) probably reflects different patient selection and diagnostic criteria.[24] These tumors are usually detected within the first two decades of life (peak incidence 8 to 18 years)[85] although they have been described in a premature infant at 31 weeks of gestation,[48] in neonates,[19,76,150,208] and in a man of 40 years.[19] There is no sex predilection.[19] Sporadic tumors are exceedingly rare[21,38,77] and some doubt their existence, suggesting that reported examples may represent a *forme fruste* of TS or that the clinical and neuroradiological data provided do not allow TS to be excluded.[6] If they do exist, sporadic examples tend to be diagnosed later in life.[41]

Tumors are almost exclusively located in the walls of the lateral ventricles, in the thalamostriate sulcus overlying the basal ganglia. They are especially common anteriorly, in the region of the foramen of Monro, which they may occlude, giving rise to hydrocephalus. Lesions also occur in the third ventricle and occasional tumors have been described within the cerebral hemispheres[77] or retina.[135] Radiologically, SGCAs show strong homogeneous enhancement on CT scans and high signal intensity on T2-weighted MRI studies.[95]

Grossly, SGCAs are smooth-surfaced masses that protrude into the ventricles and appear sharply demarcated but not encapsulated. They are well vascularized and the cut surface is gray to pinkish and may show focal hemorrhage. They are sometimes coarsely nodular and cystic[198] or may contain dilated angiomatous blood vessels, rupture of which may cause massive intratumoral and intraventricular hemorrhage.[13,223] Focal calcification is common and may be identified on plain skull x-rays or CT scans.

Pathological Findings

Microscopically, SGCAs are separated from the overlying intact ependyma by a thin layer of glial stroma[14] and are well demarcated from the surrounding brain (Figure 10A). They show considerable histological variation, but two main cell types are commonly encountered with some intermediate forms (Figure 10B). The predominant cells are large and polyhedral, globoid, or pyramidal with abundant eosinophilic hyaline cytoplasm and either coarse nonfibrillated or finer fibrillary processes (Figure 10C). Some of these processes contain Rosenthal fibers.[187] The nuclei are variably sized, usually large, and eccentric with a thin nuclear membrane, finely granular, evenly distributed chromatin and a prominent central nucleolus. Intranuclear pseudoinclusions of cytoplasm are commonly seen[75,184] and true intranuclear inclusions have been described.[200] There are numerous bi- and multinucleated forms and giant cells with vesicular nuclei, which superficially resemble dysplastic neurons; however, no Nissl substance or neurites are demonstrable on histochemical staining.[21] Many cells also resemble gemistocytic astrocytes.

The other main cell type consists of elongated uni- or bipolar strap cells, often arranged in broad fascicles (Figure 10D). The nuclei tend to be oval, with dense chromatin and inconspicuous or absent nucleoli. Perivascular pseudorosettes of both giant cells and spindle cells are not uncommon (Figure 10E) and may occasionally represent the predominant histological pattern.[19] Thin-walled blood vessels are frequently prominent, although endothelial hyperplasia or proliferation is not seen. Degenerative changes including areas of hemorrhage with collections of foamy lipid-laden macrophages, focal desmoplasia, thick-walled hyalinized blood vessels (Figure 11A), microcalcification (Figure 11B), or microcystic areas may be seen. Tumors may contain numerous interstitial and perivascular mast cells—a finding of unknown significance.[38,184,188] The cytomorphology of SGCA has been described.[2,6]

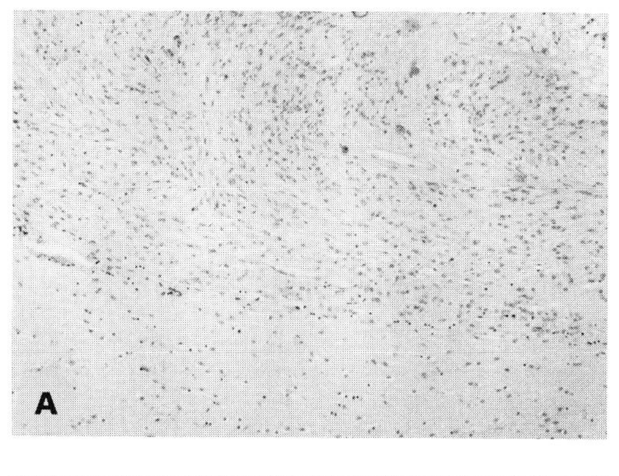

Figure 10: Photomicrographs of subependymal giant cell astrocytomas. **A)** Circumscription can be seen with no tumor infiltration into the surrounding brain. **B)** Both cell types, giant cells and fascicles of spinal cells, are demonstrated. **C)** Example of pleomorphic giant cells, with several having multiple nuclei and prominent nucleoli. Polygonal cells with abundant eosinophilic cytoplasm and eccentric nuclei resemble abnormal neurons. Despite marked pleomorphism, there are no mitoses, necrosis, or other features of malignancy. **D)** Example of fascicles of spindle cells. **E)** Spindle cells forming poorly defined perivascular pseudorosettes can be seen in some areas. (hematoxylin-eosin, Luxol fast blue, original magnification × 125 [A]; hematoxylin-eosin, original magnification × 125 [B and E] , × 500 [C])

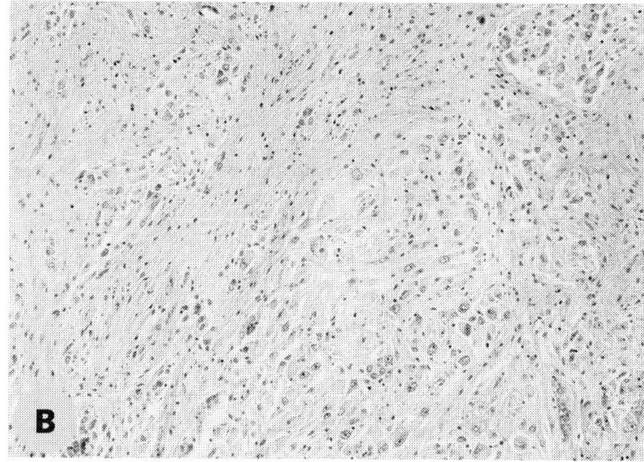

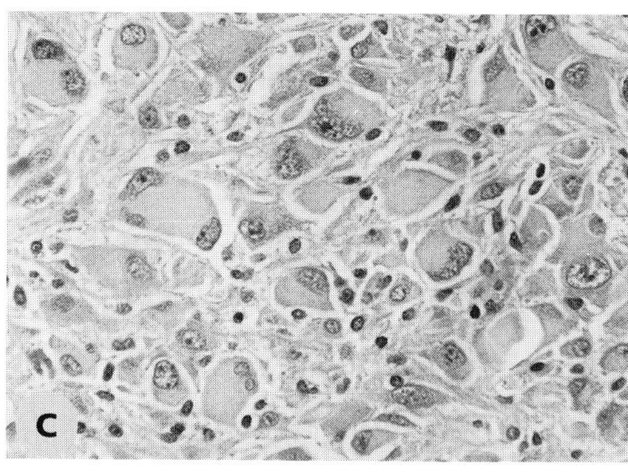

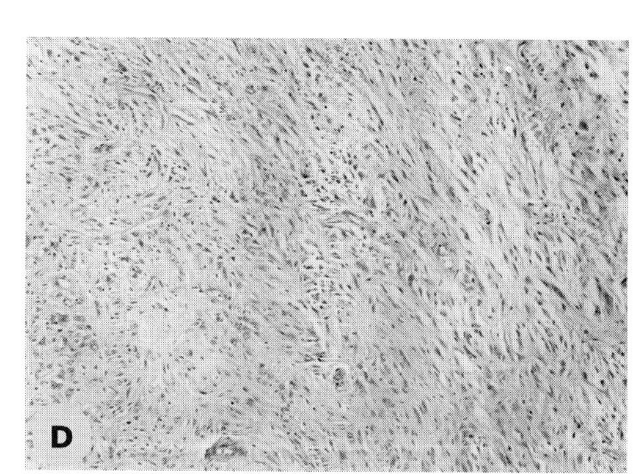

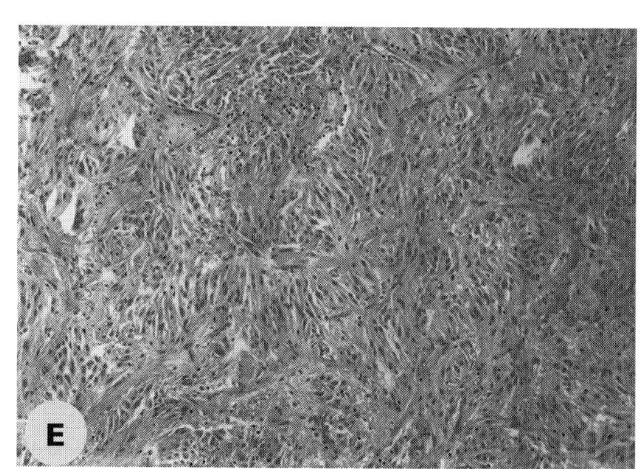

In spite of the considerable nuclear pleomorphism, other features of malignancy (such as a high nucleo-cytoplasmic ratio, necrosis, or increased cell density) are uncommon. Most reports stress the rarity or absence of mitotic figures in SGCA.[46,142] However, in occasional examples, focal necrosis[14,38] and readily identifiable mitoses may be seen; in one series, up to 5 mitoses/10 hpf were identified in eight of 13 cases.[184] The presence of mitoses and necrosis does not appear to affect prognosis. Although data are limited, most (12 of 13) SGCAs are diploid by flow cytometry with only one of 13 containing a polyploid population.[184] An S-phase fraction of <1% has been described in one case[144] and an SGCA with a bromodeoxyuridine labeling index of 1.5% has been reported.[160] This tumor, in a 4-year-old child, recurred 8 months after resection and showed similar histology with a labeling index of <1%.

Electron microscopy confirms the astrocytic nature of most cells,[142,166,187,213] but also demonstrates evidence of neuronal differentiation with occasional dense-core granules[21,46,187] and synap-

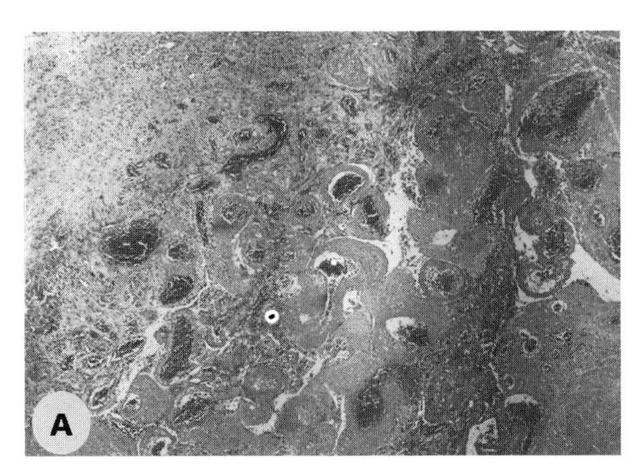

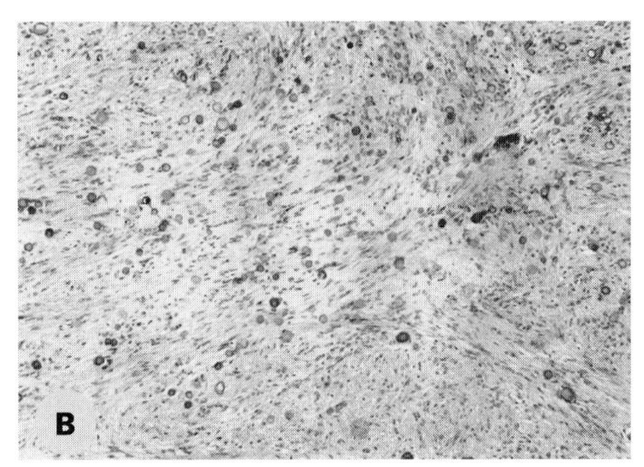

Figure 11: Photomicrographs of degenerative changes in subependymal giant cell astrocytomas. **A)** Vessels are prominent, and thick-walled hyalinized vessels with numerous engorged thin-walled blood vessels are present. Rarely, these may rupture resulting in massive intratumoral and intraventricular hemorrhage. **B)** Numerous round foci of calcification can be seen scattered throughout the tumor. This may also be seen on plain skull x-rays and CT scans. (hematoxylin-eosin, original magnification × 50 [A]; hematoxylin-eosin, Luxol fast blue, original magnification × 125 [B])

tic structures.[141] Individual tumor cells may show features that can be interpreted as supporting both neuronal and astocytic differentiation.[14]

Immunohistochemical studies also demonstrate heterogeneous phenotypic expression, with cells showing evidence of astrocytic, neuronal, and occasionally oligodendroglial differentiation. GFAP is demonstrable in nearly all tumors unassociated with TS, although the distribution and the staining intensity vary greatly. In TS-associated tumors, GFAP immunoreactivity is less intense and many cells are not labeled.[21,142] Variable immunoreactivity for vimentin,[76] neuron-specific enolase (NSE),[95,171,193,194] αB-crystallin,[94] myelin basic protein,[98] and neurofilament protein[76,144,171] has been reported, with some cells coexpressing GFAP and neurofilament protein. Factor XIIIa immunoreactivity has been demonstrated in SGCA cells as well as in other lesions associated with TS including renal angiomyolipomas and cutaneous angiofibromas.[159]

It is thought that these tumors arise from the disordered migration of a dysplastic or dysgenetic progenitor cell that has the potential for astrocytic and, to a lesser extent, neuronal differentiation—with the neuronal differentiation being incomplete.[21] They are slow growing, do not metastasize, and very rarely undergo malignant change. Recurrence following surgical resection is uncommon,[160] although Halmagyi et al[77] described a cystic parietal lobe giant cell astrocytoma that recurred twice with the same histology over a period of 47 years in a patient without TS. Occasionally, tumor enlargement has been documented on serial CT scans.[56,141] Pathological examination of these lesions shows SGCAs without atypical or malignant features.

Differential Diagnosis

The distinction between SGCAs and the multiple, small, "hamartomatous" subependymal nodules seen in TS and known as "candle gutterings" or "drippings" (from their appearance on pneumoencephalography) is largely semantic. The two lesions are separated more by clinical convention than by biological behavior, predominantly on the basis of size and associated symptoms of increased intracranial pressure.[14] Microscopically, tumors and nodules are similar, although large bizarre cells predominate in SGCAs.[19] Radiologically, they are distinguished on CT scans since SGCAs enhance while subependymal nodules do not.[111,137,142,229] The reason for this radiological difference is unknown and it is unclear whether it actually reflects a qualitative difference in the behavior of the two lesions. On MRI studies, both subependymal nodules and SGCAs may enhance following intravenous administration of contrast material.[24] Strictly speaking, the subependymal nodules seen in TS are not true hamartomas—a term that denotes an excessive focal overgrowth of mature normal cells which are abnormally arranged.[43]

The pathological differential diagnosis includes giant cell glioblastoma, gemistocytic astrocytoma, and ependymoma. Giant cell glioblastoma would be uncommon in the first two decades of life and lacks the gross circumscription and subependymal location of SGCA. Glioblastoma also demonstrates features of malignancy, with necrosis, vascular proliferation, and mitotic activity. The nuclei are more hyperchromatic and pleomorphic with coarse, unevenly distributed chromatin and irregular and thickened nuclear membranes. Gemistocytic astrocytomas are nondiscrete white matter lesions with smaller, less bizarre cells and cytological features of malignancy. Although a limited biopsy from an SGCA with prominent perivascular pseudorosettes may superficially resemble an ependymoma, giant cells and multinucleated cells with prominent cytoplasm are not features of ependymomas, and true rosettes (characteristic of ependymomas) are absent.

Desmoplastic Cerebral Astrocytoma of Infancy

Clinical Features

Only 10 cases of this rare tumor have been described,[23,47,129,203] and all were diagnosed in infants aged 1 to 14 months. CT studies demonstrate a large (10- to 13-cm), cystic, variably enhancing supratentorial mass, most commonly involving the frontal lobe. The mass is superficial and involves the cortex, leptomeninges, and dura, with or without erosion of the skull.

Macroscopically, desmoplastic cerebral astrocytoma of infancy (DCAI) presents as a grayish, white, or ivory-colored, firm, rubbery plaque-like lesion that is firmly attached to the dura and appears to be predominantly extracerebral, filling the subarachnoid space and extending into the cortex with finger-like projections. It is unencapsulated but appears relatively circumscribed with solid and cystic areas. The cystic components can be uni- or multilocular, usually extend deep to the solid parts of the tumor, and contain clear or xanthochromic proteinaceous fluid.

Pathological Findings

Microscopically, the tumor is largely composed of densely packed spindle cells in a collagenous background. The spindle cells are arranged in wide fascicles and whorls, and may assume a storiform pattern. They may be plump or thin and tapering, resembling fibroblasts. Occasionally, more polygonal cells and identifiable astrocytes, some appearing gemistocytic, are seen. In three cases, rare foci of small, poorly differentiated cells with a high nucleocytoplasmic ratio were identified, occupying less than 5% of the tumor area.[129] Special stains demonstrate abundant reticulin and collagen around both individual cells and small cell groups throughout the tumor. No differentiated mesenchyme or ganglion cells are seen. Tumor extends into the Virchow-Robin spaces and also infiltrates into brain. There is marked reactive gliosis around these areas of brain infiltration. Some cases show focal lymphocytic infiltration. Mitotic figures are rare or absent and none is abnormal. Necrosis is not seen, and there are no pleomorphic cells or bizarre giant cells. A rare cell may contain intracytoplasmic lipid. Some tumors contain focal areas of vascular prominence without endothelial proliferation. This angiomatoid pattern is more commonly seen at the periphery of the tumor.

Electron microscopy identifies a single cell type that contains numerous intermediate filaments, often arranged in bundles. The cells are surrounded by an uninterrupted basal lamina (which is focally reduplicated), and banded (type 1) collagen is present between most cells. No fibroblasts or cells showing evidence of neuronal differentiation (dense-core granules, synaptic vesicles, or conspicuous microtubules) or Schwann cell differentiation are identified.[129]

Immunohistochemical studies demonstrate strong GFAP, S100 protein, and vimentin reactivity in the majority of cells. Weak NSE reactivity was detected in two cases;[129] however, no neurofilament[204] or synaptophysin immunoreactivity has been reported. The small "undifferentiated" cells noted above do not react with antibodies to GFAP, S100 protein, NSE, or neurofilament protein. As expected from the results of reticulin staining and electron microscopy, there is strong pericellular reactivity for type IV collagen. However, pericellular fibronectin is not detected.[129]

Cytogenetic Studies

Cytogenetic analysis of one tumor, established in short-term culture, showed no clonal abnormalities but included four cells with abnormal karyotypes.[23] The significance of these nonclonal abnormalities, including partial deletion of chromosome 6, is unclear although the authors mentioned in passing a second case of DCAI with a nonclonal deletion of chromosome 6.[23] Molecular genetic analysis has been performed on two tumors. This demonstrated no loss of heterozygosity for alleles on chromosomes 10 and 17.[129]

Prognosis

No data on the proliferative potential of DCAI have been published. Physical examination of patients frequently shows rapidly increasing head size and, in one case, serial CT scans demonstrated rapid tumor growth over 3 months from a small area of hypodensity, initially thought to be an infarct, to a large complex cystic mass.[23]

The prognosis is good following gross total or even subtotal removal, with or without postoperative radiotherapy. Apart from one early postoperative death due to respiratory failure, all nine reported patients have developed normally. Most are neurologically normal and none shows evidence of recurrence with 11 months to 5.5 years of follow-up.

Differential Diagnosis

The differential diagnosis of DCAI includes a cellular mesenchymal tumor, such as a meningeal sarcoma, PXA, or desmoplastic infantile ganglioglioma. All four of these tumors have features in common. They all present as firm, superficial neoplasms involving the meninges. All contain spindle cells and are reticulin-rich. The lack of mitotic figures, pleomorphism, and necrosis and the presence of GFAP staining, pericellular basal lamina, and intracytoplasmic 10-nm intermediate filaments exclude meningeal sarcoma. PXA is uncommon in infants, being found predominantly in the second and third decades of life. It is rarely attached to the dura and contains numerous highly pleomorphic lipidized cells.[109] Even lipid-poor examples of PXA contain more lipid than DCAI.

Desmoplastic ganglioglioma of infancy[216,217] appears to be closely related to DCAI. Both tumors occur in infancy, are supratentorial, appear similar macroscopically with dural involvement and cyst formation, and share a relatively good prognosis following surgical resection. Microscopically, they both contain astrocytic spindle cells and abundant collagen and reticulin. Unlike DCAI, desmoplastic ganglioglioma of infancy contains heterogeneous neuronal elements, including atypical ganglion cells and smaller, polygonal, poorly differentiated primitive neuroectodermal cells. Some of these small cells are positive for either glial or neuronal markers.[217] The neuronal elements vary in abundance and distribution and are most frequently seen in areas with less exuberant extracellular matrix. It is possible that, in a small biopsy, neuronal elements might not be included. Frequently, neuronal differentiation is apparent only on immunohistochemical studies and or with silver impregnation techniques.[158] Occasional examples of desmoplastic gangliogliomas of infancy showing Schwann cell differentiation by electron microscopy have been described.[61,143] In view of their similar clinical behavior and pathological appearance it has been suggested that DCAI and desmoplastic ganglioglioma of infancy should be classified together as desmoplastic supratentorial neuroepithelial tumors of infancy.[158,217]

VandenBerg[216] suggests that a common precursor of both the astrocytic and neural lineages may persist in the cerebral subpial granular zone[28] and may normally differentiate into the specialized subpial astrocytes. Following neoplastic transformation, this precursor could differentiate along one or both lineages, resulting in a purely astrocytic tumor (DCAI) or a mixed astrocytic/neural tumor (desmoplastic ganglioglioma of infancy). It is possible that the small, poorly differentiated cells noted above as a minor component of several DCAI represent these precursor cells. An analogous argument could be proposed to explain the occasional examples of pleomorphic tumors (PXAs) which contain atypical neurons. These have been variously designated PXA,[117] "atypical" PXA,[132] ganglioglioma with PXA,[60,124] or cerebral ganglioglioma.[191] An example of an otherwise unremarkable PXA with scattered tumor cells showing neurofilament immunoreactivity has also been described.[84]

GLIOFIBROMA

The term "gliofibroma" was first used by Friede[55] to describe a "peculiar neoplasm of collagen forming glia-like cells." This tumor was found in the medulla of a 3-year-old girl and consisted in part of an extremely firm, round, grayish, ill-defined 12-mm nodule. Microscopically, it was a sharply delineated mass composed of well-differentiated astrocytes. Most cells were widely separated although some small clusters were present. The nuclei were large, rounded, oval, or irregular, and somewhat vesicular with sparse chromatin granules. Some cells had tapering eosinophilic processes that merged with a homogeneous, dense, eosinophilic fibrillary interstitium. Residual medullary neurons and myelinated axons were scattered throughout the tumor. No Rosenthal fibers or mitoses were identified and there was no microcystic degeneration. A Holzer stain for glial fibers and a trichrome stain demonstrated intimately interwoven collagen and glial fibers, which were often congruent with pre-existing fiber tracts. Electron microscopy demonstrated a single cell population and confirmed the admixture of collagen fibers and glial processes. The glial processes were partly covered by a basal lamina which was absent where glial processes apposed collagen fibers. No definite fibroblasts were identified and Friede suggested that the collagen was produced by a modified clone of glia-like cells rather than by admixed mesenchymal cells.

The subsequent literature is somewhat confusing, as the term "gliofibroma" has been extended to include astrocytic tumors in which collagen is synthesized by mesenchymal cells.[22,31,90,170,179,190] Cerda-Nicolas and Kepes,[36] in a recent review of gliofibromas and gliosarcomas, discussed the presence of mesenchymal elements in gliomas. They proposed that tumors in which collagen or basement membrane material is produced by neoplastic mesenchymal cells should be called "mixed glioma-fibromas" (if benign) or "gliosarcoma/sarcogliomas" (if malignant) and that the term "gliofibroma" (or desmoplastic astrocytoma) should be restricted to benign tumors in which collagen is synthesized by neoplastic astrocytes. The malignant counterpart of gliofibroma is an anaplastic gliofibroma or desmoplastic glioblastoma.

With this restricted definition, gliofibromas are exceptionally rare; only four cases have been well documented. Two of these appear to be anaplastic gliofibromas;[36] one arose in a hamartoma but showed necrosis and mitotic activity,[164] and the tumor described by Friede[55] contained an area of high-grade astrocytoma.

The tumors occur in children (9 months to 16 years of age) and may present as enhancing, superficial, space-occupying lesions on CT scans. Grossly, they are whitish yellow; they are firm and may be rubbery or somewhat translucent. In some cases they may be demarcated from the surrounding brain. There is no obvious "marbling" as seen in the mixed mesenchymal and astrocytic gliosarcoma (Feigin tumor). Microscopically, interlacing bundles of spindle cells are admixed with looser areas containing round and multipolar astrocytes. GFAP staining is prominent in both spindle and round cells with some cell-to-cell variability in staining intensity.[36] Reticulin and collagen are present between the GFAP-positive cells and no convincing fibroblastic elements are appreciated, as might be seen with gliomatous infiltration of the meninges or with gliosarcoma.

Electron microscopy demonstrates numerous intracytoplasmic intermediate filaments with pericellular basal lamina and thin collagen fibers. These features are also seen in normal subpial astrocytes.[162] It is possible that gliofibroma, desmoplastic astrocytoma of infancy, and PXA are all derived from these specialized subpial astrocytes or share a common precursor. It has been suggested that PXA represents a lipidized form of DCAI, which is seen in older children and young adults.[47]

Benign mixed glial mesenchymal tumors (glioma-fibromas) are also rare, with only a handful of published reports. They may appear at any age (2 months to 45 years). Approximately 50% are spinal with the rest being cerebral or, in two cases, within the fourth ventricle.[22,170] They may be solid or solid and cystic.[89] Histologically, two distinct but intermingled components are recognizable: astrocytic elements (which are GFAP- and S100 protein-positive and do not have intercellular reticulin), and mesenchymal elements (which are GFAP-negative, variably positive for muscle-specific actin, α-1-antichymotrypsin, or the macrophage marker CD68,[179,190] and show intercellular reticulin). Electron microscopy confirms the presence of two distinct cell types.[90] It has been suggested that, in some cases, the mesenchymal component may be derived from Schwann cells.[218]

The origin of the mesenchymal elements in glioma-fibromas is unknown. They may be derived from fibroblasts or Schwann cells associated with blood vessels or perivascular nerves. Alternatively, it has been suggested that the mesenchyme represents fibroblastic metaplasia of neoplastic glial cells.[170] This suggestion is supported by the occasional demonstration of cartilaginous differentiation in astrocytomas.[108] If this latter hypothesis is correct, then gliofibromas, glioma-fibromas, DCAIs, desmoplastic infantile gangliogliomas, and possibly PXAs may arise from a common progenitor cell with the potential for astrocytic, neural, Schwann cell, and fibroblastic differentiation.[170] Indeed, three tumors designated as superficial cerebral astrocytoma, which appear similar to DCAI but contain interweaving bundles of astrocytes and fibroblasts, have been described.[170] These tumors, in infants, also contain foci of small round primitive cells which are focally immunoreactive for synaptophysin or neurofilament protein.

Both gliofibromas and mixed glioma-fibromas should be distinguished from astrocytomas infiltrating the leptomeninges. In this relatively common situation, astrocytic elements are intermixed with reticulin and collagen. However, these mesenchymal elements are formed by leptomeningeal cells rather than by astrocytes. These tumors behave like the more usual type of diffuse astrocytoma.

References

1. Afra D, Müller W, Slowik F, et al: Supratentorial lobar pilocytic astrocytomas: report of 45 operated cases, including 9 recurrences. **Acta Neurochir 81**:90-93, 1986
2. Ahluwalia CK, Chandrasoma PT: Cytomorphology of subependymal giant cell astrocytoma. A case report. **Acta Cytol 37**:197-200, 1992
3. Alitalo K, Bernstein P, Vaheri A, et al: Biosynthesis of an unusual collagen type by human astrocytoma cells *in vitro*. **J Biol Chem 258**:2653-2661, 1983
4. Allegranza A, Ferraresi S, Bruzzone M, et al: Cerebromeningeal pleomorphic xanthoastrocytoma. Report of four cases: clinical radiological and pathological features. (Including a case with malignant evolution.) **Neurosurg Rev 14**:43-49, 1991
5. Alpers CE, Davis RL, Wilson CB: Persistence in the late malignant transformation of childhood cerebellar astrocytoma. Case report. **J Neurosurg 57**:548-551, 1982
6. Altermatt HJ, Scheithauer BW: Cytomorphology of subependymal giant cell astrocytoma. **Acta Cytol 36**:171-175, 1992
7. Alvord EC, Lofton S: Gliomas of the optic nerve or chiasm. Outcome by patients' age, tumor site, and treatment. **J Neurosurg 68**:85-98, 1988
8. Aoki S, Barkovich AJ, Nishimura K, et al: Neurofibromatosis types 1 and 2: cranial MR findings. **Radiology 172**:527-534, 1989
9. Arendt A: Histopathologic vongliomrezidiven. **Zentralbl Allg Pathol 126**:499-504, 1982
10. Auer RN, Rice GPA, Hinton GG, et al: Cerebellar astrocytoma with benign histology and malignant clinical course. Case report. **J Neurosurg 54**: 128-132, 1981
11. Austin EJ, Alvord EC: Recurrences of cerebellar astrocytomas: a violation of Collin's law. **J Neurosurg 68**:41-47, 1988
12. Balestri P, Calistiri L, Vivarelli R, et al: Central nervous system imaging in reevaluation of patients with neurofibromatosis type 1. **Childs Nerv Syst 9**:448-451, 1993
13. Barbosa-Coutinho LM, Lima EL, Gadret RO, et al: Hemorragia maciça intratumoral em esclerose tuberosa. Estudo autópticodeumcaso. **Arq Neuropsiquiatr 49**:465-470, 1991
14. Bender BL, Yunis EJ: Central nervous system pathology of tuberous sclerosis in children. **Ultra-**

struct Pathol 1:287-299, 1980
15. Beppu T, Arai H, Kanaya H, et al: [Measurement of PCNA labeling index in astrocytic tumors.] **No Shinkei Geka 20**:1255-1259, 1992 (Jpn)
16. Bernell WR, Kepes JJ, Seitz EP: Late malignant recurrence of a childhood cerebellar astrocytoma. Report of two cases. **J Neurosurg 37**:470-474,1972
17. Blom Rj: Pleomorphic xanthoastrocytoma: CT appearance. **J Comput Assist Tomogr 12**:351-354, 1988
18. Bodey B, Cosgrove M, Gonzalez-Gomez I, et al: Co-expression of four intermediate filament subclasses in childhood glial neoplasms. **Mod Pathol 4**: 42-749, 1991
19. Boesel CP, Paulson GW, Kosnik EJ, et al: Brain hamartomas and tumors associated with tuberous sclerosis. **Neurosurgery 4**:410-417, 1979
20. Bognanno JR, Edwards MK, Lee TA, et al: Cranial MR imaging in neurofibromatosis. **AJR 151**: 381-388, 1988
21. Bonnin JM, Rubinstein Lj, Papasozomenos SC, et al: Subependymal giant cell astrocytoma. Significance and possible cytogenetic implications of an immunohistochemical study. **Acta Neuropathol 62**:185-193, 1984
22. Bonnin JM, Warner JC, Turner MS: Cystic gliofibroma of the fourth ventricle. **J Neuropathol Exp Neurol 49**:261, 1990 (Abstract)
23. Boop FA, Chadduck WM, Sawyer J, et al: Congenital aneurysmal hemorrhage and astrocytoma in an infant. **Pediatr Neurosurg 17**:44-47, 1991-1992
24. Braffman BH, Bilaniuk LT, Naidich TP, et al: MR imaging of tuberous sclerosis: pathogenesis of this phakomatosis, use of gadopentetate dimeglumine, and literature review. **Radiology 183**:227-238, 1992
25. Brooks WH, Markesbery WR, Gupta GD, et al: Relationship of lymphocyte invasion and survival of brain tumor patients. **Ann Neurol 4**:219-224, 1978
26. Brown JH, Chew FS: Pleomorphic xanthoastrocytoma. **AJR 160**:1272, 1993
27. Brown MT, Friedman HS, Oakes WJ, et al: Clinically aggressive pilocytic astrocytomas. **Neurology 41(Suppl 1)**:383, 1991 (Abstract)
28. Brun A: The subpial granular layer of the foetal cerebral cortex in man. Its ontogeny and significance in congenital cortical malformations. **Acta Pathol Microbiol Scand Suppl 179**:1-98, 1965
29. Bucy PC, Thieman PW: Astrocytomas of the cerebellum. A study of a series of patients operated upon over 28 years ago. **Arch Neurol 18**:14-19, 1968
30. Budka H: Partially resected and irradiated cerebellar astrocytoma of childhood: malignant evolution after 28 years. **Acta Neurochir 32**:139-146,1975
31. Budka H, Sunder-Plassmann M: Benign mixed glial-mesenchymal tumour ("glio-fibroma") of the spinal cord. **Acta Neurochir 55**:141-145, 1980
32. Burger PC: Classification, grading, and patterns of spread of malignant gliomas, in Apuzzo MLJ (ed): **Malignant Cerebral Glioma. Neurosurgical Topics Series.** Park Ridge, Ill: American Association of Neurological Surgeons, 1990, pp 3-17
33. Burger PC, Scheithauer BW, Vogel FS: **Surgical Pathology of the Nervous System and Its Coverings, 3rd ed.** New York: Churchill Livingstone, 1991, pp 242-247
34. Burger PC, Shibata T, Kleihues P: The use of the monoclonal antibody Ki-67 in the identification of proliferating cells: application to surgical neuropathology. **Am J Surg Pathol 10**:611-617, 1986
35. Casadei GP, Arrigoni GL, D'Angelo V, et al: Late malignant recurrence of childhood cerebellar astrocytoma. **Clin Neuropathol 9**:295-298, 1990
36. Cerda-Nicolas M, Kepes JJ: Gliofibromas (including malignant forms), and gliosarcomas: a comparative study and review of the literature. **Acta Neuropathol 85**:349-361, 1993
37. Chou TM, Chou SM: Tuberous sclerosis in the premature infant: a report of a case with immunohistochemistry in the CNS. **Clin Neuropathol 8**:45-52,1989
38. Chow CW, Klug GL, Lewis EA: Subependymal giant-cell astrocytoma in children. An unusual discrepancy between histological and clinical features. **J Neurosurg 68**:880-883, 1988
39. Civitello LA, Packer RJ, Rorke LB, et al: Leptomeningeal dissemination of low-grade gliomas in childhood. **Neurology 38**:562-566, 1988
40. Clark GB, Henry JM, McKeever PE: Cerebral pilocytic astrocytoma. **Cancer 56**:1128-1133, 1985
41. Cooper JR: Brain tumors in hereditary multiple system hamartomatosis (tuberous sclerosis). **J Neurosurg 34**:194-202, 1971
42. Cosgrove M, Fitzgibbons PL, Sherrod A, et al: Intermediate filament expression in astrocytic neoplasms. **Am J Surg Pathol 13**:141-145, 1989
43. Cotran RS, Kumar V, Robbins SL: **Robbins Pathological Basis of Disease, 4th ed.** Philadelphia, Pa: WB Saunders, 1989, pp 243-245
44. Cushing H: Experiences with the cerebellar astrocytomas. A critical review of seventy-six cases. **Surg Gynecol Obstet 52**:129-204, 1931
45. Daumas-Duport C, Scheithauer BW, O'Fallon J, et al: Grading of astrocytomas. A simple and reproducible method. **Cancer 62**:2152-2165, 1988
46. de Chadarévian JP, Hollenberg RD: Subependymal giant cell tumor of tuberose sclerosis. A light and ultrastructural study. **J Neuropathol Exp Neurol 38**:419-433, 1979
47. de Chadarévian JP, Pattisapu JV, Faerber EN: Desmoplastic cerebral astrocytoma of infancy. Light microscopy, immunocytochemistry, and ultrastructure. **Cancer 66**:173-179, 1990
48. DeGirolami U, Armbrustmacher VW: Juvenile pilocytic astrocytoma of the pineal region. Report of a case. **Cancer 50**:1185-1188, 1982
49. Deckert M, Reifenberger G, Wechsler W: Determination of the proliferative potential of human brain tumors using the monoclonal antibody Ki-67. **J Cancer Res Clin Oncol 115**:179-188, 1989.
50. Dinda AK, Sarkar C, Roy S: Rosenthal fibres: an immunohistochemical, ultrastructural and immunoelectron microscopic study. **Acta Neuropathol 79**:456-460, 1990
51. Dirks PB, Jay V, Becker LE, et al: Development of

anaplastic changes in low-grade astrocytomas of childhood. **Neurosurgery 34:**68-78, 1994
52. Duffner PK, Cohen ME: Isolated optic nerve gliomas in children with and without neurofibromatosis. **Neurofibromatosis 1:**201-211, 1988
53. Forsyth PA, Shaw EG, Scheithauer BW, et al: Supratentorial pilocytic astrocytomas. A clinicopathologic, prognostic, and flow cytometric study of 51 patients. **Cancer 72:**1335-1342, 1993
54. Friedberg E, Katsetos CD, Reidv J, et al: Immunolocalization of protease inhibitors α-l-antitrypsin and α-l-antichymotrypsin in eosinophilic granular bodies of cerebral juvenile pilocytic astrocytomas. **J Neuropathol Exp Neurol 50:**293, 1991 (Abstract)
55. Friede RL: Gliofibroma. A peculiar neoplasia of collagen forming glia-like cells. **J Neuropathol Exp Neurol 37:**300-313, 1978
56. Fujiwara S, Takaki T, Hikita T, et al: Subependymal giant-cell astrocytoma associated with tuberous sclerosis. Do subependymal nodules grow? **Childs Nerv Syst 5:**43-44, 1989
57. Fulham Mj, Melisi JW, Nishimiya J, et al: Neuroimaging of juvenile pilocytic astrocytomas: an enigma. **Radiology 189:**221-225, 1993
58. Fulling KH, Nelson JS: Cerebral astrocytic neoplasms in the adult: contribution of histological examination to the assessment of prognosis. **Semin Diagn Pathol 1:**152-163, 1984
59. Fults D, Brockmeyer D, Tullous MW, et al: p53 mutation and loss of heterozygosity on chromosome 17 and 10 during human astrocytoma progression. **Cancer Res 52:**674-679, 1992
60. Furuta A, Takahashi H, Ikuta F, et al: Temporal lobe tumor demonstrating ganglioglioma and pleomorphic xanthastrocytoma components. Case report. **J Neurosurg 77:**143-147, 1992
61. Gambarelli D, Hassoun J, Choux M, et al: Complex cerebral tumor with evidence of neuronal, glial, and Schwann cell differentiation. A histologic, immunocytochemical and ultrastructural study. **Cancer 49:**1420-1428, 1982
62. Garcia DM, Fulling KH: Juvenile pilocytic astrocytoma of the cerebrum in adults. A distinctive neoplasm with a favorable prognosis. **J Neurosurg 63:**382-386, 1985
63. Garcia DM, Fulling KH, Marks JE: The value of radiation therapy in addition to surgery for astrocytomas of the adult cerebrum. **Cancer 55:** 919-927, 1985
64. Garcia-Bengochea F, Collins GH: Monstrocellular sarcoma of the brain: 6-year postoperative survival. Case report. **J Neurosurg 31:**686-689, 1969
65. Gaskill Sj, Marlin AE, Saldivar V: Glioblastoma multiforme masquerading as a pleomorphic xanthastrocytoma. **Childs Nerv Syst 4:**237-240, 1988
66. Germano IM, Ito M, Cho KG, et al: Correlation of histopathological features and proliferative potential of gliomas. **J Neurosurg 70:**701-706, 1989
67. Gherardi R, Baudrimont M, Nguyen JP, et al: Monstrocellular heavily lipidized malignant glioma. **Acta Neuropathol 69:**28-32, 1986
68. Giangaspero F, Doglioni C, Rivano MT, et al: Growth fraction in human brain tumors defined by the monoclonal antibody Ki-67. **Acta Neuropathol 74:**179-182, 1987
69. Gjerris F, Klinken L: Long-term prognosis in children with benign cerebellar astrocytoma. **J Neurosurg 49:**179-184, 1978
70. Goldman JE, Corbin E: Isolation of a major protein component of Rosenthal fibers. **Am J Pathol 130:**569-578, 1988
71. Gomez JG, Garcia JH, Colon LE: A variant of cerebral glioma called pleomorphic xanthoastrocytoma: case report. **Neurosurgery 16:**703-706, 1985
72. Grant JW, Gallagher Pj: Pleomorphic xanthoastrocytoma. Immunohistochemical methods for differentiation from fibrous histiocytomas with similar morphology. **Am J Surg Pathol 10:**336-341, 1986
73. Griffin CA, Long PP, Carson BS, et al: Chromosomal abnormalities in low-grade central nervous system tumors. **Cancer Genet Cytogenet 60:** 67-73, 1992
74. Guo LX, Zhang RL: [Pleomorphic xanthoastrocytoma—a case report.] **Chung-Hua Chung Liu Tsa Chih 12:**477-478,1990 (Jpn)
75. Haberland C, Perou M: Glioma with nuclear inclusions in tuberose sclerosis. **Acta Neuropathol 16:** 73-76, 1970
76. Hahn JS, Bejar R, Gladson CL: Neonatal subependymal giant cell astrocytoma associated with tuberous sclerosis: MRI, CT, and ultrasound correlation. **Neurology 41:**124-128, 1991
77. Halmagyi GM, Bignold LP, Allsop JL: Recurrent subependymal giant-cell astrocytoma in the absence of tuberous sclerosis. Case report. **J Neurosurg 50:**106-109,1979
78. Hashimoto T, Tayama M, Miyazaki M, et al: Cranial MR imaging in patients with von Recklinghausen's disease (neurofibromatosis type I). **Neuropediatrics 21:**193-198, 1990
79. Hayostek CJ, Shaw EG, Scheithauer B, et al: Astrocytomas of the cerebellum. A comparative clinicopathological study of pilocytic and diffuse astrocytomas. **Cancer 72:**856-869,1993
80. Heiskanen O: Intracranial tumors of children. **Childs Brain 3:**69-78, 1977
81. Herndon RM, Rubinstein LJ, Freeman JM, et al: Light and electron microscopic observations on Rosenthal fibers in Alexander's disease and in multiple sclerosis. **J Neuropathol Exp Neurol 29:**524-551, 1970
82. Herpers MJH, Freling G, Beuls EAM: Pleomorphic xanthoastrocytoma in the spinal cord. Case report. **J Neurosurg 80:**564-569, 1994
83. Heyerdahl Strøm E, Skµllerud K: Pleomorphic xanthoastrocytoma: report of 5 cases. **Clin Neuropathol 2:**188-191, 1983
84. Hirato J, Nakazato Y, Ogawa A: Expression of non-glial intermediate filament proteins in gliomas. **Clin Neuropathol 13:**1-11, 1994
85. Holanda FJCS, Holanda GMP: Tuberous sclerosis—neurosurgical indications in intraventricular tumors. **Neurosurg Rev 3:**139-150, 1980
86. Hoshino T, Nagashima T, Murovic JA, et al: *In situ*

cell kinetics studies on human neuroectodermal tumors with bromodeoxyuridine labeling. **J Neurosurg 64:**453-459, 1986
87. Hosokawa Y, Tsuchihashi Y, Okabe H, et al: Pleomorphic xanthoastrocytoma. Ultrastructural, immunohistochemical, and DNA cytofluorometric study of a case. **Cancer 68:**853-859, 1991
88. Ibayashi N, Kubo S, Sekimoto T, et al: [A case of pleomorphic xanthoastrocytoma.] **No To Shinkei 38:**1151-1155, 1986 (Jpn)
89. Iglesias JR, Kraus HB, Michilli R, et al: Intracerebral gliofibroma. **Dtsch Med Wochenschr 117:** 1918-1922, 1992
90. Iglesias JR, Richardson EP, Collia F, et al: Prenatal intramedullary gliofibroma. A light and electron microscope study. **Acta Neuropathol 62:** 230-234, 1984
91. Ilgren EB, Esiri M, Stiller CA: Cerebellar astrocytomas. Part 1. Macroscopic and microscopic features. **Clin Neuropathol 6:**185-200, 1987
92. Ito S, Hoshino T, Shibuya M, et al: Proliferative characteristics of juvenile pilocytic astrocytomas determined by bromodeoxyuridine labeling. **Neurosurgery 31:**413-419, 1992
93. Iwaki T, Fukui M, Kondo A, et al: Epithelial properties of pleomorphic xanthoastrocytomas determined in ultrastructural and immunohistochemical studies. **Acta Neuropathol 74:**142-150, 1987
94. Iwaki T, Iwaki A, Miyazono M, et al: Preferential expression of αβ-crystallin in astrocytic elements of neuroectodermal tumors. **Cancer 68:**2230-2240, 1991
95. Iwasaki Y, Yoshikawa H, Sasaki M, et al: Clinical and immunohistochemical studies of subependymal giant cell astrocytomas associated with tuberous sclerosis. **Brain Dev 12:**478-481, 1990
96. James CD, He J, Carlbom E, et al: Loss of genetic information in central nervous system tumors common to children and young adults. **Genes Chromosom Cancer 2:**94-102,1990
97. Janzer RC, Friede RL: Do Rosenthal fibers contain glial fibrillary acid protein? **Acta Neuropathol 55:**75-76, 1981
98. Jenkins RB, Kimmel DW, Moertel CA, et al: A cytogenetic study of 53 human gliomas. **Cancer Genet Cytogenet 39:**253-279, 1989
99. Karamitopoulou E, Perentes E, Diamantis 1: p53 protein expression in central nervous system tumors: an immunohistochemical study with CMI polyvalent and DO-7 monoclonal antibodies. **Acta Neuropathol 85:**611-616,1993
100. Karnes PS, Tran TN, Cui MY, et al: Cytogenetic analysis of 39 pediatric central nervous system tumors. **Cancer Genet Cytogenet 59:**12-19, 1992
101. Kawano N: Pleomorphic xanthoastrocytoma: some new observations. **Clin Neuropathol 11:**323-328, 1992
102. Kehler U, Arnold H, Müller H: Long-term follow-up of infratentorial pilocytic astrocytomas. **Neurosurg Rev 13:**315-320, 1990
103. Kepes JJ: Glioblastoma multiforme masquerading as a pleomorphic xanthoastrocytoma. **Childs Nerv Syst 5:**127, 1988 (Letter)
104. Kepes JJ: Pleomorphic xanthoastrocytoma: the birth of a diagnosis and a concept. **Brain Pathol 3:** 269-273, 1993
105. Kepes JJ, Kepes M, Slowik F: Fibrous xanthomas and xanthosarcomas of the meninges and the brain. **Acta Neuropathol 23:**187-199, 1973
106. Kepes JJ, Rubinstein LJ: Malignant gliomas with heavily lipidized (foamy) tumor cells: a report of three cases with immunoperoxidase study. **Cancer 47:**2451-2459, 1981
107. Kepes JJ, Rubinstein LJ, Ansbacher L, et al: Histopathological features of recurrent pleomorphic xanthoastrocytomas: further corroboration of the glial nature of this neoplasm. A study of 3 cases. **Acta Neuropathol 78:**585-593, 1989
108. Kepes JJ, Rubinstein LJ, Chiang H: The role of astrocytes in the formation of cartilage in gliomas. An immunohistochemical study of four cases. **Am J Pathol 117:**471-483,1984.
109. Kepes JJ, Rubinstein LJ, Eng LF: Pleomorphic xanthastrocytoma: a distinctive meningocerebral glioma of young subjects with relatively favorable prognosis. A study of 12 cases. **Cancer 44:** 1839-1852, 1979
110. Kepes JJ, Whittaker CK, Watson K, et al: Cerebellar astrocytomas in elderly patients with very long pre-operative histories: report of three cases. **Neurosurgery 25:**258-264, 1989
111. Kingsley DPE, Kendell BE, Fitz CR: Tuberous sclerosis: a clinicoradiological evaluation of 110 cases with particular reference to atypical presentation. **Neuroradiology 28:**38-46, 1986
112. Kitagawa K, Yamamura T, Tsuzuki H, et al: [Studies of ophthalmic manifestations in von Recklinghausen's disease.] **Nippon Ganka Kiyo 36:**149-154, 1985 (Jpn)
113. Kleihues P, Burger PC, Scheithauer BW: **Histological Typing of Tumors of the Central Nervous System. World Health Organization.** Berlin: Springer-Verlag, 1993
114. Kleihues P, Burger PC, Scheithauer BW: The new WHO classification of brain tumours. **Brain Pathol 3:**255-268, 1993
115. Kleinman GM, Schoene WC, Walshe TM III, et al: Malignant transformation in benign cerebellar astrocytoma. Case report. **J Neurosurg 49:**111-118, 1978
116. Kocks W, Kalff R, Reinhardt V, et al: Spinal metastasis of pilocytic astrocytoma of the chiasma opticum. **Childs Nerv Syst 5:**118-120,1989
117. Kros JM, Vecht CJ, Stefanko SZ: The pleomorphic xanthoastrocytoma and its differential diagnosis: a study of five cases. **Hum Pathol 22:**1128-1135, 1991
118. Kuhajda FP, Mendelsohn C, Taxy JB, et al: Pleomorphic xanthoastrocytoma: report of a case with light and electron microscopy. **Ultrastruct Pathol 2:** 25-32, 1981
119. Kusaka H, Hirano A, Borstein MB, et al: Basal lamina formation by astrocytes in organotypic cultures of mouse spinal cord tissue. **J Neuropathol Exp Neurol 44:**295-303, 1985

120. Laws ER Jr, Taylor WF, Clifton MB, et al: Neurosurgical management of low-grade astrocytoma of the cerebral hemispheres. **J Neurosurg 61:**665-673,1984
121. Lee YY, Van Tassel P, Bruner JM, et al: Juvenile pilocytic astrocytomas: CT and MR characteristics. **AJR 152:**1263-1270, 1989
122. Lewis RA, Gerson LP, Axelson KA, et al: von Recklinghausen neurofibromatosis. II. Incidence of optic gliomata. **Ophthalmology 91:**929-935, 1984
123. Liesi P, Kaakkola S, Dahl D, et al: Laminin is induced in astrocytes of adult brain by injury. **EMBO J 3:**683-686, 1984
124. Lindboe FL, Cappelen J, Kepes JJ: Pleomorphic xanthoastrocytoma as a component of a cerebellar ganglioglioma: case report. **Neurosurgery 31:** 353-355,1992
125. Listernick R, Charrow J, Greenwald MJ, et al: Optic gliomas in children with neurofibromatosis type 1. **J Pediatr 114:**788-792, 1989
126. Loiseau H, Rivel J, Vital C, et al: Xanthoastrocytome polymorphe. A propos de 3 nouveaux cas. Revue de la littérature. **Neurochirurgie 37:**338-347, 1991
127. Lombardi D, Scheithauer BW, Piepgras D, et al: "Angioglioma" and the arteriovenous malformation-glioma association. **J Neurosurg 75:**589-596, 1991
128. Lones MA, Verity MA: Fatal hemorrhage in a cerebral pilocytic astrocytoma—adult type. **Acta Neuropathol 81:**688-690, 1991
129. Louis DN, von Deimling A, Dickersin GR, et al: Desmoplastic cerebral astrocytoma of infancy: a histopathologic, immunohistochemical, ulrastructural, and molecular genetic study. **Hum Pathol 23:**1402-1409,1992
130. Lowe J, Blanchard A, Morell K, et al: Ubiquitin is a common factor in intermediate filament inclusion bodies of diverse type in man, including those of Parkinson's disease, Pick's disease, and Alzheimer's disease, as well as Rosenthal fibres in cerebellar astrocytomas, cytoplasmic bodies in muscle, and Mallory bodies in alcoholic liver disease. **J Pathol 155:** 9-15, 1988
131. MacKenzie JM: Pleomorphic xanthoastrocytoma in a 62-year-old male. **Neuropathol Appl Neurobiol 13:**461-487, 1987
132. Maleki M, Robitaille Y, Bertrand G: Atypical xanthoastrocytoma presenting as a meningioma. **Surg Neurol 20:**235-238, 1983
133. Margo CE, Barletta JP, Staman JA: Giant cell astrocytoma of the retina in tuberous sclerosis. **Retina 13:**155-159, 1993
134. McComb RD, Moul JM, Bigner DD: Distribution of type VI collagen in human gliomas: comparison with fibronectin and glioma-mesenchymal matrix glycoprotein. **J Neuropathol Exp Neurol 46:** 623-633, 1987
135. McKeever PE, Fligiel SEG, Varani J, et al: Products of cells cultured from gliomas. VII. Extracellular matrix proteins of gliomas which contain glial fibrillary acidic protein. **Lab Invest 60:**286-295, 1989
136. McLaughlin JE: Juvenile astrocytomas with subarachnoid spread. **J Pathol 118:**101-107,1976
137. McLaurin RL, Towbin RB: Tuberous sclerosis: diagnostic and surgical considerations. **Pediatr Neurosci 12:**43-48, 1985-1986
138. Mercuri S, Russo A, Palma L: Hemispheric supratentorial astrocytomas in children. Long term results in 29 cases. **J Neurosurg 55:**170-173, 1981
139. Mishima K, Nakamura M, Nakamura H, et al: Leptomeningeal dissemination of cerebellar pilocytic astrocytoma. Case report. **J Neurosurg 77:** 788-791, 1992
140. Moran V, O'Keeffe F: Giant cell astrocytoma in tuberous sclerosis: computed tomographic findings. **Clin Radiol 37:**543-545, 1986
141. Morimoto K, Mogami H: Sequential CT study of subependymal giant-cell astrocytoma associated with tuberous sclerosis. Case report. **J Neurosurg 65:**874-877, 1986
142. Nakamura Y, Becker LE: Subependymal giant-cell tumor: astrocytic or neuronal? **Acta Neuropathol 60:**271-277, 1983
143. Ng TH, Fung CF, Ma LT: The pathological spectrum of desmoplastic infantile gangliogliomas. **Histopathology 16:**235-241, 1990
144. Nishizaki T, Orita T, Abiko S, et al: Subependymal giant cell astrocytoma associated with tuberous sclerosis: with special reference to cell kinetic studies—a case report. **Neurol Med Chir 30:**695-697, 1990
145. Obana WG, Cogen PH, Davis RL, et al: Metastatic juvenile pilocytic astrocytoma. Case report. **J Neurosurg 75:**972-975, 1991
146. Obringer AC, Meadows AT, Zackai EH: The diagnosis of neurofibromatosis-1 in the child under the age of 6 years. **Am J Dis Child 143:**717-719, 1989
147. Ohgaki H, Eibl RH, Schwab M, et al: Mutations of the p53 tumor suppressor gene in neoplasms of the human nervous system. **Mol Carcinogen 8:** 74-80, 1993
148. Ozek MM, Sav A, Pamir MN, et al: Pleomorphic xanthoastrocytoma associated with von Recklinghausen neurofibromatosis. **Childs Nerv Syst 9:** 39-42, 1993
149. Pagni CA, Giordana MT, Canavero S: Benign recurrence of a pilocytic cerebellar astrocytoma 36 years after radical removal: case report. **Neurosurgery 28:** 606-609, 1991
150. Painter MJ, Pang D, Ahdab-Barmada M, et al: Connatal brain tumors in patients with tuberous sclerosis. **Neurosurgery 14:**570-573, 1984
151. Palma L, Celli P, Maleci A, et al: Malignant monstrocellular brain tumours. A study of 42 surgically treated cases. **Acta Neurochir 97:**17-25, 1989
152. Palma L, Guidetti B: Cystic pilocytic astrocytomas of the cerebral hemispheres. Surgical experience with 51 cases and long-term results. **J Neurosurg 62:**811-815, 1985
153. Palma L, Maleci A, Di Lorenzo N, et al: Pleomorphic xanthastrocytoma with 18-year survival. Case report. **J Neurosurg 63:**808-810, 1985
154. Palma L, Russo A, Celli P: Prognosis of so-called "diffuse" cerebellar astrocytoma. **Neurosurgery 15:**315-317, 1984
155. Palma L, Russo A, Mercuri S: Cystic cerebral astrocytomas in infancy and childhood: long-term

results. **Childs Brain 10**:79-91, 1983

156. Pasquier B, Kojder I, Labat F, et al: Le xanthroastrocytome du sujet jeune. Revue de la littérature à propos de deux observations d'evolution discordante. **Ann Pathol 5**:29-43, 1985
157. Paulus W, Roggendorf W, Schuppan D: Immunohistochemical investigation of collagen subtypes in human glioblastomas. **Virchows Arch [A] 413**:325-332, 1988
158. Paulus W, Schlote W, Perentes E, et al: Desmoplastic supratentorial neuroepithelial tumours of infancy. **Histopathology 21**:43-49, 1992
159. Penneys NS, Smith KJ, Nemeth AJ: Factor XIIIa in the hamartomas of tuberous sclerosis. **J Dermatol Sci 2**:50-54, 1991
160. Prados MD, Krouwer HGJ, Edwards MSB, et al: Proliferative potential and outcome in pediatric astrocytic tumors. **J Neurooncol 13**:277-282, 1992
161. Raine CS, Wisniewski H: On the occurence of microtubules within mature astrocytes. **Anat Rec 167**:303-308, 1970
162. Ramsey Hj: Fine structure of the surface of the cerebral cortex of human brain. **J Cell Biol 26**:323-333, 1965
163. Ransom DT, Ritland SR, Kimmel DW, et al: Cytogenetic and loss of heterozygosity studies in ependymomas, pilocytic astrocytomas, and oligodendrogliomas. **Genes Chromosom Cancer** 5:348-356, 1992
164. Reinhardt V, Nahser HC: Gliofibroma originating from temporoparietal hamartoma-like lesions. **Clin Neuropathol 3**:131-138, 1984
165. Rey JA, Bello MJ, de Campos JM, et al: Chromosomal composition of a series of 22 human low-grade gliomas. **Cancer Genet Cytogenet 29**:223-237, 1987
166. Ribadeau Dumas JL, Poirier J, Escourolle R: Etude ultrastructurale des lésions cérébrales de la sclérose tubéreuse de Bourneville. A propos de deux cas. **Acta Neuropathol 25**:259-270, 1973
167. Ringertz N, Nordenstam H: Cerebellar astrocytoma. **J Neuropathol Exp Neurol 10**:343-367, 1951
168. Rippe DJ, Boyko OB, Radi M, et al: MRI of temporal lobe pleomorphic xanthoastrocytoma. **J Comput Assist Tomogr 16**:856-859, 1992
169. Rubinstein LJ: **Tumors of the Central Nervous System. Atlas of Tumor Pathology. Series 2, Fascicle 6.** Washington, DC: Armed Forces Institute of Pathology, 1972
170. Rushing EJ, Rorke LB, Sutton L: Problems in the nosology of desmoplastic tumors of childhood. **Pediatr Neurosurg 19**:57-62, 1993
171. Russell DS, Rubinstein LJ: **Pathology of Tumours of the Nervous System, 5th ed.** Baltimore, Md: Williams & Wilkins, 1989, pp 114-120
172. Sarkar C, Roy S, Bhatia S: Xanthomatous change in tumours of glial origin. **Indian J Med Res 92**: 324-331, 1990
173. Sato K, Rorke LB: Vascular bundles and wickerworks in childhood brain tumors. **Pediatr Neurosci 15**:105-110, 1989
174. Sawada T, Oinuma T, Katada H, et al: [Argyrophilic nucleolar organizer region proteins (Ag-NORs) in human central nervous tumors.] **Rinsho Byori 40**:1179-1184, 1992 (Jpn)
175. Sawyer JR, Roloson GJ, Chadduck WM, et al: Cytogenetic findings in a pleomorphic xanthoastrocytoma. **Cancer Genet Cytogen 55**:225-230, 1991
176. Sawyer JR, Thomas EL, Roloson GJ, et al: Telomeric associations evolving to ring chromosomes in a recurrent pleomorphic xanthoastrocytoma. **Cancer Genet Cytogen 60**:152-157, 1992
177. Schiller D, Giordana MT, Mauro A, et al: Immunohistochemical demonstration of vimentin in human cerebral tumors. **Acta Neuropathol 70**:209-219, 1986
178. Schisano G, Tovi D, Nordenstam H: Spongioblastoma polare of the cerebral henisphere. **J Neurosurg 20**:241-251, 1963
179. Schober R, Bayindir C, Canbolat A, et al: Gliofibroma: immunohistochemical analysis. **Acta Neuropathol 83**:207-210, 1992
180. Schwartz AM, Ghatak NR: Malignant transformation of benign cerebellar astrocytoma. **Cancer 65**:333-336, 1990
181. Scott RM, Ballantine HT Jr: Cerebellar astrocytoma: malignant recurrence after prolonged postoperative survival. Case report. **J Neurosurg 39**:777-779, 1973
182. Shapiro K, Shulman K: Spinal cord seeding from cerebellar astrocytomas. **Childs Nerv Syst 2**: 177-186, 1976
183. Shaw EG, Daumas-Duport C, Scheithauer BW, et al: Radiation therapy in the management of low grade supratentorial astrocytomas. **J Neurosurg 70**: 853-861, 1989
184. Shepherd CW, Scheithauer BW, Gomez MR, et al: Subependymal giant cell astrocytoma: a clinical, pathological, and flow cytometric study. **Neurosurgery 28**:864-868, 1991
185. Shibata T, Burger PC, Kleihues P: Ki-67 immunoperoxidase stain as marker for the histological grading of nervous system tumours. **Acta Neurochir Suppl 43**:103-106, 1988
186. Silverberg GD: Simple cysts of the cerebellum. **J Neurosurg 35**:320-327, 1971
187. Sima AAF, Robertson DM: Subependymal giant-cell astrocytoma. Case report with ultrastructural study. **J Neurosurg 50**:240-245, 1979
188. Sipe JC, Rubinstein LJ, Herman MM, et al: Ethylnitrosourea-induced astrocytomas. Morphologic observations on rat tumors maintained in tissue and organ culture systems. **Lab Invest 31**:571-579, 1974
189. Smith DA, Lantos PL: Immunocytochemistry of cerebellar astrocytomas: with a special note on Rosenthal fibres. **Acta Neuropathol 66**: 155-159,1985
190. Snipes GJ, Steinberg GK, Lane B, et al: Gliofibroma. Case report. **J Neurosurg 75**:642-646, 1991
191. Soffer D, Lach B, Constantini S: Melanotic cerebral ganglioglioma: evidence for melanogenesis in neoplastic astrocytes. **Acta Neuropathol 83**:315-323, 1992
192. Specht CS, Pinto-Lord C, Smith TW, et al: Spontaneous hemorrhage in a mixed glioma of the cerebellum: Case report. **Neurosurgery 19**:278-281, 1986

193. Stefansson K, Wollmann R. Distribution of glial fibrillary acid protein in central nervous system lesions of tuberous sclerosis. **Acta Neuropathol 52:**135-140, 1980
194. Stefansson K, Wollmann R: Distribution of the neuronal specific protein 14-3-2, in central nervous system lesions of tuberous sclerosis. **Acta Neuropathol 53:**113-117, 1981
195. Strong JA, Hatten HP Jr, Brown MT, et al: Pilocytic astrocytoma: correlation between the initial imaging features and clinical aggressiveness. **AJR 161:**369-372, 1993
196. Stuart G, Appleton DB, Cooke R: Pleomorphic xanthoastrocytoma. report of two cases. **Neurosurgery 22:**422-427, 1988
197. Sugita Y, Kepes JJ, Shigemori M, et al: Pleomorphic xanthoastrocytoma with desmoplastic reaction: angiomatous variant. Report of two cases. **Clin Neuropathol 9:**271-278,1990
198. Sugita Y, Taguchi A, Miyagi J, et al: The cystic growth of a subependymal giant-cell astrocytoma with tuberous sclerosis. **Kurume Med J 39:** 123-128, 1992
199. Sumi SM: Sudanophilic lipid accumulation in astrocytes in periventricular leukomalacia in monkeys. **Acta Neuropathol 47:**241-243,1979
200. Sumi SM, Reifel E: Unusual nuclear inclusions in astrocytoma. **Arch Pathol 92:**14-19, 1971
201. Szénásy J, Slowik F: Prognosis of benign cerebellar astrocytomas in children. **Childs Brain 10:**39-47, 1983
202. Tanaka Y, Honda Y, Kurihashi K: [Ophthalmic observation of 15 cases of neurofibromatosis (von Recklinghausen).] **Rinsho Ganka Iho 72:**691-694, 1978 (Jpn)
203. Taratuto AL, Monges J, Lylyk P, et al: Superficial cerebral astrocytoma attached to the dura. Report of six cases in infants. **Cancer 54:**2505-2512,1984
204. Taratuto AL, Sevlever G, Schultz M: Monoclonal antibodies in superficial desmoplastic astrocytoma attached to dura in infants. **J Neuropathol Exp Neurol 46:**395, 1987 (Abstract)
205. Thiel G, Losanowa T, Kintzel D, et al: Karyotypes in 90 human gliomas. **Cancer Genet Cytogenet 58:**109-120, 1992
206. Thomas C, Golden B: Pleomorphic xanthoastrocytoma: report of two cases and brief review of the literature. **Clin Neuropathol 12:**97-101, 1993
207. Tien RD, Cardenas CA, Rajagopalan S: Pleomorphic xanthoastrocytoma of the brain: MR findings in six patients. **AJR 159:**1287-1290, 1992
208. Tien RD, Hesselink JR, Duberg A: Rare subependymal giant-cell astrocytoma in a neonate with tuberous sclerosis. **AJNR 11:**1251-1252, 1990
209. Tomita T, McLone DG, Naidich TP: Mural tumors with cysts in the cerebral hemispheres of children. **Neurosurgery 19:**998-1005, 1986
210. Tomlinson FH, Scheithauer BW, Hayostek CH, et al: Atypia and malignancy in pilocytic astrocytomas of the cerebellum: a clinicopathologic and flow cytometric study. **J Neuropathol Exp Neurol 51:** 331, 1992 (Abstract)
211. Tomokane N, Iwaki T, Tateishi J, et al: Rosenthal fibers share epitopes with αB-crystallin, glial fibrillary acidic protein, and ubiquitin, but not vimentin. Immunoelectron microscopy with colloidal gold. **Am J Pathol 138:**875-885, 1991
212. Tran TN, Cui MY, Karnes PS, et al: Cytogenetic characterization of pediatric astrocytomas. **Pediatric Neurosci 15:**152, 1989 (Abstract)
213. Trombley IK, Mirra SS: Ultrastructure of tuberous sclerosis: cortical tuber and subependymal tumor. **Ann Neurol 9:**174-181, 1981
214. Tsanaclis AM, Robert F, Michaud J, et al: The cycling pool of cells within human brain tumors: *in situ* cytokinetics using the monoclonal antibody Ki-67. **Can J Neurol Sci 18:**12-17, 1991
215. Ushio Y, Arita N, Yoshimine T, et al: Malignant recurrence of childhood cerebellar astrocytoma: case report. **Neurosurgery 21:**251-255, 1987
216. VandenBerg SR: Desmoplastic infantile ganglioglioma and desmoplastic cerebral astrocytoma of infancy. **Brain Pathol 3:**275-281, 1993
217. VandenBerg SR, May EE, Rubinstein LJ, et al: Desmoplastic supratentorial neuroepithelial tumors of infancy with divergent differentiation potential ("desmoplastic infantile gangliogliomas"). **J Neurosurg 66:**58-71, 1987
218. Vazquez M, Miller DC, Epstein F, et al: Glioneurofibroma: renaming the pediatric "gliofibroma": a neoplasm composed of Schwann cells and astrocytes. **Mod Pathol 4:**519-523, 1991
219. Velasco ME, Dahl D, Roessmann U, et al: Immunohistochemical localization of glial fibrillary acidic protein in human glial neoplasms. **Cancer 45:** 484-494, 1980
220. von Deimling A, Eibl RH,Ohgaki H, et al: P53 mutations are associated with 17p allelic loss in grade II and grade III astrocytoma. **Cancer Res 52:**2987-2990, 1992
221. von Deimling A, Louis DN, Menon AG, et al: Deletions on the long arm of chromosome 17 in pilocytic astrocytoma. **Acta Neuropathol 86:**81-85, 1993
222. von Deimling A, Louis DN, von Ammon K, et al: Evidence for a tumor supressor gene on chromosome 19q associated with human astrocytomas, oligodendrogliomas, and mixed gliomas. **Cancer Res 52:**4277-4279, 1992
223. Waga S, Yamamoto Y, Kojima T: Massive hemorrhage in tumors of tuberous sclerosis. **Surg Neurol 8:**99-101, 1977
224. Wang HC, Ho YS: Clinicopathological evaluation of 78 astrocytomas in Taiwan with emphasis on a simple grading system. **J Neurooncol 13:**265-276, 1992
225. Weldon-Linne C, Victor TA, Groothis DR, et al: Pleomorphic xanthoastrocytoma. Ultrastructural and immunohistochemical study of a case with a rapidly fatal outcome following surgery. **Cancer 52:**2055-2063, 1983
226. Westergaard L, Gjerris F, Klinken L: Prognostic parameters in benign astrocytomas. **Acta Neurochir 123:**1-7, 1993
227. Whittle IR, Gordon A, Misra BK, et al: Pleomorphic xanthoastrocytoma. Report of four cases. **J Neurosurg 70:**463-468, 1989

228. Winston K, Gilles FH, Leviton A, et al: Cerebellar gliomas in children. **J Natl Cancer Inst 58:**833-838, 1977
229. Winter J: Computed tomography in diagnosis of intracranial tumors versus tubers in tuberous sclerosis. **Acta Radiol (Diagn) 23:**337-344, 1982
230. Ye Z, Wu JK, Darras BT: Loss of heterozygosity for alleles on chromosome 10 in human brain tumours. **Neurol Res 15:**59-67, 1993
231. Yoshino MT, Lucio R: Pleomorphic xanthastrocytoma. **AJNR 13:**1330-1332, 1992
232. Yoshitake H, Oshima T, Katsumi O, et al: Ocular manifestations in von Recklinghausen's disease during childhood. **Rinsho Ganka 37:**953-957, 1983
233. Yoshizumi MO: Neuro-ophthalmologic signs in a recurrent cerebellar asrtocytoma after 48 years. **Ann Ophthalmol 11:**1714-1719, 1979
234. Zorzi F, Facchetti F, Baronchelli C, et al: Pleomorphic xanthoastrocytoma: an immunohistochemical study of three cases. **Histopathology 20:**267-269, 1992
235. Zuber P, Hamou MF, de Tribolet N: Identification of proliferating cells in human gliomas using the monoclonal antibody Ki-67. **Neurosurgery 22:** 364-368,1988
236. Zülch KJ: **Histological Typing of Tumors of the Central Nervous System.** Geneva: World Health Organization, 1979
237. Zülch KJ, Wechsler W: Pathology and classification of gliomas. **Prog Neurol Surg 2:**21-84, 1968

CHAPTER 4

THE PATHOLOGY OF OLIGODENDROGLIOMAS

M. BEATRIZ S. LOPES, MD, SCOTT R. VANDENBERG, MD, PHD, AND
BERND W. SCHEITHAUER, MD

DESCRIPTION OF OLIGODENDROGLIOMA

In most series, oligodendrogliomas represent approximately 5% to 15% of intracranial gliomas.[38,63] The figure approaches 25% in institutions that specialize in seizure surgery. Although these tumors are not uncommon in children and adolescents (up to 6% of oligodendrogliomas),[38,51] the majority arise in adults, with a peak incidence in the fourth and fifth decades of life.[38,51,63] Both sexes are affected, with a male-to-female ratio between 2:1 and 3:2.[38,51] Oligodendrogliomas most frequently affect the cerebral hemispheres, particularly the frontotemporal region, but can arise in any part of the neuraxis. Because their incidence in any region is somewhat proportional to the volume of white matter, the cerebellum, brain stem, and spinal cord are infrequently affected.[15] Not uncommonly, oligodendrogliomas involve multiple lobes,[51] and bilaterality is noted in about 20% of cases.[38] The great majority of tumors exhibit a slow clinical evolution and are associated with a long history of seizures, the latter being a feature in up to 88% of cases.[51] Nonetheless, otherwise histologically typical oligodendrogliomas occasionally behave more aggressively, presenting with rapidly progressive symptoms as they enlarge, with enhancement on neuroimaging studies.[5]

The histopathological features of oligodendrogliomas suggest that these tumors are derived from cells with oligodendroglial genotypes. The normal cytogenesis of oligodendrocytes is still incompletely understood. In classical neuropathology terms, macroglial cells (which include astrocytes, oligodendroglia, and ependymal cells) were defined on the basis of their morphology and staining qualities. Oligodendrocytes, when compared with astrocytes, have less prominent and shorter cell processes, ones that do not form perivascular or subpial endfeet and are readily identified by the silver impregnation method of del Rio-Hortega.[46] At present, macroglial cells are more specifically characterized on the basis of ultrastructural features, as well as their biochemical and physiological properties, such as manifestations of cytoskeletal and membrane protein gene expression.

During the past 10 years, a great deal of new information regarding the development of macroglial cells has been obtained by in vitro and in vivo studies of the developing rat optic nerve.[32,37,44,60] On the basis of these results, macroglial cells are divided into three classes, namely oligodendrocytes and type-1 and type-2 astrocytes.[44] These three forms of glial cells arise at different stages of development and appear to be derived from two different progenitor cells. Type-1 astrocytes develop from one form of precursor cell, whereas type-2 astrocytes and

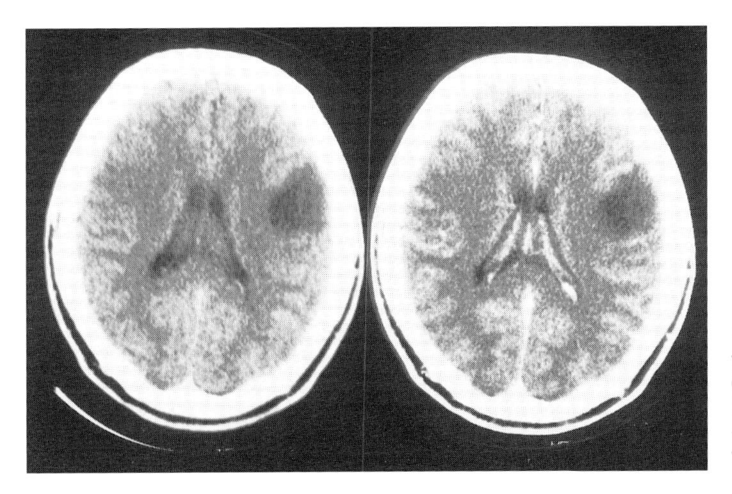

Figure 1: Oligodendroglioma as visualized on CT scans without **(left)** and with **(right)** contrast enhancement. The lesion is relatively demarcated and involves not only white matter but also cortex.

oligodendrocytes arise from a single progenitor cell termed the "oligodendrocyte-type-2 astrocyte" (O-2A) progenitor cell (see reviews by Watkins et al[57] and Cameron and Rakic[6]). The regional distribution and morphological features of these different macroglial cells within the central nervous system (CNS) appear to be greatly influenced by variations in the brain's microenvironment occurring during their lineage determination and maturation.[11] Although the precise identification of these cell types and the characterization of their role in human CNS development have not been entirely defined, the likely existence of a common progenitor cell of oligodendrocytes and of a subset of astrocytes (type-2 astrocytes) may provide a key to understanding the histogenesis of both oligodendrogliomas and mixed oligoastrocytomas.

Pathological Features

Macroscopic Appearance

Oligodendrogliomas are macroscopically soft gelatinous masses, often relatively demarcated from the adjacent brain (Figures 1 and 2). By extending from the white to gray matter, such le-

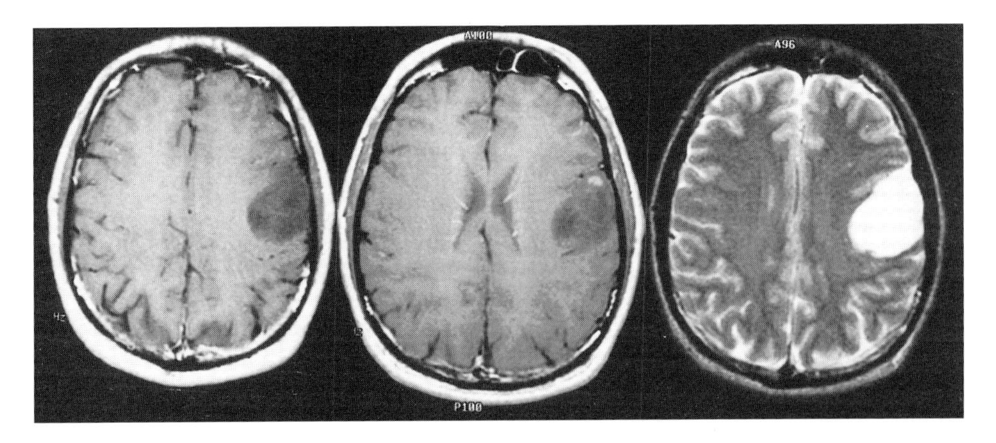

Figure 2: Oligodendroglioma as visualized in the sequence of MRI scans (same case as illustrated in Figure 1). **Left)** A nonenhanced T1-weighted image showing the well-demarcated lesion with gray and white matter involvement. **Center)** A T1-weighted image with gadolinium enhancement showing a minute focus of enhancement, which was not evident on the CT scan. **Right)** A T2-weighted image showing a strong signal limited to the volume noted on the T1-weighted images.

sions typically obliterate the gray-white matter junction and even show a tendency to focally infiltrate leptomeninges. Areas of cystic degeneration may be seen in large tumors. Although not as apparent on gross inspection, conglomerate calcification, either random or gyriform (Figure 3), may be identified by neuroimaging methods in up to 70% of cases.[22] Oligodendrogliomas are well vascularized, and occasionally exhibit spontaneous hemorrhage. As a rule, necrosis is limited to high-grade tumors.

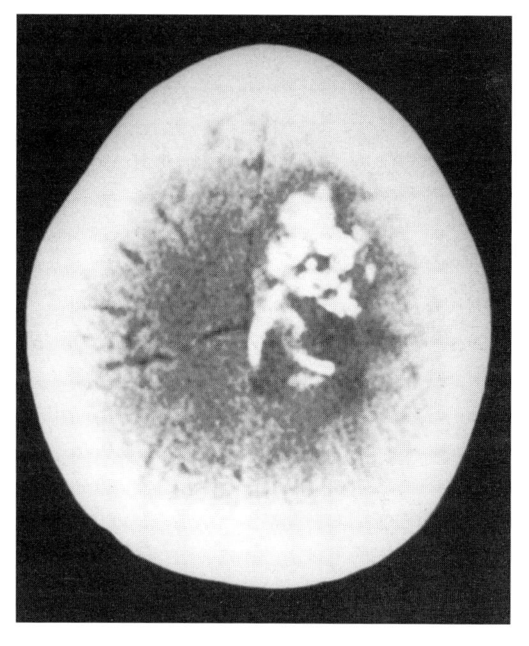

Figure 3: CT scan of an oligodendroglioma showing coarse calcifications arrayed in a gyriform pattern.

Histological Features

Although the microscopic appearance of most oligodendrogliomas is highly distinctive, such tumors may demonstrate a wide variety of histological patterns. In optimally fixed specimens, the tumor cells have scant albeit defined cytoplasm and are rather uniformly distributed, lacking cohesion, within a poorly fibrillated matrix (Figure 4). The nuclei are characteristically round and uniform. Increases in nuclear size and/or nuclear hyperchromatism are infrequently seen in tumors that have not undergone anaplastic progression. Cells are most commonly arranged in a diffuse or pseudolobulated pattern, the latter resulting from subdivision of

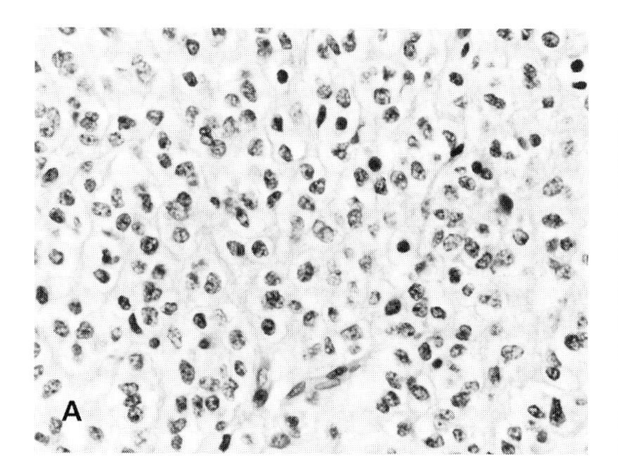

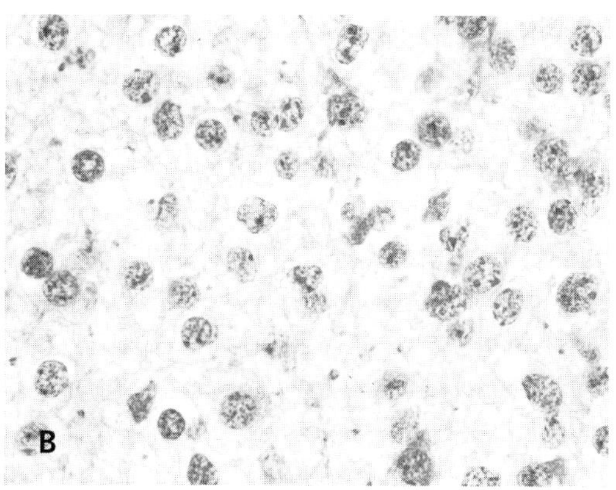

Figure 4: Photomicrographs of oligodendrogliomas. **A)** Oligodendroglioma demonstrating the commonly uniform cell population with round nuclei and conspicuous perinuclear halos, an artifact due to delayed fixation. Note that the intercellular matrix has an ill-defined quality and lacks the distinct fibrillary appearance commonly seen in these astrocytomas. **B)** Example of a grade II lesion revealing no perinuclear halos, due to prompt fixation. Note coarse chromatin and the presence of chromocenters. The background between neoplastic nuclei consists primarily of intact parenchyma rather than neoplastic cell processes. (hematoxylin-eosin)

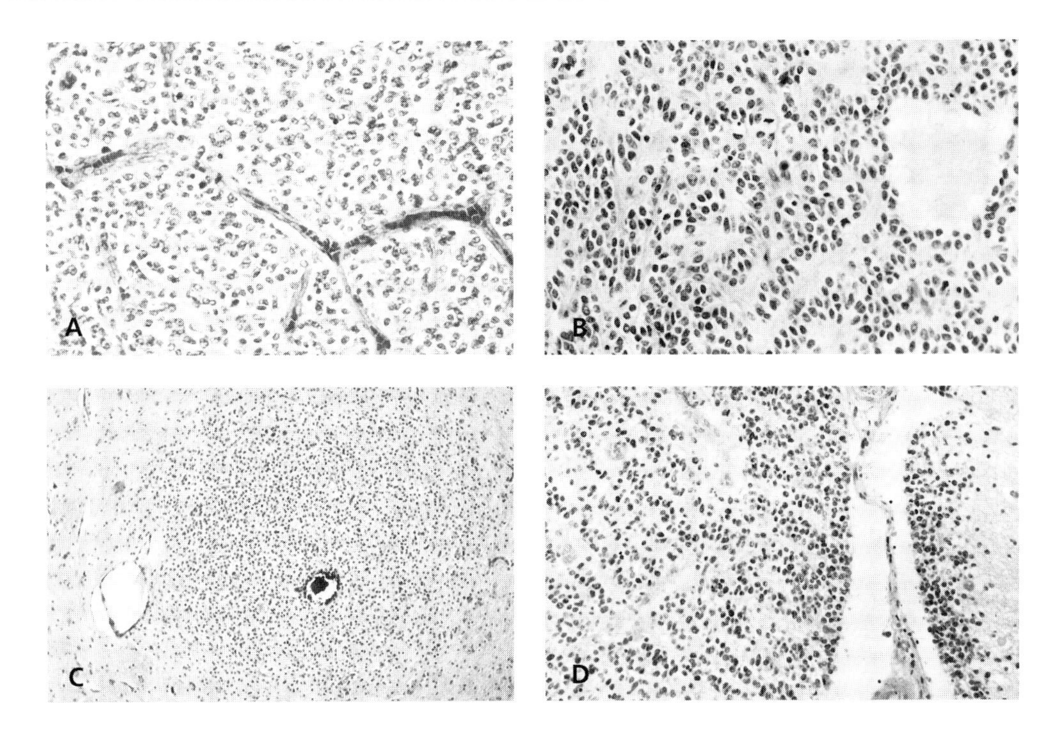

Figure 5: Oligodendrogliomas: histological patterns commonly seen in low-grade tumors. **A)** Example of the delicate arcuate vasculature. **B)** Visualization of mucin deposition and microcystic formation. **C)** Occasional nodule formations are seen in ordinary oligodendrogliomas such as this example. These tend to be patternless compared to nodules of dysembryoplastic neuroepithelial tumor. The "specific component" of the latter is also lacking. **D)** Example of parallel rows of cells arranged in palisades. Subpial accumulation of tumor cells is another characteristic feature of these tumors. (hematoxylin-eosin)

the tumor into smooth contoured groups surrounded by delicate, geometric branching vessels (Figure 5A). This highly characteristic vascular configuration is often referred to as a "chicken wire" pattern. Other cellular arrangements include: 1) sheets interrupted by numerous microcysts (Figure 5B); 2) the formation of ill-defined patternless nodules, differing from those of dysembryoplastic neuroepithelial tumor (DNT) (Figure 5C); 3) parallel rows of cells with somewhat fusiform nuclear outlines arranged in palisades (Figure 5D) mimicking those of spongioblastoma polare, a rare embryonal neuroepithelial tumor;[50] and 4) a pattern of dehiscence in which tumor cells adhere to and surround adjacent blood vessels forming somewhat papillary, perivascular pseudorosettes.

Mucin deposition, often erroneously attributed to degeneration of tumor cells, may be observed in oligodendrogliomas, particularly in low-grade examples. Such mucin with microcoalescence forms the basis of microcysts. The often complex pattern of vascularization, one in which thin-walled capillaries are lined by a single layer of endothelium, is not to be confused with endothelial proliferation. Degenerative features such as hyalinization of vessels and calcium deposition may also occur (Figure 6A). Reactive astrocytes are often found scattered throughout the tumor, preferentially around blood vessels. The cellular proliferative activity in oligodendrogliomas is not high, but mitotic figures can be observed in low numbers. Oligodendrogliomas often diffusely infiltrate the cerebral cortex with a characteristic pattern of perineuronal satellitosis (Figure 6B). Leptomeningeal infiltration, although not common, is a well known feature of oligodendrogliomas; when extensive, the process may mimic meningioma on neuroimaging studies. An accompanying desmoplastic reaction is occasionally seen, one that produces histological resemblance to metastatic carcinoma.[47]

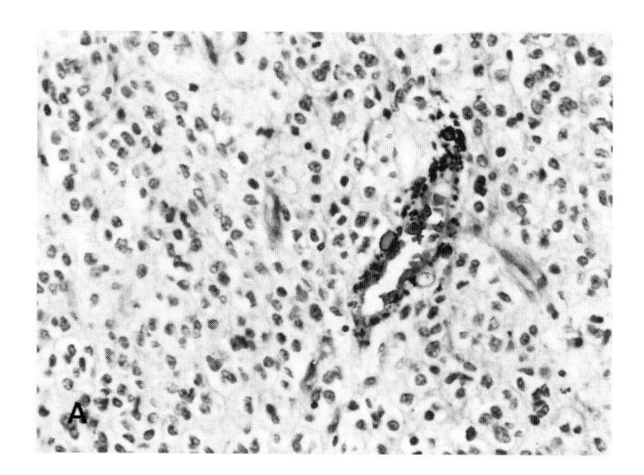
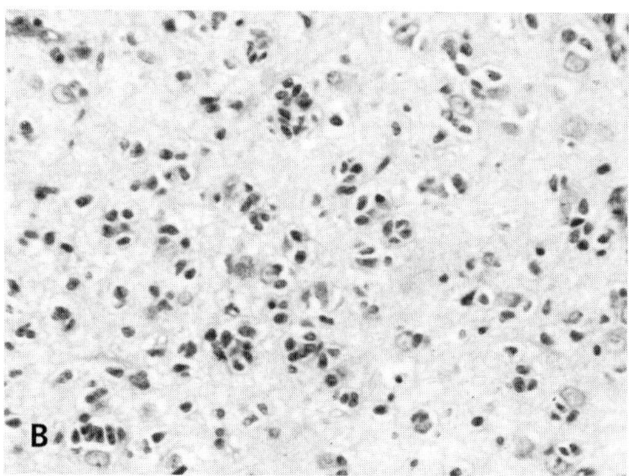

Figure 6: Oligodendrogliomas: common findings. **A)** Calcification can be seen in the vessel walls. **B)** Example of diffuse infiltration of the cerebral cortex with perineuronal satellitosis. (hematoxylin-eosin)

Cytological Considerations

Smear preparations are characterized by cellular uniformity (Figure 7). Tumor cells possess a small skirt of defined cytoplasm and, lacking cohesion, are randomly distributed in an eosinophilic matrix composed of residual parenchyma. Nuclei are typically round with a delicate particulate chromatin pattern. Nucleoli and multiple chromatin nodes may be more readily observed than in astrocytomas. The absence of a conspicuous fibrillary matrix of neoplastic cell processes serves to distinguish oligodendrogliomas from astrocytomas, as does the presence of an often conspicuous, delicate geometric microvasculature. Calcifications may be detected and, in some instances, interfere with making a satisfactory smear.

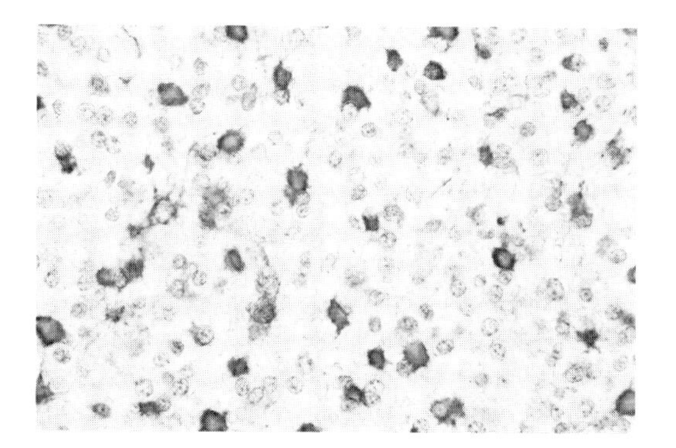

Figure 7: Smear preparation of an oligodendroglioma demonstrating uniform nuclei with relatively inapparent cytoplasm. Note the somewhat coarse chromatin and chromocenters. Also note the presence of a reactive astrocyte with a large nucleus, more open chromatin, relatively abundant cytoplasm, and radiating elongate cytoplasmic processes. (Morris stain)

Immunohistochemical Features

The identification of oligodendrogliomas has been largely based upon recognition of a few salient morphological features. Until the present, no specific immunocytochemical marker of neoplastic oligodendrocytes has been available for the purpose of diagnosis and tumor classification. The majority of proteins and other antigenic markers that are expressed by developing and mature oligodendrocytes are inconstantly exhibited by neoplastic oligodendrocytes and are unsatisfactory for characterizing oligodendrogliomas.[26,40] Among others, such antigens have included myelin basic protein (MBP) and proteolipid protein, major components of CNS myelin.[30] Although there are reports of MBP immunoreactivity in neoplastic oligodendrocytes,[14] the results of such investigations are quite variable;[39] furthermore, MBP immunoreactivity has also been detected in neoplastic astrocytes.[14] Myelin-associated glycoprotein, a protein present in normal myelin in smaller amounts than MBP, has been demonstrated in a limited number of oligodendrogliomas.[43] Conflicting results have also been reported in studies analyzing the expression of galactocerebroside (GalC), believed to be an oligodendrocyte-specific lipid.[41] Whereas Kennedy et al[26] were unable to demonstrate GalC expression in a study of seven oligodendrogliomas and four mixed oligoastrocytomas, de la Monte[10] described immunoreactivity in 27 of 28 oligodendrocytic tumors. It is notable that, in all mixed oligoastrocytomas in the latter series, GalC immunoreactivity was observed in both the oligodendrocytes and astrocytes. Kennedy et al reported similar results from cultured astrocytomas in which variable numbers of cells showed GalC immunoreactivity.

The monclonal antibody Leu-7 (also designated HNK-1), a marker for natural killer cells,[1] identifies a carbohydrate epitope associated with myelin.[34,49] Its presence has been demonstrated by immunochemical methods in the majority of oligodendrogliomas.[43] Unfortunately, this surface antigen is not reliable in discriminating between oligodendrogliomas and other gliomas, both astrocytic and ependymal.[43]

The expression of intermediate filaments in neoplastic glial cells serves to discriminate between the different gliomas. Vimentin, an intermediate filament protein with a relatively wide cellular distribution, is not expressed in the majority of oligodendrogliomas;[23] however, it is expressed in normal and neoplastic astrocytes and in ependymal cells, a property useful in discriminating between oligodendrogliomas and astrocytomas or ependymomas. Anaplastic oligodendrogliomas, on the other hand, are more likely to show vimentin expression.[9]

Neoplastic oligodendrocytes with a varying quantity of eccentric cytoplasm, ranging from the so-called "gliofibrillary oligodendrocytes" to full-bodied "mini-gemistocytes,"[21,27,58] commonly show intense glial fibrillary acidic protein (GFAP) immunoreactivity (Figure 8).[27,28] Such cells are present in a significant proportion of oligodendrogliomas.[21,39] Ultrastructurally, gliofibrillary oligodendrocytes and mini-gemistocytes contain skeins or whorls of intermediate filaments within their cytoplasm, a pattern differing from the random distribution of short intermediate filaments noted in classic gemistocytes in astrocytic tumors.[27] Tumors containing gliofibrillary and mini-gemistocytic cells are considered oligodendrogliomas. As such, they must be distinguished from true mixed oligodendroglioma-astrocytomas, lesions with a less favorable prognosis.[28] The latter, also termed "oligoastrocytomas," contain ordinary fibrillary or gemistocytic astrocytes.

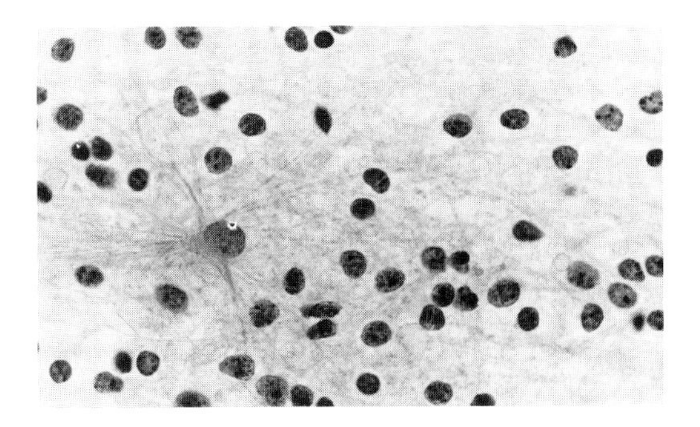

Figure 8: GFAP preparation demonstrating the presence of gliofibrillary oligodendrocytes in oligodendroglioma. Such cells possess a small quantity of fibril-containing cytoplasm which is immunoreactive. Note many of the cells lack GFAP staining. (GFAP-ABC immunoperoxidase with hematoxylin counterstain)

The occurrence of GFAP immunoreactivity in neoplastic oligodendrogliomas, a reflection of glial filament production, appears to recapitulate the transient expression of GFAP seen in immature oligodendrocytes prior to normal myelinogenesis.[7] The histogenesis of tumors containing GFAP-positive cells is not yet clear. One theory suggests that they represent a group of oligodendrogliomas in which the neoplastic counterparts of the rat optic nerve O-2A progenitor cells persist and develop into GFAP-immunoreactive lineages (type-2 astrocytes). In the rat experimental model, an epitope defined by antibody A2B5 distinguishes the O-2A progenitor cells from differentiated glial lineages, including oligodendroglia.[44] Recently, A2B5-immunoreactive cells were detected in oligodendrogliomas and in oligoastrocytomas, associated with both astrocytic and oligodendroglial elements.[3,10] These findings suggest that neoplastic GFAP-immunoreactive oligodendrocytes may originate from an O-2A-like progenitor cell population that is present in both pure and mixed oligodendrogliomas. In our experience, however, A2B5 is also expressed in low-grade astrocytomas that do not have an oligodendroglial component. Another possible explanation for GFAP immunoreactivity in

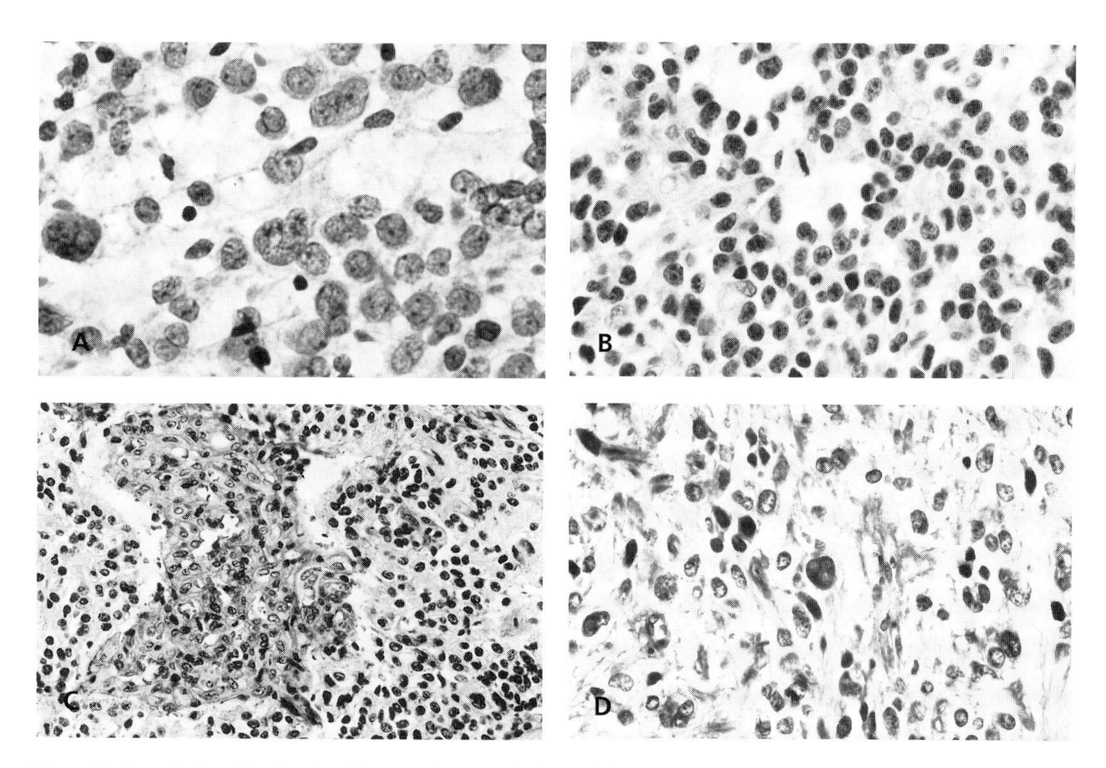

Figure 9: Anaplastic oligodendrogliomas: characteristics and histological features. **A and B)** Characteristics include hypercellularity, cellular pleomorphism, mitotic figures (A), and endothelial proliferation (B). **C)** The generally round nuclei of the well-differentiated lesion are retained and demonstrated in this smear preparation. The nuclear pleomorphism and high cell density suggest a high-grade neoplasm. **D)** Example of a grade III lesion showing not only ample mitotic activity but also considerable nuclear pleomorphism. Note the acquisition of small quantities of cytoplasm, a feature not uncommon in high-grade lesions. (hematoxylin-eosin [A, B, & D]; Morris stain [C])

oligodendrogliomas is that it represents cross-reactivity with common polypeptide sequences of cytokeratins.[25]

Anaplastic Progression

As in the case of other gliomas, both astrocytic and ependymal, oligodendrogliomas exhibit a spectrum of differentiation. Most are well differentiated, although a subset behaves aggressively and follows a clinical course similar to that of the malignant astrocytomas.[5] Only a minority of oligodendrogliomas are anaplastic, with a 3.5% incidence among new malignant gliomas in one series.[5] Such tumors either evolve from low-grade oligodendrogliomas by a process of anaplastic transformation or appear de novo. Anaplastic oligodendrogliomas are characterized by histopathological features similar to those accompanying anaplasia in diffusely infiltrating astrocytomas, including high cellularity, nuclear atypia and pleomorphism, brisk mitotic activity, endothelial proliferation, and necrosis (Figure 9).[4,38,52] It is of note that GFAP-positive cells often increase in number with anaplastic progression.[21,28] Not only is there is no widely accepted grading system for oligodendrogliomas but, at present, there is also no consensus as to what features constitute the most significant morphological criteria that indicate anaplasia. Some authors recognize more conventional parameters such as mitotic activity and necrosis to be the most important prognostic indicators.[4] Deoxyribonucleic (DNA) flow cytometric studies have demonstrated that, although ploidy per se is of little value in predicting the biological behavior of oligodendrogliomas,[8,29] proliferative activity assessed by S-phase fraction appears to be strongly associated with survival time.[8]

CYTOGENETIC ALTERATIONS IN OLIGODENDROCYTIC TUMORS

Chromosomal abnormalities and loss of heterozygosity have been observed in a variety of brain tumors. Although cytogenetic and molecular genetic data for astrocytic tumors of all subtypes and grades are relatively abundant, few reports of oncogene activation, loss of heterozygosity of specific chromosomal regions, or inactivation of tumor suppressor genes have been described in oligodendrogliomas.

The incidence of point mutations of the p53 tumor suppression gene in oligodendrogliomas appears to be similar to that reported in other types of human cancers,[19] but is much lower than in astrocytic tumors, where the figure is 30%, regardless of tumor grade.[16,17,33] Ohgaki et al[42] reported finding p53 missense mutations in two of 17 oligodendrogliomas. Mutations and allelic loss on chromosome 10 have been associated with gliomas with more aggressive biological behavior such as glioblastomas and some anaplastic astrocytomas.[17,18,56] Indeed, allelic losses on chromosome 10 were detected in one well-differentiated oligodendroglioma, which shortly thereafter progressed to a more aggressive tumor.[61] Thus, the finding of chromosome 10 deletion may be of clinical significance, serving to identify potentially aggressive oligodendrogliomas.

Genetic abnormalities other than those affecting the p53 gene and chromosome 10 have also been observed in oligodendrogliomas. Allelic deletions have been demonstrated on chromosome 19 (19q) in a large number of oligodendrogliomas.[24,45,55] Actually, loss of chromosome 19 has also been reported in astrocytomas and mixed oligoastrocytomas, a finding suggesting that a tumor suppressor gene on chromosome 19q may be associated with such tumors.[55] Other reported alterations include abnormalities on chromosomes 1 and Y in two series of oligodendrogliomas,[24,45] as well as chromosome 22 deletions in three examples and complete loss of chromosome 22 in one.[53]

GROWTH FACTORS IN OLIGODENDROCYTIC TUMORS

The biological effects of growth factors and cytokines on glial cells is a topic of active investigation in a variety of experimental systems. In the rat O-2A culture model, studies have demonstrated that specific growth factors can either induce or preserve various proliferative differentiated states. A fundamental concept with respect to oligodendroglial differentiation is that the effect and requirement of a particular growth factor is entirely dependent on the cell type and level of differentiation.[20] Oligodendroglial differentiation from a proliferative O-2A progenitor cell pool occurs in the presence of platelet-derived growth factor (PDGF) after a transient mitotic response. Multiple growth factors significantly modify both the type and degree of cellular reaction such that, in the presence of both PDGF and basic fibroblast growth factor, the O-2A progenitors can be maintained in a proliferative state and do not undergo terminal oligodendroglial differentiation.[20,35] Transforming growth factor-β also appears to play a key integrative role with respect to other factors, acting in both autocrine or paracrine modes.[35] In addition, insulin-like growth factor 1 (IGF-1) promotes the proliferation of oligodendrocyte precursors and induces immature glial precursors to develop into oligodendrocytes.[36] Regardless of which specific factors may evoke a putative effect in vitro or in vivo, the most important concept is that the influence of growth factors and cytokines on oligodendroglial biology is complex and ranges from effects on cell proliferation and motility to differentiation and the onset of programmed cell death.

Several lines of evidence support the hypothesis that aberrant growth factor production and/or altered responses to them may be involved in the development and progression of glial neoplasms. Most of the wide variety of human nervous system tumors in which abnormal expression of growth factors and/or their receptors have been described are gliomas.[48] Epidermal growth factor receptor (EGFR), a protein that represents the cellular homolog of the viral oncogene *erb* B,[13] is expressed in low levels in about 40% of oligodendrogliomas, independent of histological grade.[12] Since EGFR gene amplification has been found at an advanced stage in astrocytomas, it appears to be associated with progression rather than glioma formation.[2,31,54,59,62] Oligodendrogliomas, however, appear to behave differently from astrocytic tumors of diffuse or fibrillary type, particularly glioblastomas, with regard to EGFR gene amplification or overexpression. The few cases of oligodendrogliomas (grade II, World Health Organization classification) and anaplastic oligodendrogliomas (grades III and IV) studied to date have lacked EGFR gene amplification.[2,54]

Differential Diagnosis

The differential diagnosis of oligodendroglioma includes both reactive and a variety of neoplastic lesions. Well-differentiated oligodendroglioma must be distinguished from normal gray matter in which as many as six to eight oligodendroglial cells may surround neurons and from white matter in which oligodendroglial cells may be seen aligned between fiber tracks or aggregated around vessels. Such cells are small, uniform, and somewhat hyperchromatic, and exhibit delicate chromatin. Attention to neuroimaging studies is of importance in that such normal variation in the distribution of oligodendrocytes is unaccompanied by CT or MRI abnormalities.

Lobectomy specimens performed for intractable seizures not infrequently show "oligodendrogliosis." In such instances, white matter appears to be condensed with resultant crowding of oligodendroglial nuclei. Accompanying astrogliosis further contributes to this misleading cellularity. Atypia is lacking.

Distinguishing well-differentiated oligodendroglioma from simple gliosis is most readily done on smear preparations. These show normal oligodendrocytes to possess little discernible cytoplasm whereas active astrocytes typically have more open chromatin, ample cytoplasm, and symmetrical, radiating as well as tapering progress.

Demyelinating disease, particularly in small specimens showing artifacts of freezing, may closely resemble oligodendroglioma. Again, smear preparations most readily permit the identification of histiocytes with their moderately abundant vacuolated cytoplasm and accompanying reactive astrocytes. Stains for myelin, coupled with the periodic acid-Schiff reaction, readily permit the identification of myelin loss and infiltrating macrophages. The latter often lie clustered about vessels in association with lymphocytes. Immunostains for macrophage markers such as KP-1 or HAM-56 also facilitate the identification of macrophages, an uncommon feature in gliomas.

Freezing artifacts create a problem in recognizing oligodendroglioma because the hyperchromasia and nuclear irregularity induced by freezing often alter their characteristic morphology. Perinuclear halos, an artifact of delayed fixation, are less apparent in previously frozen tissue and nuclei become hyperchromatic and irregular. The result is an appearance resembling astrocytoma. Freezing effects are as much a problem in high-grade as in low-grade oligodendrogliomas. Because high-grade examples not infrequently show the acquisition of astrocytic features, the prognostically important recognition of an oligodendroglial component may be obscured. As previously noted, it is our philosophy that the term "glioblastoma" should not be applied to high-grade (grade IV) oligodendrogliomas, since the prognosis of such tumors is more favorable than that of grade IV astrocytomas (glioblastomas), which are by definition astrocytic in nature.

Cortical infiltration and nuclear regularity, even the finding of spherical nuclei, may be seen in gliomatosis cerebri, a process far more widespread than most oligodendrogliomas, and one associated with a poorer prognosis. Awareness of the neuroimaging features in such cells should aid in their distinction.

Pilocytic astrocytoma, particularly appearing in the cerebellum ("cerebellar astrocytoma"), often contain small foci of oligodendrocyte-like cells. The prognosis of such lesions does not appear to differ from that of pilocytic astrocytoma.

Of particular importance is the distinction of oligodendroglioma from DNT. The latter has become a well-recognized although uncommon lesion, occurring in young patients with intractable partial complex seizures. It is largely limited to the cerebral cortex, frequently at the temporoparietal region, and consists of: 1) nodules of oligodendrocyte-like cells, often arrayed in complex patterns; 2) a diffuse increase in oligodendrocyte-like cells accompanied by accumulation of intercellular mucin, which mature or occasionally dysmorphic neurons appear to "float"; and 3) disorganization of surrounding cerebral cortex (cortical dysplasia). The highly characteristic architectural complex nodules vary considerably in morphology, a minority being composed of astrocytic cells with pilocytic features. Unlike oligodendrogliomas, the neurons within DNTs do not display neuronal satellitosis. The stereotypical features of this lesion aid in the recognition of DNT, which usually poses little problem in distinction from conventional oligodendroglioma, particularly in large representative specimens.

Ependymomas, particularly those of the "clear cell type," may also be mistaken for oligodendroglioma. The presence of perivascular pseudorosettes may aid in their identification. Their distinction from oligodendroglioma is also made easier by attention to neuroimaging data, since ependymomas are typically paraventricular, sharply circumscribed, and contrast-enhancing, both on CT and MRI. Nonetheless, in a small biopsy, electron microscopy may be required to distinguish the two lesions.

Central neurocytoma also mimics oligodendroglioma. Unlike oligodendroglioma, however, this lesion is intraventricular in location and usually attached to the septum pellucidum. The finding of cellular "clearing," arborizing vasculature, and not infrequent calcification further contributes to confusion. The unique location of neurocytoma, coupled with its immunohistochemical reactivity for synaptophysin and lack of S100 protein and GFAP staining, readily permits its identification: electron microscopy showing microtubule-containing processes, clear vesicles, secretory granules, and in some cases synapses, also distinguished neurocytomas. Similar nuclear regularity may be noted in the neuroblastic variant of medulloblastoma and in some cerebral neuroblastomas.

High-grade oligodendroglioma may also simulate metastatic carcinoma. Unlike the latter, which is solid and sharply demarcated, oligodendrogliomas infiltrate parenchyma and show gradual transition to normal tissue at their periphery. Although immunohistochemical studies usually readily permit their distinction, caution is recommended since high-grade oligodendroglioma frequently exhibits some astrocytic differentiation. Such glial fibril-containing cytoplasm may show a misleading cross-reactivity with ordinary antibodies to cytokeratin. On the other hand, stains for low-molecular-weight cytokeratin are negative in high-grade oligodendroglioma and astrocytomas and are therefore more reliable in permitting their distinction from metastatic carcinoma. Oligodendrogliomas also lack epithelial membrane antigen staining. Lastly, unlike most carcinomas, oligodendrogliomas are reactive to S100 protein (Figure 10), a rather uncommon feature of carcinomas.

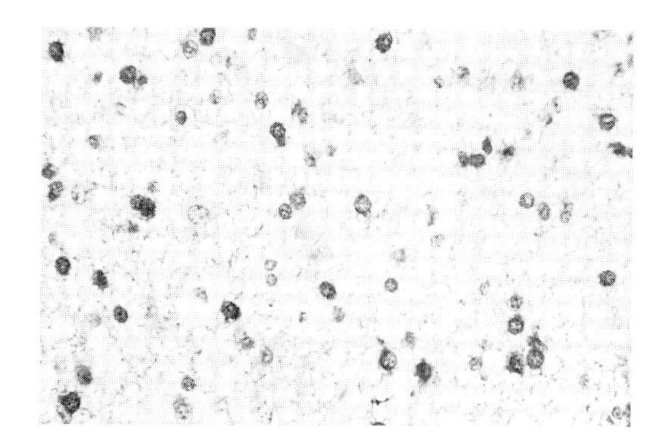

Figure 10: Oligodendroglioma: S-100 protein immunohistochemistry showing primarily nuclear staining typical but not diagnostic of oligodendrocytes. (S-100-ABC immunoperoxidase with hematoxylin counterstain)

References

1. Abo T, Balch CM: Differentiation antigen of human NK and K cells identified by a monoclonal antibody (HNK-1). **J Immunol 127:**1024-1029, 1981
2. Ahmed Rasheed BK, McLendon RE, Herndon JE, et al: Alterations of the *TP53* gene in human gliomas. **Cancer Res 54:**1324-1330, 1994
3. Bishop M, de la Monte SM: Dual lineage of astrocytomas. **Am J Pathol 135:**517-527, 1989
4. Burger PC: The grading of astrocytomas and oligodendrogliomas, in Fields WS (ed): **Primary Brain Tumors. A Review of Histologic Classification.** New York: Springer-Verlag, 1989, pp 171-180
5. Cairncross JG, Macdonald DR, Ramsay DA: Aggres-

sive oligodendroglioma: a chemosensitive tumor. **Neurosurgery 31:** 78-82, 1992
6. Cameron RS, Rakic P: Glial cell lineage in the cerebral cortex: a review and synthesis. **Glia 4:**124-137, 1991
7. Choi BH, Kim RC: Expression of glial fibrillary acidic protein in immature oligodendroglia. **Science 223:**407-408, 1984
8. Coons SW, Johnson PC, Pearl DK, et al: Prognostic significance of flow cytometry deoxyribonucleic acid analysis of human oligodendrogliomas. **Neurosurgery 34:**680-687, 1994
9. Cruz-Sanchez FF, Haustein J, Rossie ML, et al: Ependymoblastoma: a histological, immunohistochemical and ultrastructural study of five cases. **Histopathology 12:**17-27, 1988
10. de la Monte SM: Uniform lineage of oligodendrogliomas. **Am J Pathol 135:**529-540, 1989
11. de los Monteros AE, Zhang MS, de Vellis J: O-2A progenitor cells transplanted into the neonatal rat brain develop into oligodendrocytes but not astrocytes. **Proc Natl Acad Sci USA 90:**50-54, 1993
12. Di Carlo A, Mariano A, Macchia PE, et al: Epidermal growth factor receptor in human brain tumors. **J Endocrinol Invest 15:**31-37, 1992
13. Downward J, Yarden Y, Mayes E, et al: Close similarity of epidermal growth factor receptor and the v-*erb*-B oncogene protein sequences. **Nature 307:**521-527, 1984
14. Figols J, Iglesias-Rozas JR, Kazner E: Myelin basic protein (MBP) in human gliomas: a study of twenty-five cases. **Clin Neuropathol 4:**116-120, 1985
15. Fortuna A, Celli P, Palma L: Oligodendrogliomas of the spinal cord. **Acta Neurochir 52:**305-329, 1980
16. Frankel R H, Bayona W, Koslow M, et al: p53 mutations in human malignant gliomas: comparison of loss of heterozygosity with mutation frequency. **Cancer Res 52:**1427-1433, 1992
17. Fults D, Brockmeyer D, Tullous MW, et al: p53 mutation and loss of heterozygosity on chromosomes 17 and 10 during human astrocytoma progression. **Cancer Res 52:**674-679, 1992
18. Fults D, Pedone CA, Thomas GA, et al: Allelotype of human malignant astrocytoma. **Cancer Res 50:**5784-5789, 1990
19. Gaidano G, Ballerini P, Gong JZ, et al: p53 mutations in human lymphoid malignancies: association with Burkitt's lymphoma and chronic lymphocytic leukemia. **Proc Natl Acad Sci USA 88:**5413-5417, 1991
20. Hart IK, Richardson WD, Bolsover SR, et al: PDGF and intracellular signaling in the timing of oligodendrocyte differentiation. **J Cell Biol 109:**3411-3417, 1989
21. Herpers MJHM, Budka H: Glial fibrillary acidic protein (GFAP) in oligodendroglial tumors: gliofibrillary oligodendroglioma and transitional oligoastrocytoma as subtypes of oligodendroglioma. **Acta Neuropathol 64:**265-272, 1984
22. Huk WJ, Gademannn G, Friedmann G: **Magnetic Resonance Imaging of the Central Nervous System Diseases.** Berlin: Springer-Verlag, 1990, p 237
23. Jagadha V, Halliday WC, Becker LE: Glial fibrillary acidic protein (GFAP) in oligodendrogliomas: a reflection of transient GFAP expression by immature oligodendroglia. **Can J Neurol Sci 13:**307-311, 1986
24. Jenkins RB, Kimmel DW, Moertel CA, et al: A cytogenetic study of 53 human gliomas. **Cancer Genet Cytogenet 39:**253-279, 1989
25. Kashima T, Tiu SN, Merrill JE, et al: Expression of oligodendrocyte-associated genes in cell lines derived from human gliomas and neuroblastomas. **Cancer Res 53:**170-175, 1993
26. Kennedy PGE, Watkins BA, Thomas DGT, et al: Antigenic expression by cells derived from human gliomas does not correlate with morphological classification. **Neuropathol Appl Neurobiol 13:** 327-347, 1987
27. Kros JM, de Jong AAW, van der Kwast TH: Ultrastructural characterization of transitional cells in oligodendrogliomas. **J Neuropathol Exp Neurol 51:**186-193, 1992
28. Kros JM, Van Eden CG, Stefanko SZ, et al: Prognostic implications of glial fibrillary acidic protein containing cell types in oligodendrogliomas. **Cancer 66:**1204-1212, 1990
29. Kros JM, van Eden CG, Vissers CJ, et al: Prognostic relevance of DNA flow cytometry in oligodendroglioma. **Cancer 69:**1791-1798, 1992
30. Less MB, Brostoff SW: Proteins of myelin, in Morell P (ed): **Myelin, 2nd ed.** New York: Plenum Press, 1984, pp 197-224
31. Libermann TA, Nusbaum HR, Razon N, et al: Amplification, enhanced expression and possible rearrangement of EGF receptor gene in primary human brain tumours of glial origin. **Nature 313:**144-147, 1985
32. Lillien LE, Raff MC: Differentiation signals in the CNS: type-2 astrocyte development *in vitro* as a model system. **Neuron 5:**111-119, 1990
33. Louis DN, von Deimling A, Chung RY, et al: Comparative study of p53 gene and protein alterations in human astrocytic tumors. **J Neuropathol Exp Neurol 52:**31-38, 1993
34. McGarry RC, Helfand SL, Quarles RH, et al: Recognition of myelin-associated glycoprotein by the monoclonal antibody HNK-1. **Nature 306:**376-378, 1983
35. McKinnon RD, Piras G, Ida JA Jr, et al: A role for TGF-β in oligodendrocyte differentiation. **J Cell Biol 121:**1397-1407, 1993
36. McMorris FA, Mozell RL, Carson MJ, et al: Regulation of oligodendrocyte development and central nervous system myelination by insulin-like growth factors. **Ann NY Acad Sci USA 692:**321-334, 1993
37. Miller RH, French-Constant C, Raff MC: The macroglial cells of the rat optic nerve. **Annu Rev Neurosci 12:**517-534, 1989
38. Mørk SJ, Lindegaard KF, Halvorsen TB, et al: Oligodendroglioma: incidence and biological behavior in a defined population. **J Neurosurg 63:**881-889, 1985
39. Nakagawa Y, Perentes E, Rubinstein LJ: Immunohistochemical characterization of oligodendrogliomas: an analysis of multiple markers. **Acta Neuropathol 72:**15-22, 1986
40. Noble M, Ataliotis P, Barnett SC, et al: Development, regeneration and neoplasia of glial cells in the

central nervous system. **Ann NY Acad Sci 633:** 35-47, 1991

41. Norton WT, Cammer W: Isolation and characterization of myelin, in Morell P (ed): **Myelin, 2nd ed.** New York: Plenum Press, 1984, 147-195
42. Ohgaki H, Eibl RH, Wiestler OD, et al: p53 mutations in nonastrocytic human brain tumors. **Cancer Res 51:**6202-6205, 1991
43. Perentes E, Rubinstein LJ: Recent applications of immunoperoxidase histochemistry in human neuro-oncology. **Arch Pathol Lab Med 111:**796-812, 1987
44. Raff MC, Miller RH, Noble M: A glial progenitor cell that develops *in vitro* into an astrocyte or an oligodendrocyte depending on culture medium. **Nature 303:**390-396, 1983
45. Ransom BR: Vertebrate glial classification, lineage, and heterogeneity. **Ann NY Acad Sci 633:**19-26, 1991
46. Ransom DT, Ritland SR, Kimmel DW, et al: Cytogenetic and loss of heterozygosity studies in ependymomas, pilocytic astrocytomas, and oligodendrogliomas. **Genes Chromosomes Cancer** 5:348-356, 1992
47. Russell DS, Rubinstein LJ: **Pathology of Tumours of the Nervous System, 5th ed.** Baltimore, Md: Williams & Wilkins, 1989, pp 172-187
48. Rutka JT, Trent JM, Rosenblum ML: Molecular probes in neuro-oncology: a review. **Cancer Invest 8:**425-438, 1990
49. Sato S, Baba H, Tanaka M, et al: Antigenic determinant shared between myelin-associated glycoprotein from human brain and natural killer cells. **Biomed Res 4:**489-494, 1983
50. Schiffer D, Cravioto H, Giordana MT, et al: Is polar spongioblastoma a tumor entity? **J Neurosurg 78:** 587-591, 1993
51. Shaw EG, Scheithauer BW, O'Fallon JR, et al: Oligodendrogliomas: the Mayo Clinic experience. **J Neurosurg** 76:428-434, 1992
52. Smith MT, Ludwig CL, Godfrey AD, et al: Grading of oligodendrogliomas. **Cancer 52:**2107-2114, 1983
53. Thiel G, Losanowa T, Kintzel D, et al: Karyotypes in 90 human gliomas. **Cancer Genet Cytogenet 58:** 109-120, 1992
54. Torp SH, Helseth E, Ryan L, et al: Amplification of the epidermal growth factor receptor gene in human gliomas. **Anticancer Res 11:**2095-2098, 1991
55. von Deimling A, Louis DN, von Ammon K, et al: Evidence for a tumor suppressor gene on chromosome 19q associated with human astrocytomas, oligodendrogliomas, and mixed gliomas. **Cancer Res 52:**4277-4279, 1992
56. Watanabe K, Nagai M, Wakai S, et al: Loss of constitutional heterozygosity in chromosome 10 in human glioblastoma. **Acta Neuropathol 80:**251-254, 1990
57. Watkins B, Bevan K, Venter D, et al: Glial cell markers in the study of CNS development and human gliomas, in Thomas DGT (ed): **Neuro-oncology. Primary Malignant Brain Tumours.** Baltimore, Md: Johns Hopkins University Press, 1990, pp 40-50
58. Wondrusch E, Huemer M, Budka H: Production of glial fibrillary acidic protein (GFAP) by neoplastic oligodendrocytes: gliofibrillary oligodendroglioma and transitional oligoastrocytoma revisited. **Brain Tumor Pathol 8:**11-15, 1991
59. Wong AJ, Bigner SH, Bigner DD, et al: Expression of the epidermal growth factor receptor gene in malignant gliomas is invariably associated with gene amplification. **Proc Natl Acad Sci USA 84:**6899-6903, 1987
60. Wren D, Wolswijk G, Noble M: *In vitro* analysis of the origin and maintenance of O-2A^{adult} progenitor cells. **J Cell Biol 116:**167-176, 1992
61. Wu JK, Folkerth RD, Ye Z, et al: Aggressive oligodendroglioma predicted by chromosome 10 restriction fragment polymorphism analysis. Case study. **J Neurooncol** 15:29-35, 1992
62. Yamazaki H, Fukui Y, Ueyama Y, et al: Amplification of the structurally and functionally altered epidermal growth factor receptor gene (c-erbB) in human brain tumors. **Mol Cell Biol 8:**1816-1820, 1988
63. Zülch KJ: **Brain Tumors. Their Biology and Pathology, 3rd ed.** New York: Springer-Verlag, 1986

CHAPTER 5

The Pathology of Benign Ependymomas

Ignacio Gonzalez-Gomez, MD, and Floyd H. Gilles, MD

Ependymomas are tumors of cells that exhibit morphological or immunophenotypic differentiation toward each or both of the two components of the ventricular wall: the ependymal cells and subependymal astroglia. This cytogenetic definition assumes the existence of embryonal precursor(s) for both cell types. However, there is no agreement whether the progenitor cell(s) should include the primitive neural tube lining cell, the ependymal spongioblast, the polar ependymoglioblast,[126] or the primitive ependymoglial cell or tanycyte.[21,30] From a practical viewpoint, whether or not the definition requires identification of a progenitor cell, these are tumors that contain differing proportions of two cell types, ependymal cells and astrocytes. The tumor, with both of its neuroglial and ependymal components, was first recognized by Virchow.[123] Nevertheless, the presence of differing proportions of ependymal cells and astroglia in individual ependymal tumors resulted in various diagnostic names in use today that reflect these different histological components, ranging from designations that emphasize the ependymal component (e.g., "ependymoma," used in the World Health Organization (WHO) classification[62]) to those that include the astroglial component (e.g., astroependymoma[92]).

In 1899, the ependymomas were set apart from the gliosarcomas (a term in common use during the last half of the 19th century[115]) by Störch,[114] who recognized that this entity was different from many other gliosarcomas because it had distinct boundaries (he thought) and might be amenable to resection. The notion that ependymomas are frequently encapsulated is still met.[28,111] Störch recognized the main histological components that we use as the diagnostic histological criteria, namely the perivascular pseudorosette, the ependymal rosette, and sheets of ependymal cells. A few years later, Mallory[70] reported three gliomas of ependymal origin. He recognized intracytoplasmic blepharoplasts (basal bodies), attributing their identification in normal ependymal cells to Weigert. Mallory emphasized the glial fiber content of these tumors, but not the perivascular pseudorosettes. Bailey[4] presented six cases of infratentorial tumors, in two of which there were solid masses of polygonal cells (sheets) with glial fibrils. Two patients had perivascular pseudorosettes and four had a tongue of tumor extending through the foramen to the arch of the atlas. He recognized blepharoplasts in both the solid and true rosette-containing portions in all six cases. He also recognized sheets, true rosettes, and perivascular pseudorosettes. Unfortunately, he castigated "foreign writers" for not quoting the American literature (e.g., Mallory's 1902 paper on tumors of ependymal origin), but failed to mention Virchow's or Störch's papers.

Ependymal Cells

Ependymal cells are low cuboidal epithelial cells that line the ventricular system or, in a few locations, are buried deep to the ventricular wall as ependymal tubules or rosettes (e.g., near the angle of the fourth ventricle or in front of the aqueduct). Virchow[123] attributed their recognition to Purkinje. The cells initially lining the ventricular cavities in the embryo are undifferentiated germinal cells that become ependymal cells during the late embryonic or fetal period. For some parts of the ventricular system (e.g., the lining epithelium overlying the germinal matrix of the ganglionic eminence of the lateral ventricle), ependymal cells do not appear until early in the second half of gestation; in other regions of the ventricular system ependymal cells differentiate at various other times. Subsequently, ependymal cells line most of the ventricular surfaces with a few major exceptions. Ependymal epithelium covers most parts of the ventricular system by the end of gestation, but some regions of the lateral ventricles either lose their ependymal cells or fail to develop them. These include portions of the occipital horn, the lateral ventricle roof in the frontal horn, and the temporal horn ventricular surface overlying sectors CA_2 of the hippocampal formation.[33] Tumors incorporating these cells may be found in any location that embryologically included a ventricle, ranging from the embryonic and fetal ventricle of the olfactory bulb of the lateral ventricle to the terminal ventricle of the filum terminale.

Many early authors recognized the intimate relationship between the subependymal astroglia and the ependymal layer lining the ventricle.[4,37,70] The subependymal astroglia cells provide a structural support for the layer of ependymal cells (without an intervening basement membrane as in the choroid plexus) and create a dense glial fibrillary network that lasts throughout life, unlike astroglia elsewhere except those in the spinal cord and brain stem. Ependymal cells and immediately subependymal cells are similar in cytoplasmic and nuclear structure and probably differ in form only because of their position.[129] In fact, the three types of normal neuroglial cells are not sharply distinct from each other except for prototype cells that differ in form and staining properties. There are many transitional forms among the three varieties. The corresponding three broad categories of glioma are not always distinct from each other.

Ependymomas

Types of Ependymoma

Ependymomas form a heterogeneous group of neuroglial tumors. According to the WHO classification, the "benign" ependymomas include the regular ependymoma, its myxopapillary variant, and the subependymoma. The regular ependymomas include the "cellular," "papillary," and "clear" cell varieties.[62] The idea of a "benign" ependymoma was supported by Fokes and Earle[29] who felt that subtentorial ependymomas were "static." The malignant forms include the anaplastic ependymoma and ependymoblastoma.[62] The ependymal rosettes in ependymoblastoma contain a multilayered epithelium in contrast to the anaplastic ependymoma rosettes.

Incidence

The incidence in different series varies from 2% to 6% of all gliomas, except for cases in Thailand, Japan, and India, where these tumors constitute a larger proportion of brain tumors (up to 13.7%).[108] Ependymomas are predominantly tumors of children and adolescents, in whom they account for 9%[22,66,79] or 11%[13] of brain tumors.* Age and gender also influence incidence and location.[108]

* Childhood Brain Tumor Consortium (CBTC). At several places we will refer to the CBTC database. The database of the CBTC contains extensive data on each of 3291 children collected from 10 North American institutions. The data include demographic, anamnestic, and operative data, WHO brain tumor diagnoses, histological feature information, and postoperative and long-term follow-up data. The data were collected independently by consortium members, reliability was measured, and rates, proportions, and survival probabilities were provided by the CBTC data analysis team. Many of these data are unpublished.

Tumor Location

Ependymomas potentially arise near any part of the ventricular system. The exceptional development of ependymomas and ependymoblastomas apparently unrelated to either a ventricular cavity or the spinal canal presumably results from the neoplastic transformation of ectopic ependymal elements.[98] More than two-thirds of cases occur below the tentorium, with the fourth ventricle being the most common site;[79] however, in India there is no difference between the rates of supratentorial and infratentorial ependymomas and in Japan supratentorial ependymomas are more common.[108] In the above reports, the majority of intracranial ependymomas occurred in children, whereas most intraspinal tumors were in adults. The intraspinal ependymomas were equally divided between medullary and cauda equina locations. The lumbosacral segments were most frequently involved. The rate of spinal ependymomas is much smaller in children.[22] Multiple intramedullary spinal ependymomas and ependymomas associated with syringomyelia are notably associated with von Recklinghausen's neurofibromatosis.[47] Kernohan et al[56] believed that a disproportionate number occurred in the cerebellopontine angle. Prevalence varies by anatomical location. About one-half of spinal cord tumors are ependymomas,[57,111] but in children they represent only about 20%.[13] Two-thirds of tumors in the cauda equina are ependymomas.[55] While rare, ependymomas of the filum terminale have been reported in children.[8,32]

The distributions of tumors at the cervicomedullary junction differ significantly from those that occupy only the spinal or the infratentorial compartment.[34] Ependymoma is a childhood brain tumor likely to occupy more than one compartment at the time of presentation. Children with multicompartmental ependymomas (i.e., those occupying two or three compartments at presentation) differ clinically and pathologically from children whose tumor is confined to one compartment. In the CBTC population, 30% of all ependymal tumors occupied two or more compartments at the time of presentation.

Ependymomas are one of the few neuroglial tumors to occur elsewhere in the body. They have been found in a subcutaneous sacral location,[4] the ovary,[40] soft tissue,[59] lung,[17] sacrococcygeal location associated with a glomus,[72] mediastinum,[84] and a sacrococcygeal extradural location in the curve of the sacrum.[65]

Macroscopic Appearance

The macroscopic appearance of the ependymomas varies considerably. The tumors protruding into the ventricular cavity or through the foramen of Luschka into the cerebellopontine angle are lobulated and soft, and exhibit a smooth surface. Those located in the parenchyma are usually well defined at one margin. They are homogeneous, gray, and granular, and large tumors may be focally or extensively cystic or contain scattered small calcifications. In the CBTC database, ependymomas were of several colors (gray/white, purple/red, or yellow/tan). They were firm or soft, vascular, or friable. About one-fifth were cystic and about the same proportion had well-defined margins. In other words, there were no distinctive gross characteristics that would separate these tumors from other glial tumors with certainty (Table 1). Although not encapsulated, ependymomas are often well circumscribed in older populations.[111,114] Tumors in the fourth ventricle, which may arise either from the roof or from the floor, often enlarge to obliterate the ventricular lumen. They tend to extend laterally into the cerebellopontine angle or through the foramen magnum, forming smooth, firm, nodular masses, sometimes containing foci of calcification that surround and compress the dorsal and lateral aspects of the medulla and upper cervical segments. All three of these extensions were present in the first case described in 1864 by Virchow.[123pp130–135] This characteristic form of growth was called "plastic ependymoma" by Courville and Broussalian.[16] Ependymomas are rarely pedunculated.[122]

Microscopic Description

Ependymomas characteristically contain epithelial (ependymal), glial, and occasionally oligodendroglial-like components; rarely, a melanotic component[93] or melanin pigment[76,132] and

TABLE 1

SURGICAL APPEARANCE OF EPENDYMOMAS IN THE CBTC DATABASE (% OF CASES)

Finding	Ependymoma	Myxopapillary	Papillary	Anaplastic	Subependymoma
Cystic	22	17	22	22	0
Gray/white	43	17	44	40	50
Firm	16	0	0	16	17
Soft	26	8	56	21	17
Well-defined margins	18	25	11	14	17
Purple/red	35	67	44	25	17
Calcified	3	0	0	4	17
Yellow/tan	23	8	11	21	0
Vascular	24	33	44	23	0
Friable	13	33	22	7	0

mesenchymal elements such as cartilage, bone, or rhabdomyosarcomatous or paragangliomatous components are present, constituting a small part of the tumor.[8,75,120] The proportions of the first three components and the cellularity of a given tumor vary from case to case, vary in tumors located within different compartments (Table 2), and vary within the same tumor. Consequently, diagnosis rests on the identification of each of the components and their histological patterns of growth.

The histopathological examination reveals distinctive features involving mostly the epithelial component that recapitulates the normal ependyma. These features are seen both at structural (histological) and cellular (cytological) organizational levels. They include: ependymal rosettes, perivascular pseudorosettes, ependymal surfaces, tubules and/or clefts, papillae, ependymal sheets, and clear cells. The true rosettes or ependymal tubules contain cilia that are seen in the lumina of the tubules and blepharoplasts, in the apical portion of these cells. In compact cellular areas, blepharoplasts are present in juxtanuclear positions. Blepharoplasts are not present in the cells forming perivascular pseudorosettes. Typically, neoplastic ependymal cells lie on a fibrillated glial pad. Any combination of features may be seen, particularly in ependymomas in the pediatric population. Sometimes fresh or old hemorrhage is present.[26,74]

Ependymal rosettes or true rosettes (Figure 1A and B), while characteristic of ependymomas, are found only in a small proportion (which varies between compartments) of cases. They consist of closely packed and radially oriented polygonal cells with distinctive cell boundaries. Their apical cytoplasms define a central lumen, with their nuclei usually distant from it. Ependymal rosettes may be complexly arranged with multiple layers of tumor cells ("ependymoblastic") (Figure 1C) or they may be made up of a single layer or two of tumor cells forming a small lumen (Figure 1A and B). In the CBTC database, they were present in 13% of supratentorial tumors, 38% of infratentorial tumors, and 22% of spinal ependymomas (Table 2). Even when present, areas with ependymal rosettes may be exceedingly sparse. Occasionally, ependymomas exhibit ependymal surfaces, clefts, and cavities of varying size lined by tall columnar epithelium (Figure 2). These tumor cells are not ciliated and blepharoplasts are located between the nucleus and the base of the cell.

Perivascular pseudorosettes (a term coined by Bailey and Cushing[5]) (Figure 3), although not restricted to ependymomas, are present in the majority of cases (in the CBTC database, in 67% of ependymomas in the supratentorial compartment, 87% of those in the infratentorial compartment, and 61% of those in the spinal compartment). They are readily identified as an eosinophilic nucleus-free zone around a central vascular core surrounded by a collar or crown of neoplastic nuclei. Radially arranged tapering

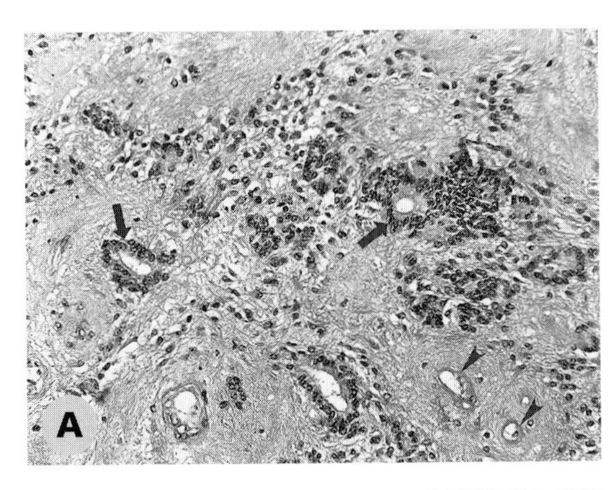

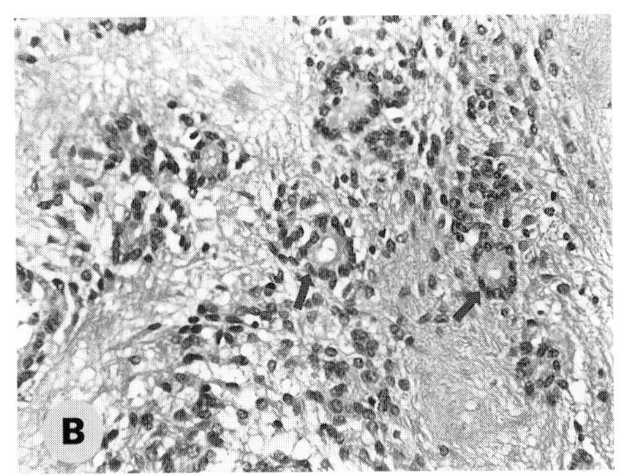

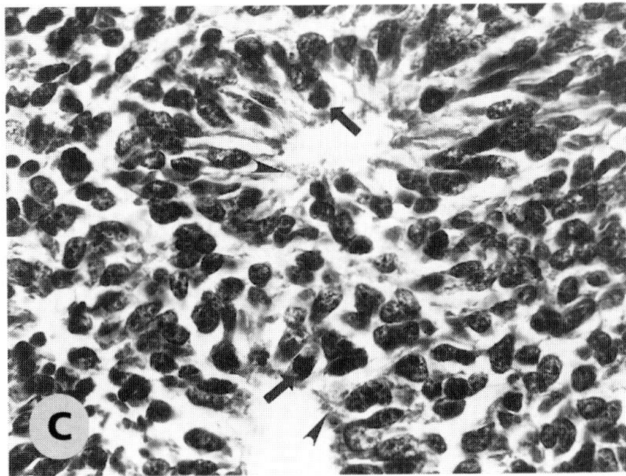

Figure 1: A) Focal areas containing ependymal rosettes *(arrows)* in otherwise typical ependymomatous areas with perivascular pseudorosettes *(arrowheads).* **B)** Ependymal rosettes (true rosettes) consisting of radially arranged tumor cells with cytoplasm forming a central lumen *(arrows)* and nuclei displaced peripherally. **C)** Ependymoblastic rosettes. There is a multilayered arrangement of tumor cells around a central lumen. Blepharoplasts are seen as granular material lining the lumen *(arrowheads).* Note the mitotic figures in the apical portions *(arrows).* (hematoxylin-eosin, original magnification × 10 [A], × 20 [B], × 40 [C])

fibrillated cytoplasmic processes of tumor cells attached to the connective tissue of the vascular wall form an eosinophilic nucleus-free zone with nuclei located distally in a collar. Homer Wright rosettes or rosettes of nuclei surrounding a central region containing a tangle of fibrils, while thought diagnostic of medulloblastoma by some, also occur in ependymomas.[35,52]

Some tumors exhibit wide cellular areas or sheets of ependymal cells (Figure 4) composed of uniform epithelial-appearing ependymal cells with little intervening glial fibrillary stroma. Sheets of ependymal cells occur with similar prevalence in all three compartments. In the CBTC database, these sheets were present in 54% of supratentorial, 68% of infratentorial, and 67% of spinal ependymomas (Table 2). Necrosis is far more common in cranial than in spinal ependymomas, and mitosis occurs much more frequently in the supratentorial than in the infratentorial compartment. A fine, delicate fibrillary stroma is common in all three locations, and astrocytes occur in significant proportions in all three compartments.

The nuclei of neoplastic ependymal cells are distinctly uniform in size, oval or round, and pale-staining, with one or more nucleoli. These nuclear characteristics change in anaplastic

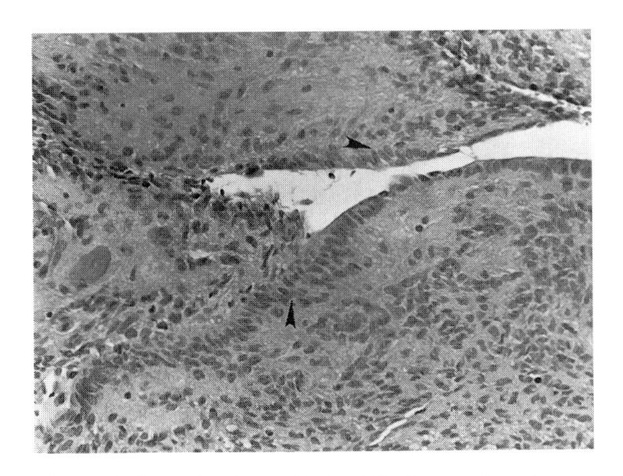

Figure 2: Neoplastic multistratified ependymal surface lining a hypocellular area *(arrowheads).* In some cases, ependymal surfaces, clefts, and tubules are conspicuous. (hematoxylin-eosin, original magnification × 4)

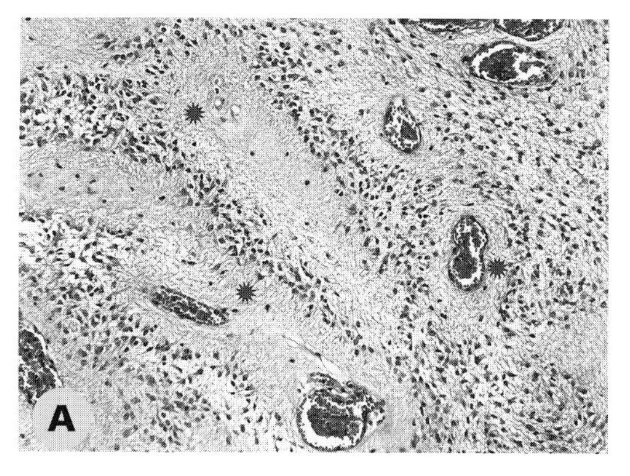

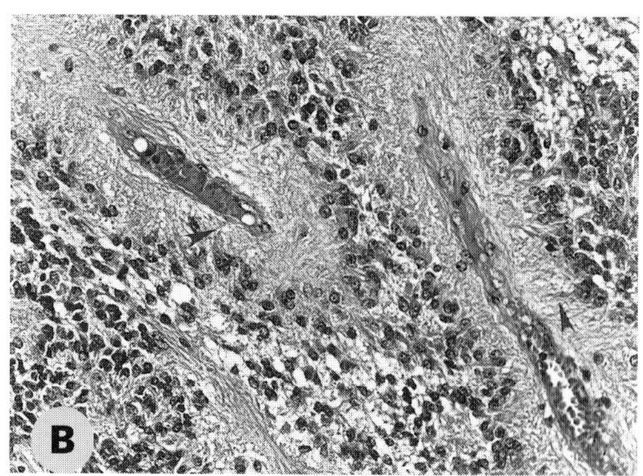

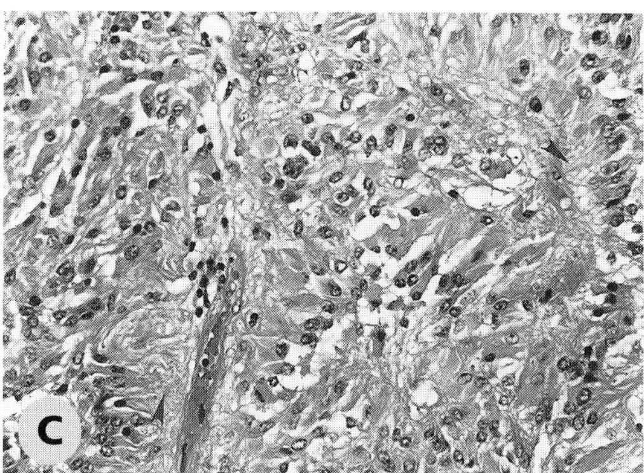

Figure 3: A) Perivascular pseudorosettes are prominent in ependymoma and are easily distinguished as perivascular nucleus-free zones. The vascular core ranges from a capillary to large ectatic vessels. **B)** Ependymoma with perivascular pseudorosettes. The neoplastic cells have a peripherally displaced nuclei and tapering fibrillary cytoplasmic processes extending to the vascular adventitial connective tissue *(arrowheads).* **C)** Occasionally the cells forming the perivascular pseudorosette are large; however, the nuclei are fairly uniform with little pleomorphism. (hematoxylin-eosin, original magnification × 10 [A], × 20 [B and C])

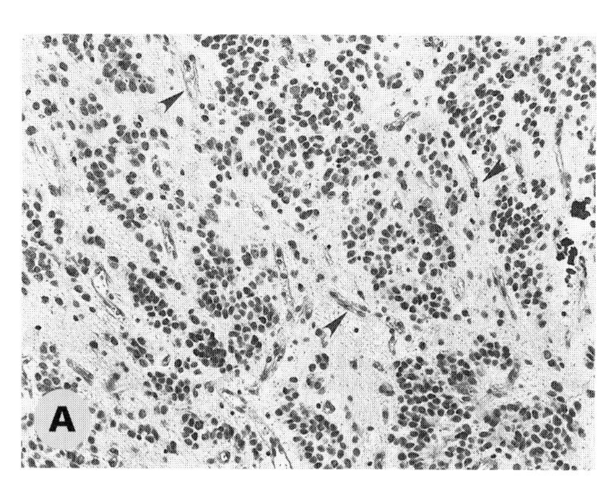

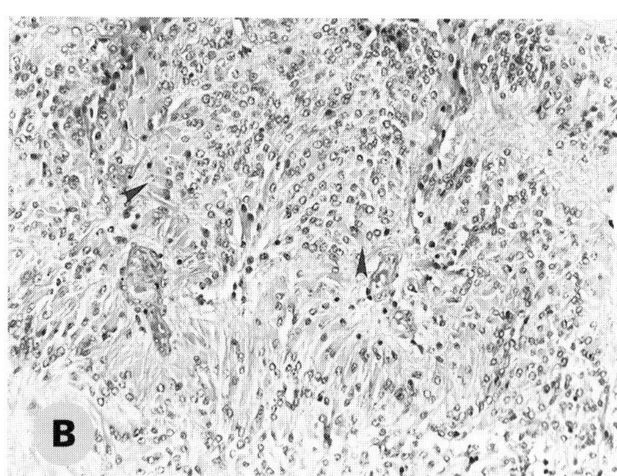

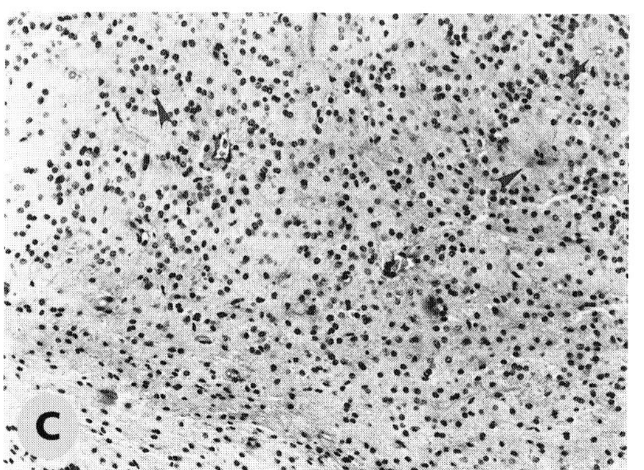

Figure 4: Sections showing sheets of ependymal cells. **A)** Characteristic areas with increased cell density and lobular arrangement circumscribed by blood vessels. **B)** The tumor cells are closely packed and exhibit an epithelioid appearance. The cytoplasm is abundant and the outer membrane distinctive. **C)** In some areas there is a diffuse uniform distribution of the tumor cells throughout the fibrillary background. The typical perivascular pseudorosettes are scanty and discrete *(arrowheads).* (hematoxylin-eosin, original magnification × 10)

TABLE 2

DISTRIBUTION OF HISTOLOGICAL FEATURES IN EPENDYMOMAS

Histological Feature	Supratentorial Ependymomas (%)	Infratentorial Ependymomas (%)**	Spinal Ependymomas (%)††
Perivascular pseudorosettes			
Large	67 *	87	61
Small	67 *	—	42
Sheets of ependymal cells	54 *	68	67
Ependymal rosettes	13 *	38	22
Necrosis	62 †	64	16
Mitosis	60 ‡	39	20
Prominent nucleoli	9 ‡	—	5
Small nuclei	—	—	100
Intermediate-sized nuclei	42	—	55
Large nuclei	9	—	15
Hyperchromic nuclei	—	57	—
Pleomorphic nuclei	9	35	70
Oval nuclei	—	90	—
Elongated nuclei			
With cytoplasm	24	30	53
Without cytoplasm	22	36	47
Irregular nuclei	—	41	—
Astrocytic regions	28	40	10
Giant cells	9		10
High cell density	—	96	90
Very high cell density	67	70	70
Low cell density	59	89	80
Very low cell density	24	66	50
Microcysts	15	10	21
Vacuoles	27	23	58
Fine stroma	87	93	80
Coarse stroma	8	12	20
Astrocytes	28	40	10
Oligodendroglial foci	13	—	—
Parenchymal calcification	32	—	—

* These histological features were unreliably identified in tumors in the supratentorial compartment.
† Significantly more frequent in ependymomas.
‡ Significantly more frequent in anaplastic ependymomas.
** There were no significant differences in the distributions of any histological features between anaplastic and nonanaplastic ependymomas.
†† The reliability of histological features in spinal tumors has not been tested. The mean age of children with spinal ependymomas is 10.6 years.
— = Too frequent or infrequent in this location to test reliability, or less than eight cases.

areas. When present, blepharoplasts are useful (but not necessary) for the diagnosis of ependymoma; they represent the basal bodies in which the cilia shafts terminate in the cytoplasm. They are seen best with oil immersion and a phosphotungstic acid hematoxylin (PTAH) stain, in which they are seen as dots or rods in the apical cytoplasmic portion of the ependymal cells bordering ependymal rosettes or canals or in a juxtanuclear position in the more compact cellular areas (Figure 1C).

Occasionally (0.3% of the CBTC database), the predominant pattern of growth is papillary, and this variant is referred to as "papillary ependymoma." The stroma of each papilla is scanty and is formed by fibrillary neuroglia

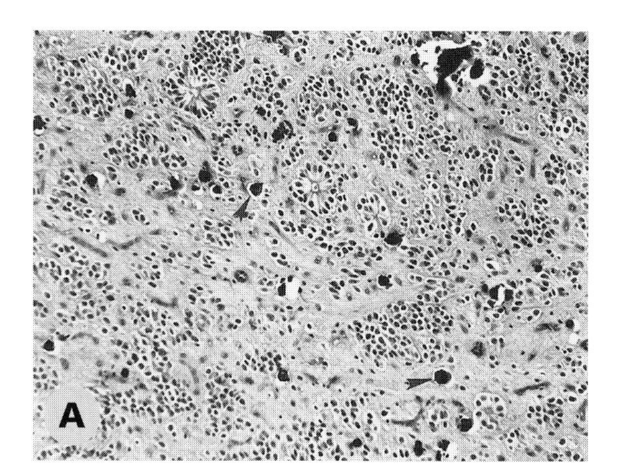

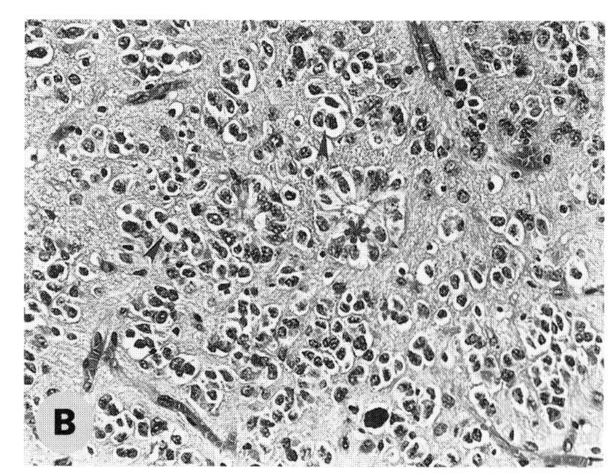

Figure 5: A) Areas containing clusters of clear cells separated by abundant fine stroma with delicate blood vessels. Note the numerous calcifications. **B)** Small patches of cells with darkly stained nuclei and clear cytoplasm forming a perinuclear "halo," thus resembling oligodendrocytes. Some of these cells are forming ependymal rosettes. (hematoxylin-eosin, original magnification × 10 [A], × 20 [B])

(unlike the choroid plexus papilloma with its collagenous stroma); it usually contains central vascular tissue covered with a single or sometimes stratified layer of cuboidal or low columnar epithelium, which can be pseudostratified or arranged in several layers. Stromal myxomatous change is sometimes present in these areas. The papillary variant is more commonly found in the cauda equina; however, it may originate in other locations. There is focal formation of ependymal tubules. The papillary ependymoma is distinguished from the choroid plexus papilloma by the frequent arrangement of cells in multiple layers, the additional formation of tubules, and the presence of a neuroglial stroma. The papillae of a choroid plexus papilloma never contain a neuroglial stroma.

Clear cells (Figure 5) may be found in ependymomas. Clear cells with a centrally located round nucleus and an empty-appearing cytoplasm form clusters or are scattered among the fibrillated glial stroma; classically, they have been considered oligodendrocytes on light microscopy;[54] however, Kawano et al[53] found ependymal features in these cells ultrastructurally. In the CBTC database, they were recognized as oligodendroglial foci only in supratentorial ependymomas and then in only 13% of tumors.

The stroma in ependymomas consists of glial cells and is inversely proportional to that of the epithelial component. A fine delicate stroma is present in the majority of ependymomas, no matter which compartment. Frankly astrocytic regions, on the other hand, were present in 40% of infratentorial ependymomas and in a smaller proportion of ependymomas located elsewhere in the central nervous system. Scattered calcifications (Figure 6) are frequent and in some studies are associated with a worsened survival probability.[130]

Smears from ependymomas disclose a highly papillary pattern, with the characteristic arrangement of the perivascular pseudorosettes. Individual cells with abundant cytoplasm and well-defined cytoplasmic membranes are seen in less papillary areas. Ependymal tubules or surfaces are rarely present.[1]

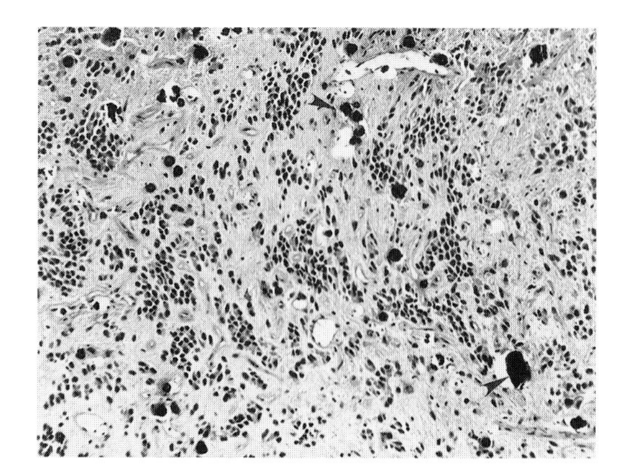

Figure 6: Irregular calcification of variable size is a conspicuous finding in ependymoma, usually occurring in the central, less cellular portion of the tumor. (hematoxylin-eosin, original magnification × 10)

Ultrastructure

Electron microscopic studies of ependymomas and anaplastic ependymomas reveal a variable number of basal bodies, cilia, cell junctions, and intracellular intermediate filaments, which are normal components of the non-neoplastic ependymal cell.[39] A characteristic ultrastructural feature is the finding of microrosettes formed by concentrically oriented cells with apical intercellular junctional complexes (gap junctions) (Figure 7).[118] The luminal surfaces of these cells have abundant microvilli and few cilia; occasionally, their number is exaggerated and they entirely fill the lumen of the microrosette. The cilia may display either the normal 9 + 2 configuration of the axial filament complex or various internal configurations.[42,63] Cytoplasmic intermediate filaments measuring 8 to 10 nm in diameter have been repeatedly demonstrated in neoplastic ependymal cells, consistent with the glial fibrillary acidic protein (GFAP) positivity.

Immunohistochemical Features

Ependymomas are frequently positive for GFAP and vimentin. This is expected, since ependyma and subependymal neuroglia may have the same cellular precursor. Ependymal cells transiently express GFAP at the time that cilia appear during fetal development.[91] The cells forming perivascular pseudorosettes and the fibrillary stroma are positive for GFAP. Vimentin and S100 protein usually correlate with the GFAP positivity.[50,58,83,117] Monoclonal antibody Leu-7 (HNK-1) and keratin give inconsistent positive staining in scattered cells.[20,70] Occasional cells forming the ependymal rosettes and tubules are positive for GFAP.

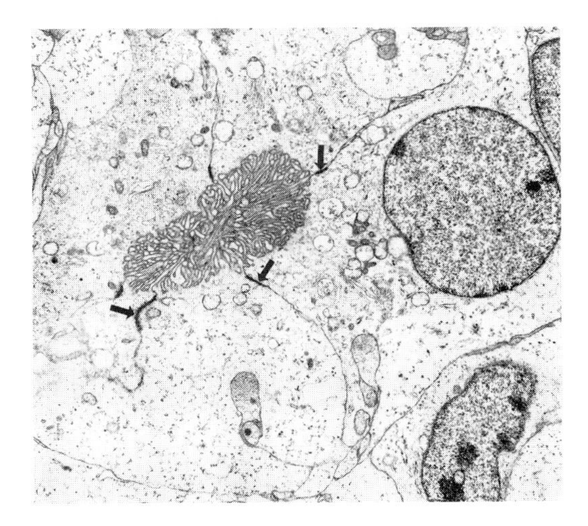

Figure 7: Ultrastructural appearance of an ependymal rosette. The lumen is filled with numerous microvilli. Note the intercellular junctions (zonulae adherens) in the apical region of the participating cells. (hematoxylin-eosin, original magnification × 15,000)

Genetic Studies

Although no consistent clonal abnormality is reported in ependymoma, major chromosomal abnormalities have been described[87,121] involving chromosome 22,[38,127] chromosome 11,[99] and the short arm of chromosome 1 in a myxopapillary ependymoma.[102] Abnormalities of p53 were found in some ependymomas.[51,77,85] Ependymomas and choroid plexus tumors can be induced in rodents by inoculating them intracerebrally or intravenously with the BK,[15] JC,[67] or SV40 or adenovirus 7[23,24,60,61,86] viruses. Ependymomas and choroid plexus tumors of childhood sometimes contain deoxyribonucleic acid (DNA) sequences similar to those of SV40.[6]

SUBEPENDYMOMAS

Subependymomas, usually located in the fourth ventricle as small rounded or lobulated tumors, were first described by Scheinker,[103] who believed that the predominant cell was astrocytic. Shortly after, Kuhlenbeck[64] added more details. Mitotic figures, giant cells, and areas of necrosis were absent. The name "subependymal glomerate astrocytoma" was introduced by Boykin et al.[7] Although usually single, these tumors may be multiple.[11]

Subependymomas are insidious tumors that typically exhibit a noninvasive slow growth. Three theories have been suggested regarding the histogenesis of this tumor. 1) Ho[43] proposed an association between subependymomas, sometimes multiple, and the presence of heterotopic leptomeningeal neuroglial tissue. Both lesions have occurred in identical twins.[14] 2) Reactive processes (e.g., granular ependymitis) could also explain the multiplicity of some subependymomas. Ho et al[46] reported a third

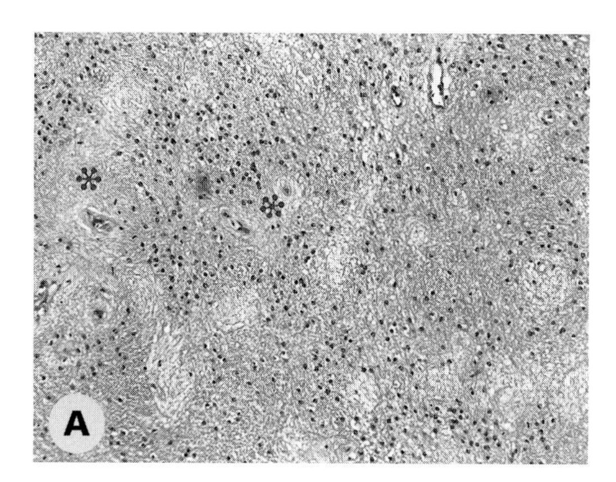

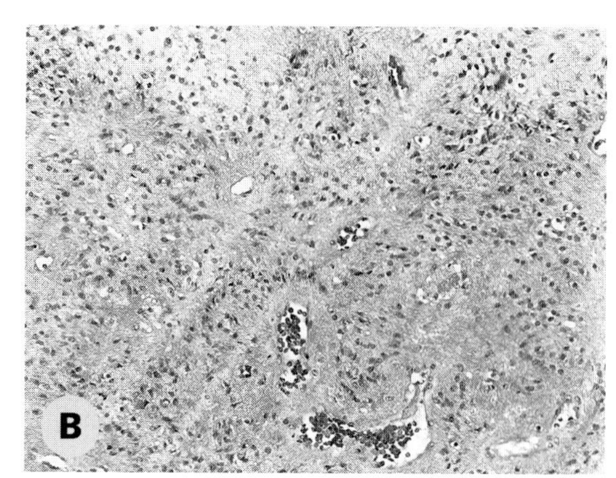

Figure 8: Appearance of a subependymoma. **A)** The cellularity concentrates irregularly throughout the tumor. This tumor exhibits abundant fibrillary stroma. The perivascular arrangement of tumor cells is maintained despite the relatively low vascularity *(asterisks).* **B)** The tumor cells are fairly uniform in size and shape, and mitotic figures are absent. The blood vessels are for the most part delicate capillaries; however, areas containing large ectatic sinusoidal vessels are a frequent occurrence, explaining why hemorrhage is often a presenting sign. (hematoxylin-eosin, original magnification × 5 [A], × 10 [B])

ventricular subependymoma occurring after 18 years in a patient with a craniopharyngioma. This patient had received radiation to the suprasellar region 15 years earlier. 3) Moss[81] proposed a precursor ependymoglial cell persisting in the adult subependymal layer as the cell of origin for subependymomas. However, the tumor cells do not exhibit the primitive embryonal cellular features expected in such cases.[96] They are occasionally associated with gliosarcoma (vascular)[69] and are sometimes symptomatic.[104]

Incidence

Many subependymomas are asymptomatic and are only identified as incidental autopsy findings (usually <1 cm in diameter). They are most frequently found in male patients from the fifth to the eighth decades of life, with a mean of about 60 years.[11,104] Symptomatic tumors have an earlier presentation, with some diagnosed in the first decade of life. These tumors usually contain ependymomatous areas with increased cellularity.

Location

Subependymomas are distinctive for their paraventricular location, two-thirds of them occurring near the fourth ventricle or lateral recesses.[104] They may arise at any level of the ventricular system, but are exceptionally rare in the spinal cord.

Macroscopic Appearance

The tumors are frequently multiple and lobulated, and present a sharp demarcation from the adjacent neural tissue. They are occasionally pedunculated.[122] Commonly, these tumors are small (<1.5 cm in diameter). The larger specimens usually exhibit cystic changes, hemorrhage, and calcifications.

Microscopic Description

Subependymomas are hypocellular neoplasms with unevenly scattered ependymal cells that form ependymal rosettes, perivascular pseudorosettes, or small clumps with no particular orientation (Figure 8). Blepharoplasts are present in the epithelial component. The characteristic predominant feature of this neoplasm is the proliferation of fibrillary subependymal astrocytes. The astroglial component varies from case to case and is maximal in the incidental cases. Ependymal cellular features have been confirmed ultrastructurally, by tissue culture, and by the not infrequent existence of transitional or mixed forms in which the histological pictures of typical ependymoma and subependymoma are juxtaposed.[104] The ependymal cells rest upon a layer of subependymal glia. In many instances, the subependymal glia are the preponderant component.

Ultrastructure

The ependymal nature of the epithelial cells in subependymoma is usually confirmed.[2,31] Scheithauer[104] described typical astrocytic, ependymal, and transitional cellular elements in subependymoma and mixed subependymoma and ependymoma.

Myxopapillary Ependymomas

Myxopapillary ependymomas occur mostly in patients in the third or fourth decade of life,[57] although they may also present in childhood.[10]

Location

These tumors are virtually restricted to the region of the cauda equina and originate from the conus medullaris or the filum terminale.[57] In this region, the typical epithelial, cellular, or papillary patterns of ependymoma may also occur.[111] Myxopapillary ependymomas may originate in other areas of the ventricular system including the cerebrum.[74,101,125] In the CBTC population, one case was located in the fourth ventricle.

Macroscopic Appearance

Myxopapillary ependymomas vary in size and present as well-defined sausage-shaped growths with smooth or irregularly nodular surfaces. Notably they have a gelatinous appearance and may envelop and compress the spinal cord and nerve roots of the cauda equina. In these circumstances, the determination of their origin from the filum terminale or the conus medullaris may not always be possible at surgery. Exceptionally, the tumor infiltrates the spinal rootlets so diffusely that surgical removal is not feasible. With more massive growth, adjacent bone may be deformed or even eroded. Several examples have developed remote metastasis. These tumors are highly vascular and evidence of antecedent spontaneous hemorrhage is common.

Microscopic Description

The myxopapillary ependymoma may exhibit several separate morphological patterns or a combination of them. The typical histological feature is a myxopapillary structure consisting of a perivascular arrangement of tumor cells (perivascular pseudorosettes), accompanied by myxoid stromal degeneration, and microcyst formation between papillae and individual epithelial cells (Figure 9). Mucinous change is typical of myxopapillary ependymomas and may be attributed to myxoid degeneration of the collagenous stroma or mucin secretion from the tumor cells themselves. The unusual character of the supporting stroma in the myxopapillary ependymomas is determined by the special features of the filum terminale, which contains pia mater, nerve fibers, neurons, and various neuroglial elements, among which ependymal cells are conspicuous.[78,119] Tumor cells range from elongated fibrillated cells with long fine processes attached to vascular walls to columnar or cuboidal cells, depending on the extent of myxoid change. The vascular cores are thin and delicate in myxopapillary areas and occasionally they undergo fibrinoid degeneration. In areas with less myxoid change the vascular framework is prominent, with a single layer of small tumor cells surrounding individual blood vessels. In some cases, the connective tissue of the papillae exhibits severe thickening and hyalinization with obliteration of scattered vascular lumens. The myxoid and hyalinized areas are metachromatic and positive for mucin. Between the perivascular pseudorosettes are irregular sheets formed of closely united polygonal cells of variable size. True ependymal rosettes, tubules, and clefts lined with low columnar cells and resting on a collagenous basement membrane are an uncommon finding. In our experience, the demonstration of blepharoplasts is usually not possible. This tumor can easily be diagnosed in smears when the basic architecture and the papillary patterns are preserved. Occasionally, the tumor is composed of scattered stellate cells in a metachromatic myxoid matrix. These appearances may be difficult to distinguish from those of chordoma. Clinicopathological correlations usually relate to location.[112]

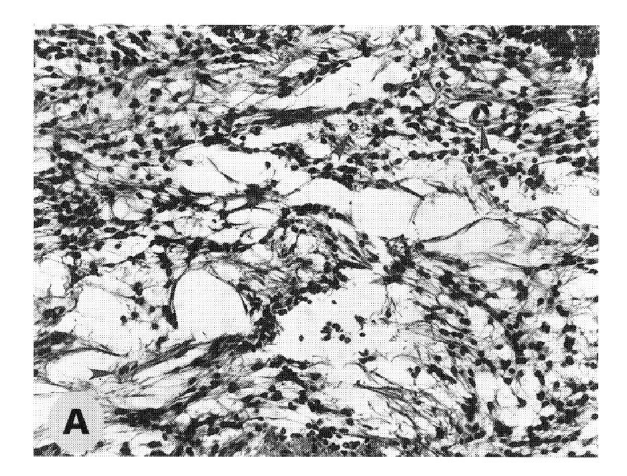

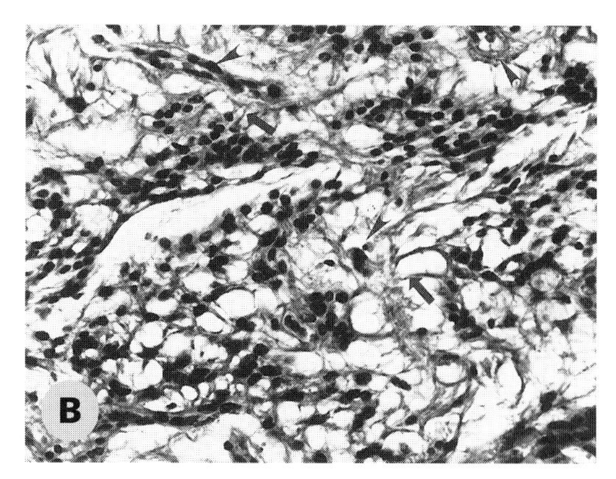

Figure 9: A) Myxopapillary ependymoma exhibiting the characteristic myxomatous stromal change that separates masses of tumor cells from delicate fibrovascular cores *(arrowheads)*. **B)** Perivascular pseudorosettes in a myxopapillary ependymoma. The tumor cells exhibit marked cytoplasmic vacuolation which appears as filamentous processes *(arrows)* attached to the adventitia of a delicate vascular core *(arrowheads)*. (hematoxylin-eosin, original magnification × 10 [A], × 20 [B])

Ultrastructure

Ultrastructurally, cells in myxopapillary ependymomas have many features of the conventional ependymal cell but also basement membranes (Figure 10), which some believe mimic the normal subpial position of ependymal cells in the filum terminale.[89,90] The ependymal cells in these tumors have many similarities to choroid plexus epithelium, and contain relatively few cilia. There are complex cellular interdigitations and abundant basement membrane material often topographically related to collagen fibrils and microtubular aggregates and junctions.[44,45] Some of these features are probably related to the normal structure of the filum terminale and conus medullaris where ependymal cells may be directly apposed to connective tissue derived from the leptomeninges instead of resting on the neuropil.[113]

Figure 10: Electron micrograph of a myxopapillary ependymoma showing the interdigitating cytoplasmic processes of several cells *(arrowheads)* separated by microcystic spaces *(asterisks)*. These processes are attached to a well-defined basal membrane *(arrows)* lying on the adventitial layer of a capillary. The endothelial cell is labeled with a star. (original magnification × 18,900)

Immunohistochemical Features

The glial nature of the fibrils is easily confirmed with special stains for neuroglia.

Anaplastic and Nonanaplastic Ependymomas

Several methods of classification of ependymomas have been described. Only a very few authors (e.g., Sutton el al[116]) have defined the criteria used for the diagnosis of anaplastic ependymoma. The strict criteria for anaplastic ependymoma according to the revised WHO scheme[92] are the presence of many mitoses and anaplasia with the characteristic rosettes. Tumors with increased cellularity, rare mitotic figures, and mixed tumors with low-grade glial elements constitute "benign" ependymomas;[116] however, in the CBTC database there was no difference in survival data between anaplastic and nonanaplastic ependymomas. Older children tended to have longer survival but the differences between older and younger patients were not significant. Supratentorial or infratentorial location had no effect. Extent of surgery was an important determinant of survival time. Survival did not differ significantly between anaplastic and nonanaplastic ependymomas in the series of Schiffer et al,[106] who found shortened survival associated only with cell density and many mitoses.

Anaplastic varieties of ependymoma and papillary ependymoma have been recognized since the descriptions early in this century. Great variation in survival was recognized by Bailey and Cushing[5] in their classification in 1926 and by Kernohan's group.[111] Confusion about the role of the subclass of ependymoblastoma existed from the time of its first description. The WHO classification[92] clearly recognizes both forms and separates the anaplastic variety by the presence of high mitotic activity. Minor amounts of nuclear atypia and even foci of necrosis may occur, but ". . . are not necessarily indicative of malignancy."[62] The anaplastic variety requires high cellularity, variable nuclear atypia, marked mitotic activity, and often prominent vascular proliferation. Ependymoblastomas in the WHO classification are rare malignant embryonal tumors composed of ". . . undifferentiated cells, accompanied by numerous, surprisingly well-formed ependymoblastic rosettes. The latter are multilayered, true rosettes with a lumen. . . . Ependymoblastomas are further characterized by high cellularity, marked mitotic activity and occasional areas of necrosis." These are thought to be childhood tumors, but none were encountered in the CBTC database.

In the CBTC study, separate teams of neuropathologists classified each of the tumors into a WHO category or sought the individual histological features. In practice, the use of the above criteria must have differed between the teams. In supratentorial anaplastic ependymomas, mitoses and prominent nucleoli were the only histological features that were significantly increased; necrosis was not. In infratentorial ependymomas there were no significant differences in histological features between anaplastic and nonanaplastic ependymomas (Table 2). The mean age of children with anaplastic ependymomas was significantly less than that of children with ependymomas in both supratentorial and infratentorial compartments. The mean ages of children with both varieties were less when the tumor was located in the infratentorial compartment.

The term "ependymoblastoma" has had different meanings since it was first applied. In 1924, Bailey[4] named the group of tumors resembling ependymal cells "ependymomas" but made no attempt to separate ependymoblastoma from ependymoma. By 1926, he and Cushing[5] recognized a tumor of that name but thought it no more malignant than ependymoma; however, they did not separate tumors by anaplastic histological features, and felt that both of these varieties, with an "average survival" of 32 months, were "benign." They did recognize a great variation in survival times. By the 1950s, survival time was recognized as being quite variable, and this has been repeatedly confirmed by Kernohan's group.[111,131]

Bailey and Cushing[5] used both "ependymoblastoma" and "ependymoma" in their classification of the brain tumors. This division was based on cellular architectural differences only, and for practical purposes the terms were interchangeable. Microscopically, ependymoblastoma was a tumor composed of ependymal spongioblasts forming perivascular pseudorosettes that contained fibrillary cytoplasmic processes in the nucleus-free zone stained positive with PTAH and blepharoplasts. Mitotic figures were almost never found. Similarly, ependymoma cells also displayed blepharoplasts but differed in that they were polygonal and had no tail (tapering fibrillary cytoplasmic process attached to a vascular wall). Occasionally, spongioblasts were found in this last tumor. The separation of this variant was later considered insignificant as it had little difference in biological behavior.[5] The term "ependymoblastoma" has been used as a synonym of malignant ependymoma.[22,54] Ependymoblastoma as described by Mørk and Rubinstein[80,97] meets the original description of Bailey and Cushing in the sense that it exhibits ependymal differentiation represented by spongioblasts and rosette formation. It meets also Willis' suggestion[129] that the "blastoma" suffix be applied to tumors reproducing to some extent the embryonic blastema. Ependymoblastoma is then a distinctive primitive tumor composed of a neuroepithelial precursor committed to ependymal differentiation resembling the ependymoblast, a cell type that represents a stage in the differentiation of the ventricular cell to mature ependyma. Central primitive neuroectodermal tumors (PNETs) are multipotential and may exhibit differentiation toward glial or neuronal cells or a combination of both cell lineages. However, exclusive ependymal differentiation is rare, and those cases qualify for the term "ependymoblastoma."

Most ependymoblastomas occur early, within the first 5 years of life;[80] they range from congenital forms[25,68,82] to occasional cases occurring in late childhood, adolescence, and adulthood. There is no sex predominance. Similar to PNETs, they have a short clinical history of signs and symptoms usually related to increased intracranial pressure and mass effect on the adjacent cerebral structures. The case reported by Shyn et al[110] is of particular interest because the presenting symptoms were related to spinal cord compression due to a metastatic lesion. Survival is similar to that for PNET. Extracranial metastasis follows the metastatic pattern of ependymomas, e.g., to the lungs.[9,36,80] There is a 3:1 supratentorial predominance in the cases reported and they may or may not be related to the ventricular system.[18,80] Most cases have originated as primary intracranial brain tumors and there is frequent leptomeningeal invasion. Unique cases of primary leptomeningeal ependymoblastoma and a sacral subcutaneous ependymoblastoma without bone involvement or spinal canal abnormality have been reported.[82,124] Ependymoblastomas present as massive, soft, friable, circumscribed growths. Frequently, cystic degeneration is present with yellow-brown fluid, which contrasts with the clear fluid found in cystic astrocytomas. Areas of necrosis and hemorrhage are common.

Microscopically, the criteria for diagnosis were established by Rubinstein,[97] and several reports have followed that support his findings.[18,19,80,100] Ependymoblastoma contains a characteristic regular pattern of growth-forming, thick, densely cellular anastomosing cords or sheets among thin-walled blood vessels (Figure 11). Areas with rosettes and tubules are characteristic. There are abundant mitotic figures and scattered cell necrosis. The tumor cells are primitive and small, constituting a uniform population possessing a dark round or oval nucleus; the cytoplasm is scanty. Rosettes are the microscopic sign of ependymal differentiation; however, their number varies from case to case and sometimes they are only seen ultrastructurally. Although most rosettes in ependymoblastoma are of ependymoblastic type, ependymal rosettes are also present. The latter are represented by scattered cells putting out a fine polar fibrillated cytoplasmic process directed toward a vascular wall. This cytoplasmic process is positive on PTAH and silver impregnation staining, resembling spongioblasts or glioblasts. A portion of cells including those forming ependymal rosettes contains granules positive on PTAH staining that correspond to blepharoplasts. Stains for neural fibrils (Bielschowsky and Bodian) are consistently negative. The majority of rosettes are composed of a multistratified cell layer and feature abundant mitoses at their juxtaluminal portion, thus resembling the primitive neural tube. These rosettes have been labeled ependymoblastic, and differ from ependymal rosettes in that later mitotic activity is absent and they are formed by

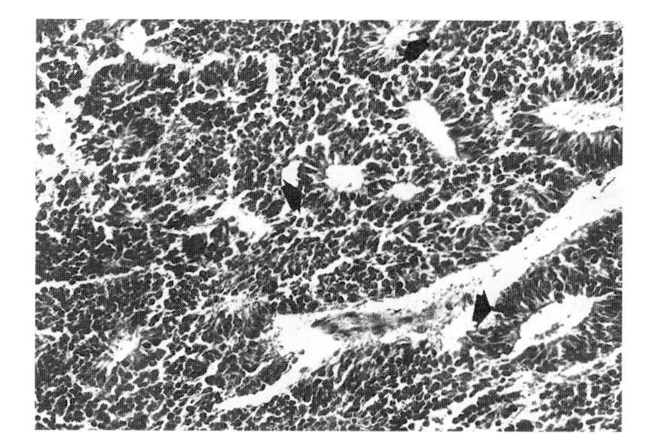

Figure 11: Photomicrograph of an ependymoblastoma showing dense proliferation of primitive-appearing cells separating multilayered rosettes of ependymoblastic type *(arrows).* Vascularity is sparse. (hematoxylin-eosin, original magnification × 10)

only one or two layers of radially oriented cells. Both types of rosettes exhibit cilia and juxtaluminal blepharoplasts. Minimal vascular or endothelial proliferation is typical of this tumor. Irregular areas of necrosis are a common finding in most cases. Despite the sharp edge seen grossly between tumor and adjacent neural tissue, microscopically the margin of the tumor is infiltrative. The absence of pleomorphism and multinucleation distinguishes ependymoblastoma from anaplastic ependymoma.[80]

Ultrastructurally, ependymoblastomas contain populations of undifferentiated primitive cells and well-differentiated ependymal cells. Abundant mitosis of primitive cells and within the rosettes is present. The nucleus is uniform, with frequent indentation of the nuclear membrane and nucleolus. The chromatin is dense and sometimes marginated. The undifferentiated cells have scanty cytoplasmic organelles. The ependymal cells form rosettes with lumina of varying sizes in which rudimentary or mature-structured cilia and microvilli project. There is apposition of the lateral cell surfaces with formation of cellular attachments (zonulae adherentes) at the apical portions of the cells. There is no basal lamina at the luminal surface of these cells. The apical cytoplasm contains abundant cellular organelles. Scattered cells contain perinuclear bundles of intermediate filaments (7.5 to 10 nm). In perivascular regions, the basal cytoplasm of the tumor cells forms labyrinths lined by basal lamina rarely connecting with that of the capillary. The cytoplasmic processes forming perivascular pseudorosettes frequently have a basal lamina and end near the endothelial cell. Intermediate cell forms, suggesting varying lines of differentiation, are not present. Immunohistochemically, the pattern of staining correlates with the primitive microscopic appearance.

Are Ependymomas "Benign"?

Clearly, some ependymomas are relatively benign in that they are associated with prolonged postoperative survival or are often simple masses discovered incidentally at autopsy. The myxopapillary ependymoma and the subependymoma (subependymal glomerate astrocytoma) fall into this category. However, even these two tumors may prove difficult to resect when they become symptomatic.

Predicting the clinical behavior of the remaining subclasses of ependymoma is difficult because of the many confounding characteristics of this group of tumors. Clinical behavior differs depending upon tumor site,[73] patient age, and extent of surgical resection,[116] and should depend upon diagnosis. Many problems with diagnostic criteria have ensured that the rates of anaplastic ependymomas and ependymoblastomas have varied widely among institutions. The anaplastic type varies in many series between 40% and 94%, hence this diagnostic category may have been based on variable criteria.[128] Some authors have found no difference in survival times between anaplastic ependymoma and ependymoma.[95,106] The majority of studies of prognosis do not use appropriate mathematical models of survival that simultaneously consider important confounding variables such as patient age, tumor location, extent of surgical resection, other treatments, or specific histological feature content, but merely use the name of the tumor. One problem is that specific operational defining criteria have not been agreed upon by neuropathologists. The result is that when the reproducibility of diagnostic categories is measured, reliability may fall short of clinical expectation. For instance, in the only evaluation to date of the reliability of the WHO diagnoses as applied to childhood brain tumors, ependymoma was considered a diagnosis reliably made, while the diagnosis of anaplastic ependymoma was not.[12]

Ependymomas in children generally have a poor outlook relative to those in adults[109,130] despite the WHO classification of ependymoma as grade I or II. Infratentorial tumors were associated with lower mean ages and with significantly shorter median survival times than supratentorial or spinal tumors.[88] Sutton et al[116] believed that tumor location had little effect on survival in children, but that the extent of surgery was the most important prognostic factor. Histological degree of malignancy had no influence on survival. They concluded that adjuvant chemotherapy with CCNU (lomustine), vincristine, and cisplatin does not improve the period of progression-free survival.

Operative mortality for infratentorial ependymomas is twice that for supratentorial ependymomas.[27] In the CBTC database, postoperative mortality (death within the first postoperative month) for 1930 to 1979 was 7% for patients with supratentorial and 30% for infratentorial ependymomas. It was slightly easier to "totally" remove supratentorial ependymomas (32%) than infratentorial ependymomas (19%) (P=.02). Ilgren et al[48,49] believed that patients with infratentorial tumors had a shorter disease-free interval and were likely to live for a shorter time than those with tumors of the cauda equina, and that younger patients died sooner if the tumor was in the infratentorial compartment. There was no difference in survival time between ependymoma and anaplastic ependymoma.[95,105]

Histology seems of limited value for prognosis.[79,95,106] High mitotic index and tumor cell number were not correlated with the length of survival and, in the infratentorial compartment, rosette-bearing tumors had a poor prognosis[48,49] (in contrast to the contention of Willis[129]). Thus, standard histology[105] and supplemental studies such as of nucleolar organizing regions have not been associated with length of postoperative survival.[28,94,95] Estimates of the growth potential with Ki-67, such as by Schröder et al,[107] have not yet been tested in separate populations.

In the CBTC database, children with ependymomas in the infratentorial compartment have a 50% probability of surviving 2.6 years, in contrast to children with anaplastic ependymomas in whom there is a 50% probability of surviving 1.1 years. Anaplastic ependymal tumors occur in significantly younger children in the infratentorial compartment (3.5 vs. 4.9 years; P< .05) as well as in the supratentorial compartment (5.1 vs. 7.1 years; P<.05). Anaplastic ependymomas are more common in the supratentorial compartment (31% vs. 15%; P= .003). Some have maintained that the presence of true ependymal rosettes improves survival probability;[129] however, in the CBTC population ependymal rosettes have no influence on the outcome in appropriate mathematical models of prognosis. Children with supratentorial anaplastic and nonanaplastic ependymal tumors have indistinguishable survival probabilities, and furthermore, there is no difference in the survival probability between supratentorial and infratentorial ependymomas. Therefore, children with infratentorial anaplastic ependymomas have a significantly (P< .05) worse survival probability than do children with a tumor of the same name in the supratentorial compartment. Irradiation improves survival significantly in appropriate proportional hazards models (P<.005), as has been repeatedly observed by others, such as Healey et al.[41]

Conclusion

Ependymomas remain a challenge to the neuro-oncologist, neurosurgeon, and pathologist. Until we understand the underlying biology of these tumors, we need to develop a set of reliably recognized diagnostic categories useful for providing homogeneous groups of patients for clinical trials of putative therapeutic agents.

References

1. Adams JH, Graham DI, Doyle D: **Brain Biopsy. The Smear Technique for Neurosurgical Biopsies.** Philadelphia, Pa: JB Lippincott, 1981
2. Azzarelli B, Rekate HL, Roessmann U: Subependymoma. A case report with ultrastructural study. **Acta Neuropathol 40:**279-282, 1977
3. Bailey P: Histologic atlas of gliomas. **Arch Pathol Lab Med 4:**871-921, 1927
4. Bailey P: A study of tumors arising from ependymal cells. **Arch Neurol Psychiatry 11:**1-27, 1924
5. Bailey P, Cushing H: **A Classification of the Tumors of the Glioma Group on a Histogenetic Basis with a Correlated Study of Prognosis.** New York, NY: Sentry Press, 1926
6. Bergsagel DJ, Finegold MJ, Butel JS, et al: DNA sequences similar to those of simian virus 40 in ependymomas and choroid plexus tumors of childhood. **N Engl J Med 326:**988-993, 1992
7. Boykin FC, Cowen D, Iannucci CAJ, et al: Subependymal glomerate astrocytomas. **J Neuropathol Exp Neurol 15:**30-49, 1954
8. Caccamo DV, Ho KL, Garcia JH: Cauda equina tumor with ependymal and paraganglionic differentiation. **Hum Pathol 23:**835-838, 1992
9. Campbell AN, Chan HSL, Becker LE, et al: Extracranial metastases in childhood primary intracranial tumors. A report of 21 cases and review of the literature. **Cancer 53:**974-981, 1985
10. Chan HSL, Becker LE, Hoffman HJ, et al: Myxopapillary ependymoma of the filum terminale and cauda equina in childhood: report of seven cases

and review of the literature. **Neurosurgery 14**:204-210, 1984
11. Chason JL: Subependymal mixed gliomas. **J Neuropathol Exp Neurol 15**:461-470, 1956
12. Childhood Brain Tumor Consortium: Intraobserver reproducibility in assigning brain tumors to classes in the World Health Organization diagnostic scheme. **J Neurooncol 7**:211-244, 1989
13. Childhood Brain Tumor Consortium: A study of childhood brain tumors based on surgical biopsies from ten North American institutions: sample description. **J Neurooncol 6**: 9-23, 1988
14. Clarenbach P, Kleihues P, Metzel E, et al: Simultaneous clinical manifestation of subependymoma of the fourth ventricle in identical twins. Case report. **J Neurosurg 50**:655-659, 1979
15. Corallini A, Altavilla G, Cecchetti MG, et al: Ependymomas, malignant tumors of pancreatic islets, and osteosarcomas induced in hamsters by BK virus, a human papovavirus. **J Natl Cancer Inst 61**:875-883, 1978
16. Courville CB, Broussalian SL: Plastic ependymomas of the lateral recess. Report of eight verified cases. **J Neurosurg 18**:792-799, 1961
17. Crotty TB, Hooker RP, Swensen SJ, et al: Primary malignant ependymoma of the lung. **Mayo Clin Proc 67**:373-378, 1992
18. Cruz-Sanchez FF, Haustein J, Rossi ML, et al: Ependymoblastoma: a histological, immunohistological and ultrastructural study of five cases. **Histopathology 12**:17-27, 1988
19. Cruz-Sanchez FF, Rossi ML, Hughes JT, et al: Differentiation in embryonal neuroepithelial tumors of the central nervous system. **Cancer 67**:965-976, 1991
20. Cruz-Sanchez FF, Rossi ML, Hughes JT, et al: An immunohistological study of 66 ependymomas. **Histopathology 13**:443-454, 1988
21. Deck JH, Eng LF, Bigbee J, et al: The role of glial fibrillary acidic protein in the diagnosis of central nervous system tumors. **Acta Neuropathol 42**:183-190, 1978
22. Dohrmann GJ, Farwell JR, Flannery JT: Ependymomas and ependymoblastomas in children. **J Neurosurg 45**:273-283, 1976
23. Eddy BE: Tumors produced in hamsters by SV40. **Fed Proc 21**:930-935, 1962
24. Eddy BE, Borman GS, Berkeley WH, et al: Tumors induced in hamsters by injection of rhesus monkey cell extracts. **Proc Soc Exp Biol Med 107**:191-197, 1961
25. Ehret M, Jacobi G, Hey A, et al: Embryonal brain neoplasms in the neonatal period and early infancy. **Clin Neuropathol 6**:218-223, 1987
26. Ernestus RI, Schröder R, Klug N: Spontaneous intracerebral hemorrhage from an unsuspected ependymoma in early infancy. **Childs Nerv Syst 8**:357-360, 1992
27. Ernestus RI, Wilcke 0, Schröder R: Intracranial ependymomas: prognostic aspects. **Neurosurg Rev 12**:157-163, 1989
28. Figarella-Branger D, Gambarelli D, Dollo C, et al: Infratentorial ependymomas of childhood. Correlation between histological features, immunohistological phenotype, silver nucleolar organizer region staining values and post-operative survival in 16 cases. **Acta Neuropathol 82**:208-216, 1991
29. Fokes EC Jr, Earle KM: Ependymomas: clinical and pathological aspects. **J Neurosurg 30**:585-594, 1969
30. Friede RL, Pollak A: The cytogenetic basis for classifying ependymomas. **J Neuropathol Exp Neurol 37**:103-118, 1978
31. Fu YS, Chen ATL, Kay S, et al: Is subependymoma (subependymal glomerate astrocytoma) an astrocytoma or ependymoma? A comparative ultrastructural and tissue culture study. **Cancer 34**:1992-2008, 1974
32. Gagliardi FM, Cervoni L, Domenicucci M, et al: Ependymomas of the filum terminale in childhood: report of four cases and review of the literature. **Childs Nerv Syst 9**:3-6, 1993
33. Gilles FH: **The Developing Human Brain.** Littleton, Mass: John Wright, 1983, pp 59-86
34. Gilles FH, Leviton A, Hedley-Whyte ET, et al: Childhood brain tumors that occupy more than one compartment at presentation. Multiple compartment tumors. **J Neurooncol 14**:45-56, 1992
35. Gilles FH, Leviton A, Hedley-Whyte ET, et al: Childhood brain tumor update. **Hum Pathol 14**:834-845, 1987
36. Glasauer FE, Yuan RHP: Intracranial tumors with extracranial metastasis. Case report and review of the literature. **J Neurosurg 20**:474-493, 1963
37. Globus JH, Kuhlenbeck H: The subependymal cell plate (matrix) and its relationship to brain tumors of the ependymal type. **J Neuropathol Exp Neurol 3**:1-35, 1944
38. Griffin CA, Long PP, Carson BS, et al: Chromosome abnormalities in low-grade central nervous system tumors. **Cancer Genet Cytogenet 60**:67-73, 1992
39. Guccion JG, Saini N. Ependymoma: ultrastructural studies of two cases. **Ultrastruct Pathol 15**: 159-166,1991
40. Guerrieri C, Jarlsfelt I: Ependymoma of the ovary. A case report with immunohistochemical, ultrastructural, and DNA cytometric findings, as well as histogenetic considerations. **Am J Surg Pathol 17**: 623-632, 1993
41. Healey EA, Barnes PD, Kupsky WJ, et al: The prognostic significance of postoperative residual tumor in ependymoma. **Neurosurgery 28**:666-671, 1991
42. Ho KL: Abnormal cilia in a fourth ventricular ependymoma. **Acta Neuropathol 70**:30-37, 1986
43. Ho KL: Concurrence of subependymoma and heterotopic leptomeningeal neuroglial tissue. **Arch Pathol Lab Med 107**:136-140, 1983
44. Ho KL: Intercellular septate-like junction of neoplastic cells in myxopapillary ependymoma of the filum terminale. **Acta Neuropathol 79**:432-437, 1990
45. Ho KL: Microtubular aggregates within rough endoplasmic reticulum in myxopapillary ependymoma of the filum terminale. **Arch Pathol Lab Med 114**:956-960, 1990
46. Ho KL, Meyer G, Caya J, et al: Craniopharyngioma and "reactive" subependymoma of the third ventricle—a case report. **Clin Neuropathol 6**:12-15, 1987
47. Hope DG, Mulvihill JJ: Malignancy in neurofibromatosis. **Adv Neurol 29**:33-56, 1981
48. Ilgren EB, Stiller CA, Hughes JT, et al: Ependymo-

mas: a clinical and pathologic study. Part I. Biologic features. **Clin Neuropathol 3:**113-121, 1984
49. Ilgren EB, Stiller CA, Hughes JT, et al: Ependymomas: a clinical and pathologic study. Part II. Survival features. **Clin Neuropathol 3:**122-127, 1984
50. Kaneko Y, Takeshita I, Matushima T, et al: Immunohistochemical study of ependymal neoplasms: histological subtypes and glial and epithelial characteristics. **Virchows Arch [A] 417:**97-103, 1990
51. Karamitopoulou E, Perentes E, Diamantis I: P53 protein expression in central nervous system tumors: an immunohistochemical study with CM1 polyvalent and DO-7 monoclonal antibodies. **Acta Neuropathol 85:**611-616, 1993
52. Kawano N, Ito H, Yagishita S: Homer Wright rosettes in ependymoma. **J Neurooncol 11:**269-273, 1991
53. Kawano N, Yada K, Yagishita S: Clear cell ependymoma. A histological variant with diagnostic implications. **Virchows Arch [A] 415:**467-472, 1989
54. Kernohan JW, Fletcher-Kernohan EM: **Tumors of the Nervous System.** Baltimore, Md: Williams & Wilkins, 1937, pp 182-209
55. Kernohan JW, Woltman HW, Adson AW: Gliomas arising from the region of the cauda equina. Clinical, surgical and histologic considerations. **Arch Neurol Psychiatry 29:**287-307, 1933
56. Kernohan JW, Woltman HW, Adson AW: Gliomas of the cerebellopontine angle. **J Neuropathol Exp Neurol 7:**349-367, 1948
57. Kernohan JW, Woltman HW, Adson AW: Intramedullary tumors of the spinal cord. A review of fifty-one cases, with an attempt at histologic classification. **Arch Neurol Psychiatry 25:**679-701, 1931
58. Kimura T, Budka H, Soler-Federsppiel S: An immunocytochemical comparison of the glia-associated proteins glial fibrillary acidic protein (GFAP) and S-100 protein (S100P) in human brain tumors. **Clin Neuropathol 5:**21-27, 1986
59. King P, Cooper PN, Malcolm AJ: Soft tissue ependymoma: a report of three cases. **Histopathology 22:**394-396, 1993
60. Kirschstein RL, Gerber P: Ependymomas produced after intracerebral inoculation of SV40 into newborn hamsters. **Nature 195:**299-300, 1962
61. Kirschstein RL, Rabson AS, O'Conor GT: Ependymomas produced in Syrian hamsters by adenovirus 7 and SV40. **Proc Soc Exp Biol Med 120:**484-487, 1965
62. Kleihues P, Burger PC, Scheithauer BW: **Histological Typing of Tumours of the Central Nervous System, 2nd ed.** Berlin: Springer-Verlag, 1993
63. Kubota T, Ishise J, Yamashima T, et al: Abnormal cilia in a malignant ependymoma. **Acta Neuropathol 71:**100-105, 1986
64. Kuhlenbeck H: Neoplastic transformation of the subependymal cell plate in the floor of the fourth ventricle (subependymal spongioblastoma). With a clinicopathologic case report. **J Neuropathol Exp Neurol 6:**139-151, 1947
65. Lemberger A, Stein M, Doron J, et al: Sacrococcygeal extradural ependymoma. **Cancer 64:**1156-1159, 1989
66. Liu HM, Boogs J, Kidd J: Ependymomas in childhood. I. Histological survey and clinicopathological correlation. **Childs Brain 2:**92-110, 1976
67. London WT, Houff SA, Madden DL, et al: Brain tumors in owl monkeys inoculated with a human polyomavirus (JC virus). **Science 201:**1246-1249, 1978
68. Lorentzen M, Hägerstrand I: Congenital ependymoblastoma. **Acta Neuropathol 49:**71-74, 1980
69. Louis DN, Hedley-Whyte ET, Martuza RL: Sarcomatous proliferation of the vasculature in a subependymoma. **Acta Neuropathol 78:**332-335, 1989
70. Mallory FB: Three gliomata of ependymal origin: two in the fourth ventricle, one subcutaneous over the coccyx. **J Med Res 8:**1-11, 1902
71. Mannoji H, Becker LE: Ependymal and choroid plexus tumors. Cytokeratin and GFAP expression. **Cancer 61:**1377-1385, 1988
72. Marchadour FL, Pasquier B: Subcutaneous sacrococcygeal ependymoma with incidental glomus coccygeum. **Histopathology 18:**570-572, 1991
73. Marks JE, Adler SJ: A comparative study of ependymomas by site of origin. **Int J Radiat Oncol Biol Phys 8:**37-43, 1982
74. Maruyama R, Koga K, Nakahara T, et al: Cerebral myxopapillary ependymoma. **Hum Pathol 23:**960-962, 1992
75. Mathews T, Moossy J: Gliomas containing bone and cartilage. **J Neuropathol Exp Neurol 33:**456-471, 1974
76. McCloskey JJ, Parker JC Jr, Brooks WH, et al: Melanin as a component of cerebral gliomas. The melanotic cerebral ependymoma. **Cancer 37:**2373-2379, 1976
77. Metzger AK, Sheffield VC, Duyk G, et al: Identification of a germ-line mutation in the p53 gene in a patient with an intracranial ependymoma. **Proc Natl Acad Sci 88:**7825-7829, 1991
78. Miller C: The ultrastructure of the conus medullaris and filum terminale. **J Comp Neurol 132:**547-566, 1968
79. Mork SJ, Loken AC: Ependymoma. A follow-up study of 101 cases. **Cancer 40:**907-915, 1977
80. Mørk SJ, Rubinstein LJ: Ependymoblastoma. A reappraisal of a rare embryonal tumor. **Cancer 55:**1536-1542, 1985
81. Moss TH: Observations on the nature of subependymoma: an electron microscopic study. **Neuropathol Appl Neurobiol 10:**63-75, 1984
82. Murphy MN, Dhalla SS, Diocee M, et al: Congenital ependymoblastoma presenting as a sacrococcygeal mass in a newborn: an immunohistochemical, light and electron microscopic study. **Clin Neuropathol 6:**169-173, 1987
83. Nakamura Y, Becker LE, Marks A: Distribution of immunoreactive S-100 protein in pediatric brain tumors. **J Neuropathol Exp Neurol 42:**136-145, 1983
84. Nobles E, Lee R, Kircher T: Mediastinal ependymoma. **Hum Pathol 22:**94-96, 1991
85. Ohgaki H, Eibl RH, Wiestler OD, et al: P53 mutations in nonastrocytic human brain tumors. **Cancer Res 51:**6202-6205, 1991
86. Rabson AS, O'Conor GT, Kirschstein RL, et al: Papil-

lary ependymomas produced in *Rattus (Mastomys) natalensis* inoculated with vacuolating virus (SV40). **J Natl Cancer Inst 29**:765-787, 1962

87. Ransom DT, Ritland SR, Kimmel DW, et al: Cytogenetic and loss of heterozygosity studies in ependymomas, pilocytic astrocytomas, and oligodendrogliomas. **Genes Chromosome Cancer 5**:348-356, 1992
88. Rawlings CE III, Giangaspero F, Burger PC, et al: Ependymomas: a clinicopathologic study. **Surg Neurol 29**:271-281, 1988
89. Rawlinson DG, Herman MM, Rubinstein LJ: The fine structure of a myxopapillary ependymoma of the filum terminale. **Acta Neuropathol 25**:1-13, 1973
90. Rawlinson DG, Rubinstein LJ, Herman MM: In vitro characteristics of a myxopapillary ependymoma of the filum terminale maintained in tissue and organ culture systems. Light and electron microscopic observations. **Acta Neuropathol 27**:185-200, 1974
91. Roessmann U, Velasco ME, Sindely SD, et al: Glial fibrillary acidic protein (GFAP) in ependymal cells during development. An immunocytochemical study. **Brain Res 200**:13-21, 1980
92. Rorke LB, Gilles FH, Davis RL, et al: Revision of the World Health Organization classification of brain tumors for childhood brain tumors. **Cancer 56**:1869-1886, 1985
93. Rosenblum MK, Erlandson RA, Aleksic SN, et al: Melanotic ependymoma and subependymoma. **Am J Surg Pathol 14**:729-736, 1990
94. Ross DA, McKeever PE, Sandler HM, et al: Myxopapillary ependymoma. Results of nucleolar organizing region staining. **Cancer 71**:3114-3118, 1993
95. Ross GW, Rubinstein LJ: Lack of histopathological correlation of malignant ependymomas with postoperative survival. **J Neurosurg 70**:31-36, 1989
96. Rubinstein LJ: Cytogenesis and differentiation of primitive central neuroepithelial tumors. **J Neuropathol Exp Neurol 31**:7-26, 1972
97. Rubinstein LJ: The definition of ependymoblastoma. **Arch Path 90**:35-45, 1970
98. Russell DS, Rubinstein LJ: **Pathology of Tumours of the Nervous System.** London: Edward Arnold, 1959
99. Sainati L, Montaldi A, Putti MC, et al: Cytogenetic t(11;17)(q 13;21) in a pediatric ependymoma. Is 11q13 a recurring breakpoint in ependymomas? **Cancer Genet Cytogenet 59**:213-216, 1992
100. Sarkar C, Roy S, Tandon PN: Primitive neuroectodermal tumours of the central nervous system—an electron microscopic and immunohistochemical study. **Indian J Med Res 90**:91-102, 1989
101. Sato H, Ohmura K, Mizushima M, et al: Myxopapillary ependymoma of the lateral ventricle. A study on the mechanism of its stromal myxoid change. **Acta Pathol Jpn 33**:1017-1025, 1983
102. Sawyer JR, Crowson ML, Roloson GJ, et al: Involvement of the short arm of chromosome 1 in a myxopapillary ependymoma. **Cancer Genet Cytogenet 54**:55-60, 1991
103. Scheinker IM: Subependymoma: a newly recognized tumor of subependymal derivation. **J Neurosurg 2**:232-240, 1945
104. Scheithauer BW: Symptomatic subependymoma. **J Neurosurg 49**:689-696, 1978
105. Schiffer D, Chiò A, Cravioto H, et al: Ependymoma: internal correlations among pathological signs: the anaplastic variant. **Neurosurgery 29**:206-210, 1991
106. Schiffer D, Chiò A, Giordana MT, et al: Histologic prognostic factors in ependymoma. **Childs Nerv Syst 7**:177-182, 1991
107. Schröder R, Ploner C, Ernestus RI: The growth potential of ependymomas with varying grades of malignancy measured by the Ki-67 labelling index and mitotic index. **Neurosurg Rev 16**:145-150, 1993
108. Shuangshoti S, Panyathanya R: Ependymomas. A study of 45 cases. **Dis Nerv Syst 34**:307-314, 1973
109. Shuman RM, Alvord EC Jr, Leech RW: The biology of childhood ependymomas. **Arch Neurol 32**:731-739, 1975
110. Shyn PB, Campbell GA, Guinto FC Jr, et al: Primary intracranial ependymoblastoma presenting as spinal cord compression due to metastasis. **Childs Nerv Syst 2**:323-325, 1986
111. Slooff JL, Kernohan JW, MacCarty CS: **Primary Intramedullary Tumors of the Spinal Cord and Filum Terminale.** Philadelphia, Pa: WB Saunders, 1964
112. Sonneland PRL, Scheithauer BW, Onofrio BM: Myxopapillary ependymoma. A clinicopathologic and immunocytochemical study of 77 cases. **Cancer 56**:883-893, 1985
113. Specht CS, Smith TW, DeGirolami U, et al: Myxopapillary ependymoma of the filum terminale. A light and electron microscopic study. **Cancer 58**: 310-317, 1986
114. Störch H: Ueber die path.-anat. Vorgange am Stutzgerust des Centralnervensystems. **Virchows Arch 157**:127-171, 197-234, 1899
115. Stroebe H: Ueber Entstehung und Bau der Gehirngliome. **Beit Pathol Anat Allg Pathol 18**: 405-486, 1895
116. Sutton LN, Goldwein J, Perilongo G, et al: Prognostic factors in childhood ependymomas. **Pediatr Neurosurg 16**:57-65, 1990-1991
117. Tabuchi K, Moriya Y, Furuta T, et al: S-100 protein in human glial tumours. Qualitative and quantitative studies. **Acta Neurochir 65**:239-251, 1982
118. Tani E, Higashi N: Intercellular junctions in human ependymomas. **Acta Neuropathol 22**:295-304, 1972
119. Tarlov IM: Structure of the filum terminale. **Arch Neurol Psychiatry 40**:1-17, 1938
120. Tomlinson FH, Scheithauer BW, Kelly PJ, et al: Subependymoma with rhabdomyosarcomatous differentiation: report of a case and literature review. **Neurosurgery 28**:761-768, 1991
121. Vagner-Capodano AM, Gentet JC, Gambarelli D, et al: Cytogenetic studies in 45 pediatric brain tumors. **Pediatr Hematol Oncol 9**:223-235, 1992
122. Vaquero J, Heffero J, Cabezudo JM, et al: Symptomatic subependymomas of the lateral ventricles. **Acta Neurochir 53**:99-105, 1980
123. Virchow R: **Die Krankhaften Geschulste.** Berlin: August Hirschwald, 1864-1865
124. Wada C, Kurata A, Hirose R, et al: Primary leptomeningeal ependymoblastoma. Case report. **J Neurosurg 64**:968-973, 1986

125. Warnick RE, Raisanen J, Adornato BT, et al: Intracranial myxopapillary ependymoma: case report. **J Neurooncol 15:**251-256, 1993
126. Wechsler W: Elektronenmikroskopischer beitrag zur Differenzierung des Ependyms am Rückenmark von Hühnerembryonen. **Z Zellforsch 74:**423-442, 1966
127. Weremowicz S, Kupsky WJ, Morton CC, et al: Cytogenetic evidence for a chromosome 22 tumor suppressor gene in ependymoma. **Cancer Genet Cytogenet 61:**193-196, 1992
128. West CR, Bruce DA, Duffner PK: Ependymomas. Factors in clinical and diagnostic staging. **Cancer 56:**1812-1816, 1985
129. Willis RA: **Pathology of Tumors, 2nd ed.** London: Butterworth, 1953
130. Winston K, Gilles FH, Leviton A, et al: Cerebellar gliomas in children. **J Natl Cancer Inst 58:**833-838, 1977
131. Woltman HW, Kernohan JW, Adson AW, et al: Intramedullary tumors of the spinal cord and gliomas of intradural portion of filum terminale. Fate of patients who have these tumors. **Arch Neurol Psychiatry 65:**378-395, 1951
132. Zimmer C, Gottschalk J, Goebel S, et al: Melanoma-associated antigens in tumours of the nervous system: an immunohistochemical study with the monoclonal antibody HMB-45. **Virchows Arch [A] 420:** 121-126, 1992

CHAPTER 6

THE PATHOLOGY OF GANGLION CELL TUMORS

MAHLON D. JOHNSON, MD, PHD

GANGLION CELL TUMORS

As a group, ganglion cell tumors include central nervous system (CNS) neoplasms with differentiated neurons and a variable, neoplastic glial component. The majority of these tumors fall within a spectrum from gangliocytomas to gangliogliomas.[41] Gangliocytomas are populated predominantly by mature neurons with a minimal glial component. Along this continuum, gangliogliomas contain a variable neuronal component, which can be quite limited; hence, in some areas, gangliogliomas may resemble a pure astrocytoma (for an excellent discussion see Russell and Rubinstein[41] and Burger et al[4]). In most series, ganglion cell tumors represent 0.3% or 0.4% of intracranial tumors;[5,49] however, an incidence of 1.2% to 7.6% has been observed in children.[23,42] Although predominantly neoplasms of the temporal lobe, ganglion cell tumors can arise anywhere in the CNS including the cerebral hemispheres, third and fourth ventricles, hypothalamus, pineal region, thalamus, cerebellum, brain stem, spinal cord, and optic nerve.[1,3,9-11,14,16,23,24,34,36,42,45] The majority of ganglion cell tumors are circumscribed, often cystic, tumors.[4,41] Focal calcification is also common.[4,9,24,41]

The diagnosis of ganglion cell tumor is contingent on recognition of neoplastic differentiated neurons, which must be distinguished from their entrapped normal counterparts.[4,41] In contrast to normal neurons, neoplastic ganglion cells exhibit a lack of appropriate orientation and uneven spacing in the cortex. The dysplastic neurons of varying shape often occur in irregular clusters (Figure 1A). Lobular organization and heterotopic location in white matter all suggest a diagnosis of ganglion cell tumor. In addition, the cytological features of ganglion cells (i.e., irregular or bizarre cytological configurations, disorganized orientation of axons and dendrites, and binucleation) differentiate neoplastic cells from normal neurons (Figure 1B). Occasionally, immature neuroblasts may accompany other more mature counterparts.[4,41] Traditionally, Nissl and silver impregnation stains have been utilized to establish the neuronal identity of dysplastic cells. However, immunohistochemical analysis with antibodies against neuron-associated epitopes now facilitates this recognition, as described below. In many tumors, the presence of atypical neurons is apparent; however, they may be obscured by the prominent neoplastic astrocytic component, microcysts, or reticulin and collagen deposition.[4,41] Neoplastic astrocytes constitute a variable proportion of the neoplasm in gangliogliomas. In some areas of these tumors, the astrocytic component may dominate the histological appearance suggesting a diagnosis of astrocytoma. Interestingly, cytological atypia within the glial component may not portend

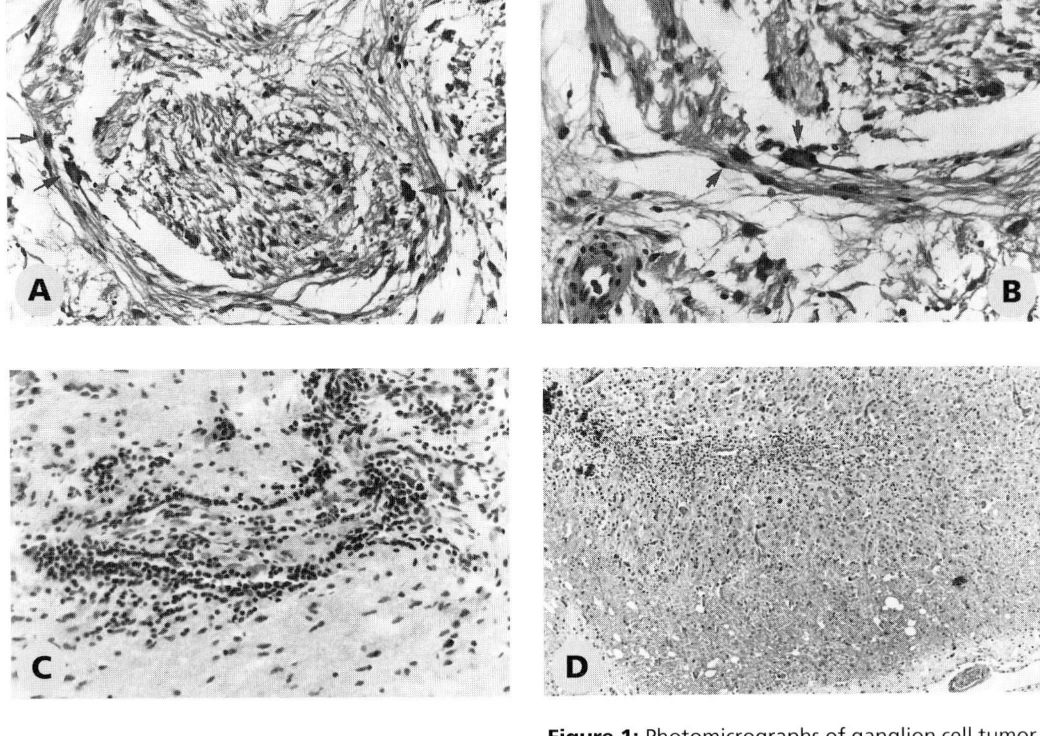

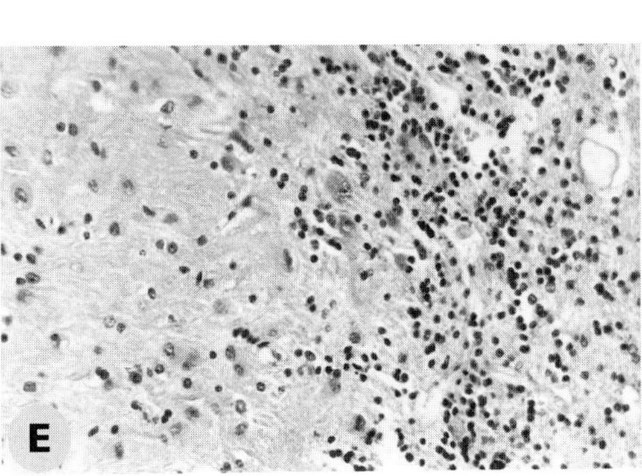

Figure 1: Photomicrographs of ganglion cell tumor. **A)** Disoriented clusters of dysplastic neurons *(arrows)* are a striking histological feature of ganglion cell tumors. **B)** Bizzare or binucleate ganglion cells *(arrows)* are of diagnostic importance. **C)** Perivascular lymphocytic infiltrates may be prominent in ganglion cell tumors. **D)** The dysplastic gangliocytoma of the cerebellum in Lhermitte-Duclos disease exhibits an expanded molecular layer and reduced granular cell layer. **E)** Abnormal neurons resembling Purkinje cells replace much of the granular cell layer. (Nissl, original magnification × 160 [A], × 240 [B]; hematoxylin-eosin, original magnification × 240 [C and E], × 60 [D])

the same poor prognosis that such features predict when associated with astrocytomas.[23,24] Neoplastic astrocytes with prominent nucleoli and variable processes reminiscent of ganglion cells can be identified, at least in some cases, through use of glial fibrillary acidic protein (GFAP) immunohistochemistry. Another histological characteristic of gangliogliomas is the prominent fibroblastic component associated with extensive reticulin deposition. The presence of mild perivascular lymphocytic infiltrates and telangiectatic blood vessels complete the classic histological pattern of a ganglioglioma (Figure 1C).[4,41]

Immunohistochemical studies with antibodies against a variety of neuronal epitopes facilitates identification of differentiating neurons among collections of dysplastic cells (Table 1). The presence of the neurofilament epitopes in ganglion cell tumors is well established. Synaptophysin immunoreactivity is also considered a marker for ganglion cell tumors.[31] These differentiated neurons have also been shown to contain chromogranin A and the neuropeptides met-enkephalin, neurotensin, vasoactive intestinal polypeptide, and the catecholaminergic marker tyrosine hydroxylase.[4,15,18,22,25,31,41]

Ultrastructural analysis can facilitate the di-

TABLE 1
GANGLION CELL TUMOR IMMUNOREACTIVITY*

Glial fibrillary acidic protein
Neurofilament[32]
Synaptophysin[31]
Chromagranin A[22]
Neuropeptides
Met-enkephalin[18,22]
Neurotensin[15]
Vasoactive intestinal polypeptide[15]
Tyrosine hydroxylase[25]

*Partial list with reference citations.

agnosis of ganglion cell tumor. In contrast to normal neurons with a few dense core granules, neoplastic ganglion cells frequently contain numerous granules in their cytoplasm.[39,40]

A notable, albeit rare, variant of a gangliocytoma can be seen in the dysplastic gangliocytoma of the cerebellum seen in Lhermitte-Duclos disease. This focal expansion of cerebellar folia produces a mass lesion with both neoplastic and malformative features.[38,41] The abnormally thickened folia possess a broad molecular layer and diminished granular layer populated by hypertrophic granule cells reminiscent of Purkinje cells (Figure 1D and 1E).[38,41]

GANGLION CELL VARIANTS

Desmoplastic Infantile Ganglioglioma

The desmoplastic infantile ganglioglioma (DIG) has recently been identified as a unique clinicopathological entity of importance to neurosurgeons. This tumor is encountered in infants at a median age of 4 months and mean age of 6 months, with both males and females at equal risk.[35,43-45] Characteristically, these are "massive" supratentorial tumors which, in over 60% of cases, involve more than one lobe.[35] Most arise from the parietal lobe, with fewer originating in the frontal, and rarely, occipital lobes (see the excellent review by VandenBerg).[44]

Desmoplastic infantile gangliogliomas arise superficially, infiltrating the leptomeninges and often the dura;[35,43-45] however, overt extension to the ventricles is not a characteristic.[4,35,43,44] Grossly, DIGs are multicystic and firm due to the desmoplasia.[35] Infiltrating borders may obscure the interface between these tumors and surrounding brain.[4,35,43,44]

Desmoplasia dominates the light microscopic appearance of DIGs. Fibroblastic cells and attendant pericellular stroma composed primarily of collagen types III, IV, and VIII but also types I and VI[4,35,45] often produce a storiform pattern (Figure 2A). As expected, special stains demonstrate dense reticulin deposition. Neoplastic astrocytes represent the predominant neuroepithelial cell type and appear more prominent in densely desmoplastic areas of the tumor.[35] Hence, astrocytes may induce the desmoplastic response (Figure 2B).[35] Within this stroma, GFAP-positive astrocytes may appear polygonal or elongated.[35]

Intermingled with the desmoplastic areas are more pleomorphic, differentiated cells with variable expanded cytoplasm. By special stains and immunohistochemical examination, these are shown to be differentiating neurons. However, definite ganglion cells may be lacking in a small sample.[45] Moreover, neuronal differentiation may be apparent only after use of immunohistochemistry or silver stains.[43,44] Hence, the ganglion cell component of this tumor can be obscure. Because neuronal antigens have been detected in other glial tumors such as giant cell and anaplastic astrocytomas, they should be interpreted within the histological context of the glioma.[2,43,44] Nonetheless, the absence of necrosis, endothelial proliferation, and significant mitotic activity in DIGs usually facilitates their differentiation from malignant gliomas.[4,35,45]

Several immunohistochemical studies have revealed the cellular distribution of glial and neuronal epitopes within neoplastic cells of DIGs. GFAP and S100 protein immunoreactivity have been demonstrated in both spindle and pleomorphic cells of this tumor. Neuronal markers, particularly neuron-specific enolase (NSE), 200 kD neurofilament, synaptophysin, and beta tubulin, have been demonstrated primarily in pleomorphic cells. Interestingly, muscle actin has also been identified in spindle cells.[44]

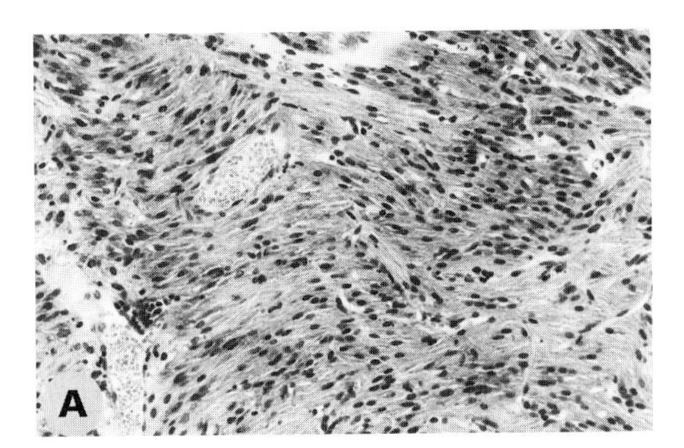

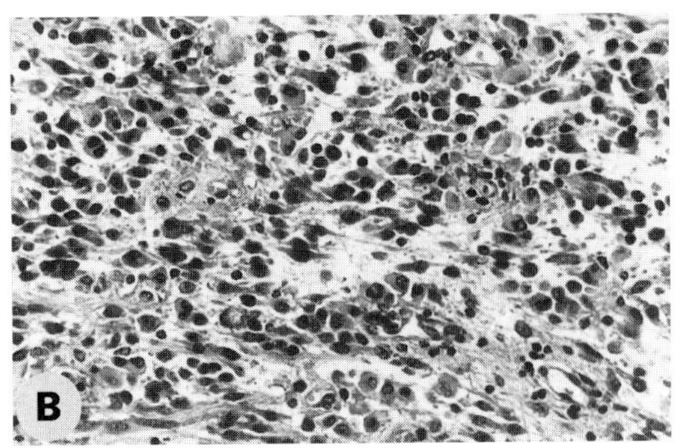

Figure 2: Desmoplastic infantile ganglioglioma. **A)** Fibroblasts and elongated astrocytes associated with a dense extracellular matrix may dominate areas of this tumor. **B)** Primitive neuroepithelial cells may be present in desmoplastic areas of the tumor. (hematoxylin-eosin, original magnification × 240)

The differential diagnosis for DIGs includes desmoplastic cerebral astrocytomas of infancy and gliofibromas.[44] Desmoplastic cerebral astrocytomas of infancy arise in an essentially identical patient population and location as DIGs. Like DIGs, the histology of these tumors is dominated by desmoplasia. However, these tumors lack the ganglion and primitive cells that are prominent in DIGs.[8,13,28] Likewise, gliofibromas (which arise in young adults) contain astrocytes, a more marked fibroblastic component, and no ganglion cells.[19,44]

Neurocytoma

The central neurocytoma was originally described by Hassoun et al[19] in 1982 as a discrete interventricular tumor histologically mimicking an oligodendroglioma or clear cell ependymoma. Since then, numerous cases have been described delineating a relatively distinct clinicopathological entity (see review by Hassoun et al[20]). Central neurocytomas present primarily in the second or third decades of life with an equal predilection for males and females.[19,20] The vast majority of these intraventricular tumors arise in the anterior half of the lateral ventricle (twice as commonly on the left), attached to the septum pellucidum adjacent to the foramen of Monro. Central neurocytomas have also been identified in the retina, corpus callosum, hypothalamus, and spinal cord.[19,20,30] These tend to be circumscribed, calcified tumors.

Histologically, central neurocytomas resemble oligodendrogliomas or clear cell ependymomas. Cellular areas of the tumor appear "monotonous" due to the sheets or linear arrays of small round nuclei, surrounded by perinuclear halos or minimal eosinophilic cytoplasm (Figure 3A).[19,20] Fortunately, "clear cells" (i.e., those with perinuclear halos) usually constitute only a fraction of the tumor (Figure 3B and D).[19,20] Anuclear fibrillary zones represent a variable pattern in central neurocytomas which, when intercalated between cellular zones, may mimic the large rosettes of a pineocytoma (Figure 3C); however, true Homer Wright rosettes are rare.[20] The round or oval nuclei of neurocytomas exhibit a fine nuclear pattern with variable nucleoli.[19,20] Delicate capillaries, perhaps less conspicuous than seen in oligodendrogliomas, are also present.[20,27]

Focal necrosis, mitotic activity, and endothelial proliferation are not typically seen in central neurocytomas although they have been reported in four tumors designated "anaplastic."[20,48] Two patients received radiation therapy. Follow-up revealed no evidence of recurrence at up to 4 years, suggesting that anaplastic features may not portend aggressive behavior.[48] Rare neurocytomas have recurred 18 or 38 months after resection.[48] Fortunately, 37 months after reoperation and radiotherapy, one patient was tumor-free.[48] Thus, recurrence of neurocytomas appears rare. Histological evaluation of these tumors revealed no mitotic activity, necrosis, or evidence of anaplasia that might predict recurrence.[48] However, it has been suggested that those tumors with a growth fraction of greater

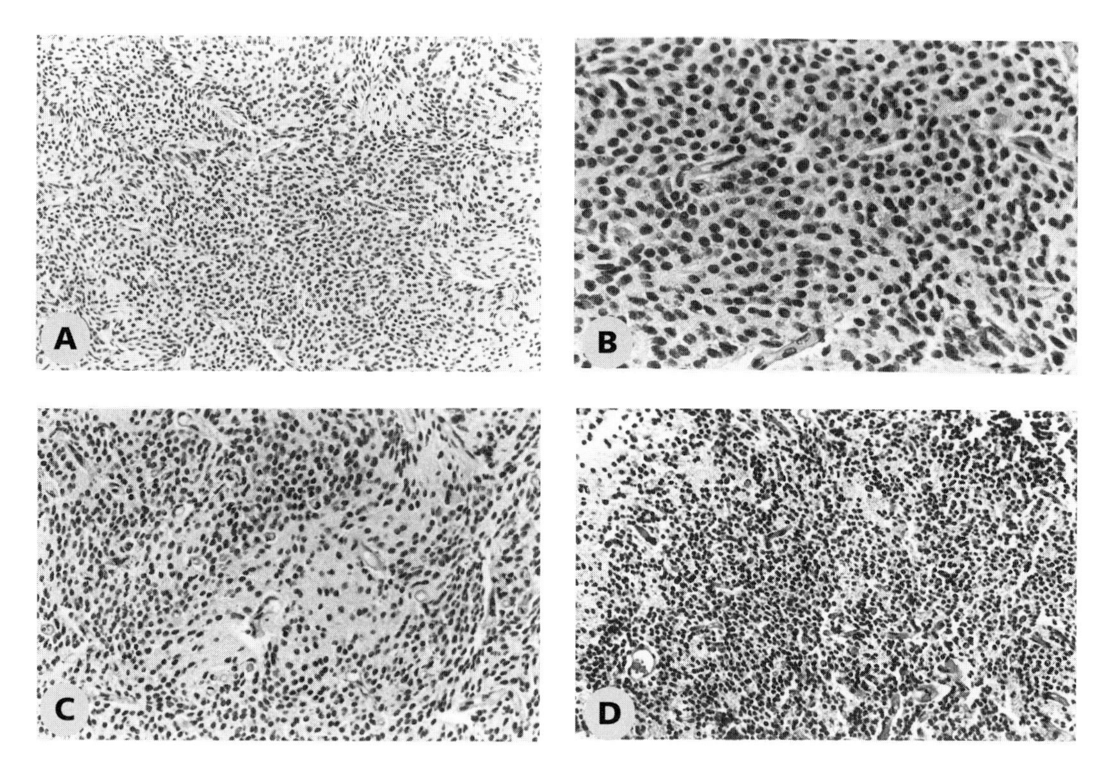

Figure 3: Central neurocytoma. **A)** Cellular uniformity is one of the histological features of neurocytomas. **B)** Round uniform nuclei in a fibrillar background are characteristic. **C)** Fibrillary zones may be prominent in some areas of the tumor. **D)** Perinuclear halos and fine capillaries may mimic the histological appearance of an oligodendroglioma. (hematoxylin-eosin, original magnification × 160 [A], × 240 [B to D])

than 2% may be more likely to recur.[20] Thus, occasional neurocytomas may exhibit more aggressive growth characteristics than are typically associated with this benign tumor.

Numerous proteins associated with neuronal differentiation have been demonstrated immunohistochemically in central neurocytomas (Table 2).[19,20,27,30,48] At present, detection of synaptophysin immunoreactivity, using commercially available antibodies, may be the most practical and reliable immunohistochemical test for neuronal differentiation.[12,17,21,26,29,33,46,47] Fortunately, some cases exhibiting no synaptophysin immunoreactivity contain other neuronal antigens. Unfortunately, these tumors also express extensive GFAP, S100 protein, and Leu-7 immunoreactivity, which is also expressed in ependymomas and oligodendrogliomas. Hence, identification of these glial markers in neurocytomas may be of little diagnostic value. Although subtle perivascular rosettes in neurocytomas may mimic the appearance in ependymomas, these structures are reportedly devoid of GFAP.

The definitive diagnosis of neurocytomas is typically made by electron microscopy. Neurocytomas exhibit neuronal differentiation with neuritic processes containing dense core secretory granules and microtubules. Their presence differentiates these tumors from ependymomas and oligodendrogliomas.[4,20,41]

The differential diagnosis for neurocytoma includes ependymoma and oligodendroglioma. Neurocytoma cell association with blood vessels may mimic the perivascular pseudorosettes of ependymomas. Moreover, perinuclear halos occur in "clear cell" ependymomas. Nonetheless, the perivascular anuclear zones in neurocytomas are often less pronounced than are those of ependymomas. Central neurocytomas should also express neural antigens such as synaptophysin, but none or little of the GFAP immunoreactivity seen in ependymomas.[19,26,46,47] Likewise, ultrastructural features such as

TABLE 2
CENTRAL NEUROCYTOMA IMMUNOREACTIVITY*

Marker	Immuno-reactivity	References
Glial proteins		
Glial fibrillary acidic protein	+	46,47
	–	19,26
S100 protein	+	12,26
	–	29,33
Myelin basic protein	–	26,33
Leu-7	+	12,26
Neuronal proteins		
Neuron-specific enolase	+	12,46
	+	21,47
Neurofilament	–	27,12
Synapsin	+	47
Synaptophysin	+	46,47
Neuron-associated b-tubulin	+	21
Tau 2	+	21
Calcineurin	+	17
Microtubule-associated protein-2	+	17,21
Vasopressin	+	29

*Partial list.

neurosecretory granules and absence of cilia help differentiate central neurocytomas from ependymomas.[20] Similarly, neurocytomas typically exhibit less prominent perinuclear halos, an absence of endothelial proliferation, and absence of myelin on electron microscopy, facilitating differentiation from an oligodendroglioma. Unfortunately, Leu-7 immunoreactivity described in oligodendrogliomas is present in neurocytomas as well.[12,26]

Dysembryoplastic Neuroepithelial Tumor

The dysembryoplastic neuroepithelial tumor (DNT) represents another recently defined distinct clinicopathological entity with ganglionic differentiation. Its recognition is particularly important in view of its benignity and tendency to mimic more aggressive tumors such as oligoastrocytomas.

DNTs are encountered in patients with longstanding partial complex seizures, often present since early childhood.[6,7,37] The mean age of presentation is 9 years, with a range of 1 to 19 years of age.[6,7,37] The majority of these tumors (approximately 62%) occur in the temporal lobe, although occurrence in the frontal lobe (31%) and parieto-occipital lobes was also noted in the original series.[7] At least one-third of patients exhibit radiographic evidence of cranial deformities (see the excellent review by Daumas-Duport[6]).

Grossly, DNTs involve and often expand the cortex, which may render the gray matter pale.[6,7] Calcification is detected in approximately one-quarter of cases.[7,37]

Histologically, these tumors resemble oligodendrogliomas or mixed oligoastrocytomas; however, they occur in gray matter or near the gray-white junction. The multinodular architecture and microcysts in DNTs produce a distinctive low-magnification appearance (Figure 4A). Higher magnification reveals the cellular heterogeneity of DNTs. The principal histological feature of simple DNTs is the "specific glioneuronal element" characterized by an alveolar or columnar pattern perpendicular to the cortical surface with oligodendrocytes accompanied by scattered neurons and astrocytes in a background of eosinophilic interstitial fluid (Figure 4B).[7] Capillaries also run throughout the element and variable numbers of neoplastic oligodendrocytes may be seen in the adjacent cortex.[7]

Complex DNTs have "specific glioneuronal elements" but also nodular oligodendroglial or astrocytic components. Nodular "oligodendrocytic components" contain round or voluminous oligodendrocyte nuclei with perinuclear halos in a solid or microcystic background (Figure 4C). Nodular "astrocytic components" often mimicking pilocytic astrocytoma may be solid or microcystic.[6,7] Areas of cortical dysplasia with loss of normal cortical lamination and neuronal atypia are also prevalent in complex DNTs (Figure 4D). Associated hamartomatous blood vessels have also been described.[7] Usually, the distinct clinical history, radiographic appearance, intercortical location, and multinodular multicystic appearance with glioneuronal elements are sufficient to make a diagnosis. However, immunohistochemical demonstration of neuronal antigens in the putative neurons populating nodular or cystic areas may facilitate the diagnosis.

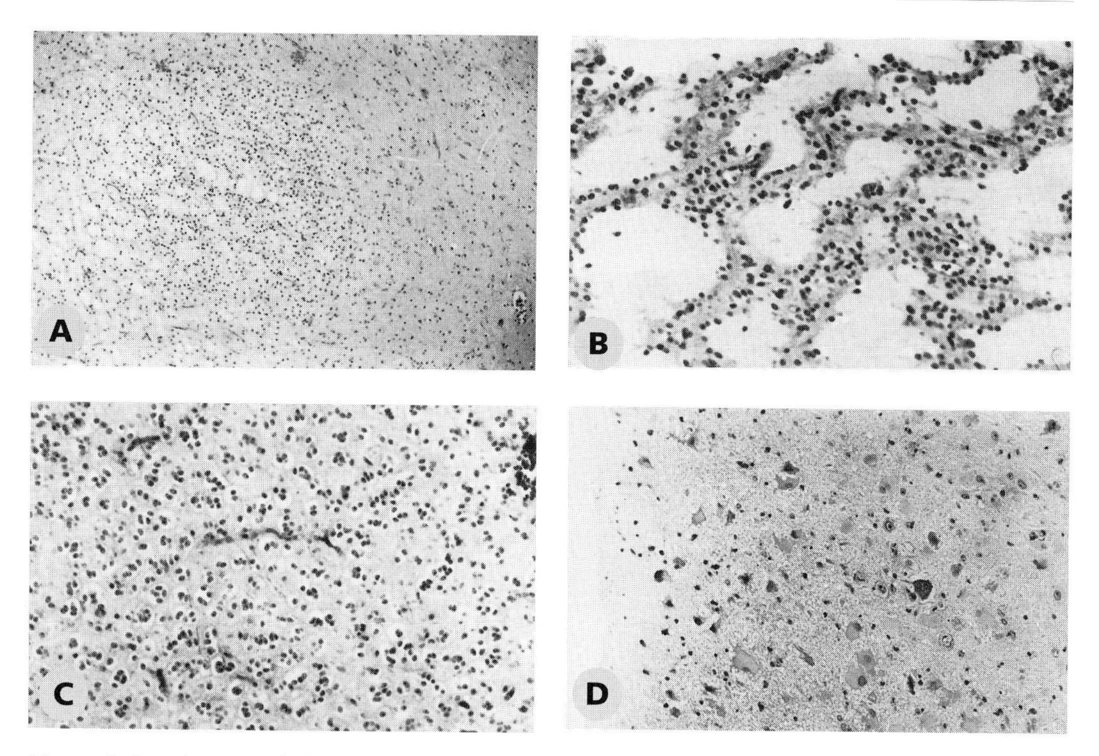

Figure 4: Complex DNT. **A)** The glial elements may impart a nodularity to this tumor. **B)** "Specific glioneuronal elements" often exhibit an alveolar pattern. **C)** Oligodendroglial elements may mimic an oligodendroglioma. **D)** Cortical dysplasia, with local disorganization of cortical lamination and slightly dysplastic neurons, can be seen adjacent to the tumor. (hematoxylin-eosin, original magnification × 160 [A and C], × 240 [B and D])

The differential diagnosis includes oligoastrocytoma and ganglioglioma.[12,29] In small, unrepresentative samples, complex DNTs might also resemble oligodendrogliomas or astrocytomas.[7] A history of long-standing partial complex seizures, radiographic evidence of overlying bone defects, intracortical location, nodularity, cortical dysplasia, and paucity of cytological atypia help to distinguish DNTs from oligoastrocytomas. However, one should be cognizant that nodular foci may be encountered in oligoastrocytomas and oligodendrogliomas. Moreover, infiltration of overlying cortex by oligoastrocytomas may suggest an intracortical origin.[6,7] DNTs lack the fine arcuate capillary pattern of oligodendrogliomas. Moreover, DNTs are also associated with cortical dysplasia. Anaplasia, endothelial proliferation, mitotic activity, and necrosis are not features of these neoplasms. In contrast to other ganglion cell tumors, neuronal atypia is not significant.[12,29,33] Differentiation from gangliogliomas should be facilitated by recognition of the multinodular architectural pattern, absence of bizarre ganglion cells, absence of fibrous stroma, and perivascular lymphocytic cuffing in DNTs.[6,7]

Conclusion

Seminal papers over the last 12 years have expanded the classification of benign neuroepithelial tumors with neuronal differentiation to include entities such as DIGs, neurocytomas, and DNTs. Knowledge of their clinical, radiographic, and pathological characteristics should facilitate early diagnosis, differentiation from higher-grade gliomas, and optimal neurosurgical management.

References

1. Bevilacqua G, Sarnelli R: Ganglioglioma of the spinal cord. A case with a long survival. **Acta Neuropathol 48**:239-242, 1979

2. Bonnin JM, Rubinstein LJ, Papasozomenos SC, et al: Subependymal giant cell astrocytoma. Significance and possible cytogenetic implications of an immunohistochemical study. **Acta Neuropathol 62:** 185-193, 1984
3. Burchiel KJ, Shaw CM, Kelly WA: A mixed functional microadenoma and ganglioneuroma of the pituitary fossa. Case report. **J Neurosurg 58:** 416-420, 1983
4. Burger PC, Scheithauer BW, Vogel FS: **Surgical Pathology of the Nervous System and Its Coverings, 3rd ed.** New York: Churchill Livingstone, 1991
5. Cushing H: **Notes Upon a Series of 2000 Verified Cases with Surgical-Mortality Percentages Pertaining Thereto.** Springfield, Ill: Charles C Thomas, 1932, pp 9-68
6. Daumas-Duport C: Dysembryoplastic neuroepithelial tumour. **Brain Pathol 3:**283-295, 1993
7. Daumas-Duport C, Scheithauer BW, Chodkiewicz JP, et al: Dysembryoplastic neuroepithelial tumor: a surgically curable tumor of young patients with intractable partial seizures. Report of 39 cases. **Neurosurgery 23:**545-556, 1988
8. De Chadarévian J-P, Pattisapu JV, Faerber EN: Desmoplastic cerebral astrocytoma of infancy. Light microscopy, immunocytochemistry and ultrastructure. **Cancer 66:**173-179, 1990
9. Demierre B, Stichnoth FA, Hori A, et al: Intracerebral ganglioglioma. **J Neurosurg 65:**177-182, 1986
10. Doyle JB, Kernohan JW: Ganglioneuroma of the third ventricle with diabetes insipidus and hypopituitarism. **J Nerv Ment Dis 73:**55-61, 1931
11. Epstein N, Epstein F, Allen JC, et al: Intractable facial pain associated with a ganglioglioma of the cervicomedullary junction: report of a case. **Neurosurgery 10:**612-616, 1982
12. Figarella-Branger D, Pellissier JF, Daumas-Duport C, et al: Central neurocytomas. Critical evaluation of a small-cell neuronal tumour. **Am J Surg Pathol 16:**97-109, 1992
13. Fried RL: Gliofibroma. A peculiar neoplasia of collagen forming glia-like cells. **J Neuropathol Exp Neurol 62:**230-234, 1978
14. Garcia CA, McGarry PA, Collada M: Ganglioglioma of the brain stem. Case report. **J Neurosurg 60:** 431-434, 1984
15. Giangaspero F, Burger PC, Budwit DA, et al: Regulatory peptides in neuronal neoplasms of the central nervous system. **Clin Neuropathol 4:**111-115, 1985
16. Gondim-Oliveira JA, Choux M: Tumeurs du tronc cérébral chez l'enfant. **Neurobiologia 45:**167-180, 1982
17. Goto S, Nagahiro S, Ushio Y, et al: Immunocytochemical detection of calcineurin and microtubule-associated protein 2 in central neurocytoma. **J Neurooncol 16:**19-24, 1993
18. Gustin T, Bachelot T, Verna JMG, et al: Immunodetection of endogenous opioid peptides in human brain tumors and associated cyst fluids. **Cancer Res 53:**4715-4719, 1993
19. Hassoun J, Gambarelli D, Grisoli F, et al: Central neurocytoma. An electron-microscopic study of two cases. **Acta Neuropathol 56:**151-156, 1982
20. Hassoun J, Soylemezoglu F, Gambarelli D, et al: Central neurocytomas: a synopsis of clinical and histological features. **Brain Pathol 3:**297-306, 1993
21. Hessler RB, Lopes MBS, Frankfurter A, et al: Cytoskeletal immunohistochemistry of central neurocytomas. **Am J Surg Pathol 16:**1031-1038, 1992
22. Hirose T, Kannuki S, Nishida K, et al: Anaplastic ganglioglioma of the brain stem demonstrating active neurosecretory features of neoplastic neuronal cells. **Acta Neuropathol 83:**365-370, 1992
23. Johannsson JH, Rekate HL, Roessmann U: Gangliogliomas: pathological and clinical correlation. **J Neurosurg 54:**58-63, 1981
24. Kalyan-Raman UP, Olivero WC: Ganglioglioma: a correlative clinicopathological and radiological study of ten surgically treated cases with follow-up. **Neurosurgery 20:**428-433, 1987
25. Kawai K, Takahashi H, Ikuta F, et al: The occurrence of catecholamine neurons in a parietal lobe ganglioglioma. **Cancer 60:**1532-1536, 1987
26. Kubota T, Hayashi M, Kawano H, et al: Central neurocytoma: immunohistochemical and ultrastructural study. **Acta Neuropathol 81:**418-427, 1991
27. Louis DN, Swearingen B, Linggood RM, et al: Central nervous system neurocytoma and neuroblastoma in adults—report of eight cases. **J Neurooncol 9:**231-238, 1990
28. Louis DN, von Deimling A, Dickersin GR, et al: Desmoplastic cerebral astrocytomas of infancy: a histopathologic, immunohistochemical, ultrastructural, and molecular genetic study. **Hum Pathol 23:**1402-1409, 1992
29. Maguire JA, Bilbao JM, Kovacs K, et al: Hypothalamic neurocytoma with vasopressin immunoreactivity: immunohistochemical and ultrastructural observations. **Endocrine Pathol 3:**99-104, 1992
30. Metcalf C, Mele EM, McAllister I: Neurocytoma of the retina. **Br J Ophthalmol 77:**382-384, 1993
31. Miller DC, Koslow M, Budzilovich GN, et al: Synaptophysin: a sensitive and specific marker for ganglion cells in central nervous system neoplasms. **Hum Pathol 21:**271-276, 1990
32. Nakazato Y, Ishida Y, Tamura M: Immunohistochemical distribution of neurofilament protein in brain tumors: localization of phosphorylated and non-phosphorylated neurofilament epitope. **Brain Tumor Pathol 6:**61-67, 1989
33. Nishio S, Tashima T, Takeshita I, et al: Intraventricular neurocytoma: clinicopathological features of six cases. **J Neurosurg 68:**665-670, 1988
34. Packer RJ, Sutton LN, Rosenstock JG, et al: Pineal region tumors of childhood. **Pediatrics 74:**97-102, 1984
35. Paulus W, Schlote W, Perentes E, et al: Desmoplastic supratentorial neuroepithelial tumours of infancy. **Histopathology 21:**43-49, 1992
36. Ponzi S, Corgiolu E, Cocchini F, et al: Apporto diagnostico dell'esame otv nella pathologia espansiva del IV ventricolo. **Min Otorinolaringol 31:**411-416, 1981
37. Prayson RA, Estes ML: Dysembryoplastic neuroepithelial tumor. **Am J Clin Pathol 97:**398-401, 1992

38. Reznik M, Schoenen J: Lhermitte-Duclos disease. **Acta Neuropathol 59**:88-94, 1983
39. Robertson DM, Hendry WS, Vogel FS: Central ganglioneuroma: a case study using electron microscopy. **J Neuropathol Exp Neurol 23**: 692-705, 1964
40. Rubinstein LJ, Herman MM: A light- and electron-microscopic study of a temporal-lobe ganglioglioma. **J Neurol Sci 16**:27-48, 1972
41. Russell DS, Rubinstein LJ: **Pathology of Tumours of the Nervous System, 5th ed.** Baltimore, Md: Williams & Wilkins, 1989, pp 289-306
42. Sutton LN, Packer RJ, Rorke LB, et al: Cerebral gangliogliomas during childhood. **Neurosurgery 13**:124-130, 1983
43. VandenBerg SR: Desmoplastic infantile ganglioglioma: a clinicopathologic review of sixteen cases. **Brain Tumor Pathol 8**:25-31, 1991
44. VandenBerg SR: Desmoplastic infantile ganglioglioma and desmoplastic astrocytoma of infancy. **Brain Pathol 3**:275-281, 1993
45. VandenBerg SR, May EE, Rubinstein LJ, et al: Desmoplastic supratentorial neuroepithelial tumors of infancy with divergent differentiation potential ("desmoplastic infantile gangliogliomas"). Report of 11 cases of a distinctive embryonal tumor with favorable prognosis. **J Neurosurg 66**:58-71, 1987
46. von Deimling A, Janzer R, Kleihues P, et al: Patterns of differentiation in central neurocytoma. An immunohistochemical study of eleven biopsies. **Acta Neuropathol 79**:473-479, 1990
47. von Deimling A, Kleihues P, Saremaslani P, et al: Histogenesis and differentiation potential of central neurocytomas. **Lab Invest 64**:585-591, 1991
48. Yasargil MG, von Ammon K, von Deimling A, et al: Central neurocytoma: histopathological variants and therapeutic approaches. **J Neurosurg 76**:32-37, 1992
49. Zülch KJ: **Atlas of Gross Neurosurgical Pathology**. Berlin: Springer-Verlag, 1975, pp 49-50

CHAPTER 7

PATTERNS OF TUMOR GROWTH AND PROBLEMS ASSOCIATED WITH HISTOLOGICAL TYPING OF LOW-GRADE GLIOMAS

CATHERINE DAUMAS-DUPORT, MD, PHD

The definition of benign gliomas and criteria used to distinguish them from their malignant counterparts remain subjects of controversy. By definition, only histological categories of glial neoplasms that naturally behave as a slow-growing process, that are resectable, and that do not recur after surgical removal should be considered benign. For the neurosurgeon confronted with therapeutic decisions, a suitable classification scheme of gliomas should provide an adequate answer to the following major questions: is the tumor resectable without a resultant deficit, will the tumor recur after surgery, and is adjuvant aggressive radio- and/or chemotherapy indicated?

Current conventional histological classification schemes of gliomas based on the predominant cell type and histoprognostic evaluation according to cell differentiation and/or nonspecific morphological features (such as cell density and mitotic activity) are quite easy to apply and satisfactory, at least for the pathologist. Unfortunately, they do not provide accurate identification of benign tumors; in addition, they are of little help in surgical decision-making for several reasons. 1) The term "low-grade glioma" is indiscriminately applied to tumors that, in fact, possess highly variable growth potential including tumors with slow and constant growth, such as pilocytic astrocytomas; tumors that may become more malignant with time, such as low-grade "ordinary" astrocytomas; and tumors that may behave as carcinologically stable lesions, such as cerebellar astrocytomas in children. 2) The growth pattern of gliomas, solid or infiltrative, is not taken into consideration in conventional routine histological interpretation. This aspect of the pathology of gliomas is, however, crucial in regard to surgical decision-making. 3) Conventional classification schemes of gliomas are based on tumors in adults and are inadequate for the characterization of a large proportion of glial tumors in children. 4) The problems of classification are also related to a long tradition of brain tumor assessment in which histology is commonly considered sufficient by itself for predicting the growth potential of gliomas.

The first part of this chapter focuses on the growth patterns of gliomas which, with the advent of imaging-based serial stereotactic biopsies, can now safely be explored in vivo. It will be shown that assessment of the structure type provides a better interpretation of imaging data and useful information for planning therapy. Next is described how the simple distinction between two patterns of tumor growth, solid or infiltrative, can provide a more accurate identi-

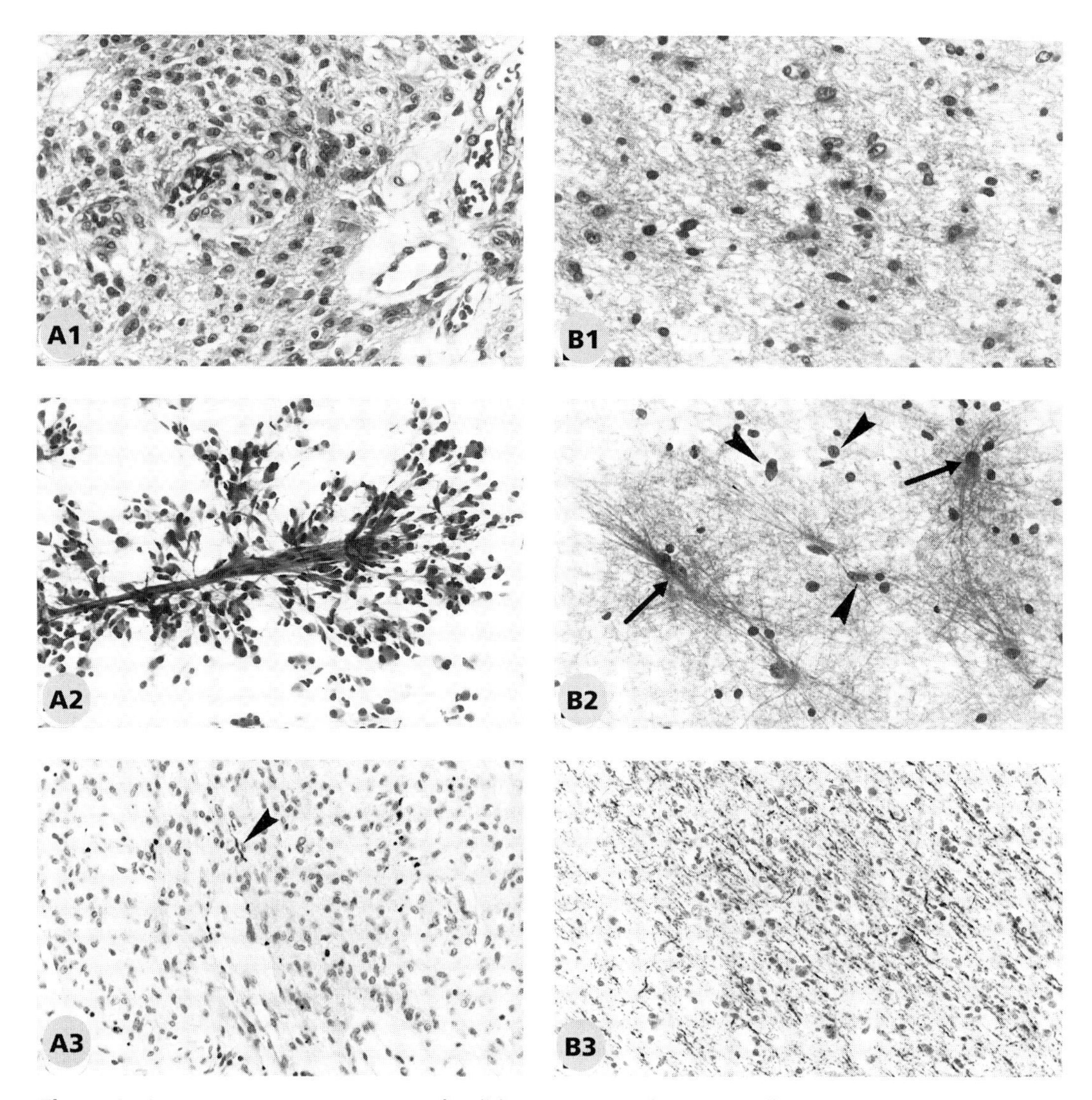

Figure 1: Astrocytoma structure type II. **A)** Solid tumor tissue. The tumor cells are crowded, possess cell processes (A2), and are associated with neovascularity (A1). Neurofilament (NF) immunostaining demonstrates a few residual axons (A3, *arrowhead*). **B)** Isolated tumor cells in white matter. The tumor cells (B1 and B2, *arrowheads*) show nuclear abnormalities and lack visible cytoplasm, the appearance being that of "naked nuclei" cells (B2). Isolated tumor cells are associated with reactive astrocytes (B2, *arrows*). Parenchyma is architecturally intact, as demonstrated by NF immunostaining (B3). Edema accompanies permeation by isolated tumor cells (B1). (hemalun-phloxine-safranin stain, original magnification × 250 [A1 and B1]; smear preparations, hemalun-phloxine, original magnification × 150 [A2], × 250 [B2]; NF immunostaining, original magnification × 200 [A3 and B3])

fication of pilocytic astrocytomas and avoid the common misdiagnosis of low-grade infiltrative oligodendrogliomas as fibrillary astrocytomas.

The second part of this chapter deals with the new concept of a dysembryoplastic neuroepithelial tumor (DNT) and its impact on the histological typing of glial tumors in children. It is shown that the categories of DNT cover a large spectrum of glial neoplasms and may histologically resemble any form of low- or high-grade gliomas but, in fact, are stable lesions. It will be stressed that, particularly in children, identification of indolent tumors and their distinction from slow-growing or malignant gliomas requires that histological, clinical, and radiological data be simultaneously taken into consideration.

Growth Pattern of Gliomas

Histological Assessment

Two distinct growth patterns are encountered in gliomas:[13,16] 1) Solid tumor tissue. In this element, tumor cells are crowded and are unaccompanied by intervening normal brain parenchyma. The tumor tissue proper possesses newly formed microscopic blood vessels (Figure 1A). 2) Isolated tumor cells (ITCs). In this tumor component, the tumor cells are not in contact with each other but permeate largely intact brain parenchyma. This pattern is not accompanied by neovascularity. The presence of ITCs is usually associated with edema (Figure 1B). These patterns of growth are easily identified on smear preparations, which preserve the entire cell and distinguish ITCs from the background parenchyma (Figures 1 and 2). It is thus recommended that smears be used in addition to paraffin-embedded sections.

In astrocytomas, the tumor tissue is predominantly composed of cells that possess visible cytoplasm and cell processes (Figure 1A), whereas ITCs usually lack visible cytoplasm, giving the appearance of "naked nuclei." Such individual tumor cells can be identified because of their distinct nuclear abnormalities; the lack of visible cytoplasm permits their differentiation from reactive astrocytes (Figure 1B). Similarly, in oligodendrogliomas, as is described later, the tumor tissue is composed of cells with a visible round cytoplasm, often showing a characteristic fried-egg appearance, whereas isolated tumoral oligodendrocytes often lack visible cytoplasm (Figure 2).

Structural Classification of Gliomas

The existence of two distinct growth patterns, solid or infiltrative, is the basis for the following structural classification of gliomas:[13,16] structure type I, solid tumor tissue only and no peripheral ITCs; structure type II, solid tumor tissue and peripheral ITCs; and structure type III, ITCs within intact brain parenchyma and no solid tumor tissue. According to our three-part classification scheme of gliomas, the structural type is indicated to complement the histological type and degree of malignancy. For example, a given neoplasm will be diagnosed as an oligodendroglioma grade 2, structure type III. The purpose of this architectural classification of gliomas is not to predict survival, but to provide a guide for surgical decision-making. Accurate determination of the structural type of a glioma requires that data be obtained as demonstrated by computed tomography (CT) and/or magnetic resonance imaging (MRI) from each of the different components including neighboring normal brain parenchyma. The structural type can thus be best determined on imaging and serial stereotactic biopsies.[12,34,35]

For the purpose of this chapter, we have evaluated the distribution of the structural type in a recent series of 166 gliomas explored by stereotactic biopsy at our institution between the years 1988 and 1992. This series comprised cases for which adequate serial biopsy sampling could be safely obtained for assessing the structure of the tumor and included 12 pilocytic astrocytomas, 78 ordinary astrocytomas, 31 oligoastrocytomas, and 45 oligodendrogliomas. As shown in Table 1, our data suggest that nearly all ordinary astrocytomas exhibit a structure type II, whereas a structure type III is encountered only in oligodendrogliomas or oligoastrocytomas. According to our restrictive criteria (see above), pilocytic astrocytomas are structure type I tumors. The recent introduction of more accurate criteria for distinguishing infiltrative oligodendrogliomas from ordinary astrocytomas and DNTs from conventional categories of gliomas accounts for the marked differences in the distribution of the stuctural type of gliomas compared to our earlier studies.[11] Improved criteria in the typing of gliomas also make it apparent that, with few exceptions, structure type II corresponds to high-grade astrocytomas or high-grade oligodendrogliomas. In addition, our recent data suggest that low-grade astrocytomas are, in fact, uncommon. Based on our histological grading system,[17] among the 78 ordinary astrocytomas included in the present series, we found only two in grade 2; eight cases were diagnosed as grade 3, and 66 as grade 4.

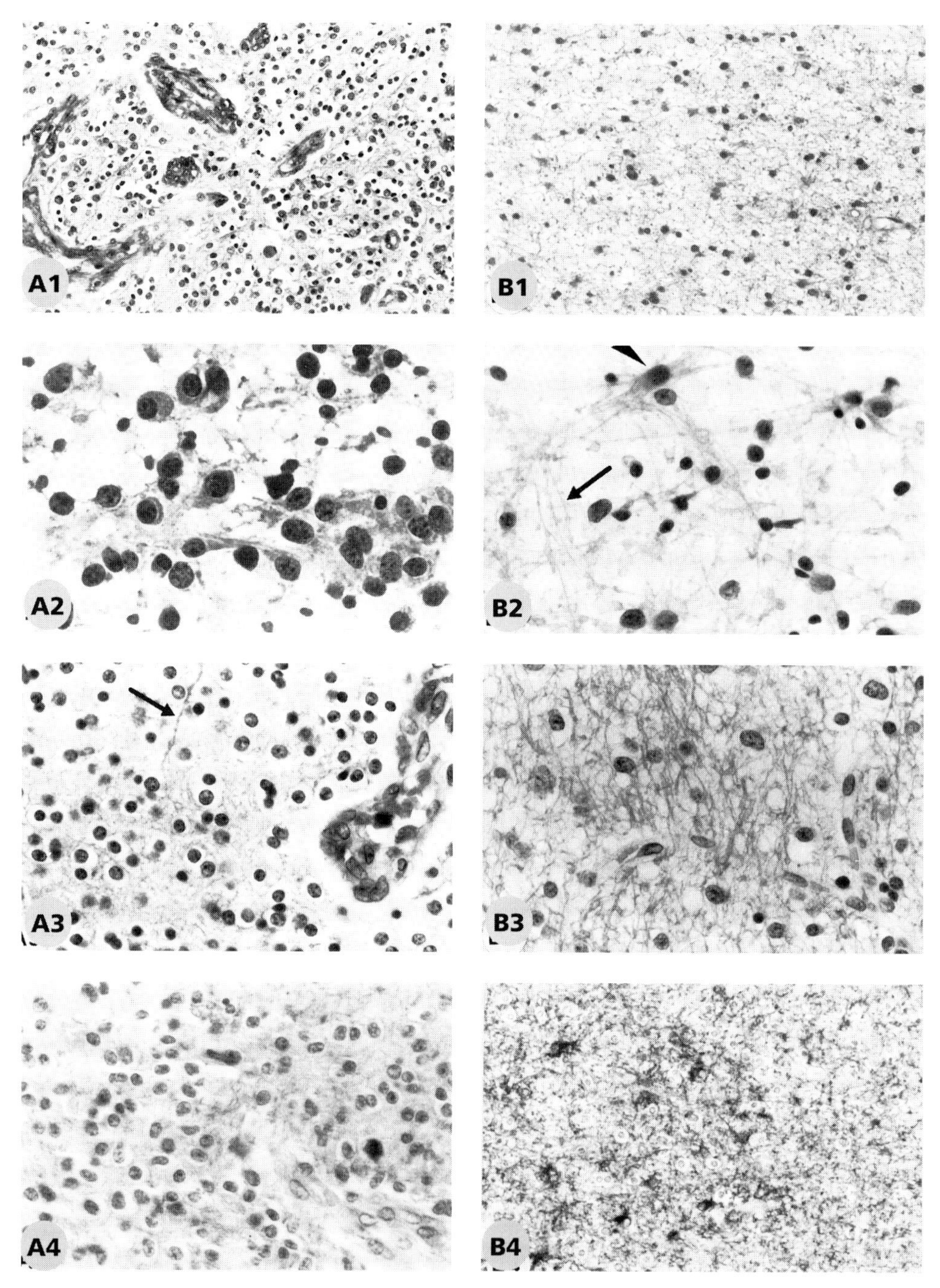

Figure 2: Oligodendroglioma structure type II. **A)** Tumor tissue. Smear preparations (A2) show that tumor cells possess a round cytoplasm.On paraffin-embedded section (A1), artifactual clearing of the cytoplasm gives the cells a characteristic "fried-egg" appearance. Tumor cells are associated with newly formed blood vessels (A1 and A3). Neurofilament (NF) immunostaining (A3) demonstrates only a few residual axons *(arrow)*. GFAP immunostaining (A4) shows only occasional positive tumor cells. **B)** Isolated tumor cell component. On the paraffin-embedded section (B1), this element has the appearance of a so-called "fibrillary astrocytoma." Smear preparations (B2) demonstrate that tumor cells lack visible cytoplasm and that the fibrillary frame is in fact made of axons *(arrow)* and of fibrillary reactive astrogliosis *(arrowhead)*. This is also apparent on NF (B3) and GFAP (B4) immunostaining. (paraffin sections, hemalun-phloxine-safranin, original magnification × 170 [A1 and B1]; smear preparations, hemalun-phloxine, original magnification × 300 [A2], × 250 [B2]; NF immunostaining, original magnification × 250 [A3 and B3]; GFAP immunostaining, original magnification × 250 [A4], × 170 [B4])

TABLE 1

TUMOR STRUCTURAL TYPE IN A SERIES OF 166 GLIOMAS EXPLORED BY SERIAL STEREOTACTIC BIOPSY*

Histological Diagnosis	No. of Tumors	Tumor Structural Type		
		I	II	III
Pilocytic astrocytoma	12	100%	0%	0%
Ordinary astrocytoma	78	1%	99%	0%
Oligoastrocytoma	31	0%	60%	40%
Oligodendroglioma	45	0%	31%	69%

*For a definition of tumor structural type see text.

Structural Types of Glioma and Imaging Correlations

There is a strong correlation between the degree of tumor microvascularity and contrast enhancement on CT[11,34,35] or MRI. Contrast enhancement depicts the solid tumor tissue, but usually does not occur in ITC components. This is explained by the fact that the solid tumor tissue possesses newly formed microscopic blood vessels whereas ITC components usually do not induce neovascularity. On the other hand, ITCs that infiltrate edematous parenchyma are shown as areas of hypodensity on CT or of hypersignal on T2-weighted MRI. Thus, a relationship is observed between the structural type of a glioma and its appearance on imaging. Contrast enhancement is always present in structure type I and in malignant gliomas with structure type II, but is absent in structure type III gliomas.[11,34,35]

Structural Types of Glioma and Surgical Decision-Making

The histological demarcation of gliomas into tumor tissue and infiltrated parenchyma is important therapeutically. Solid tumor tissue contains little or no residual brain parenchyma. This component can thus be destroyed without a resultant deficit. On the other hand, parenchyma infiltrated by ITCs is morphologically and functionally intact; thus, the area of parenchyma infiltrated by ITCs in important brain structures must not be damaged if the patient's neurological function is to be maintained.[7,13,34,35]

In structure type I gliomas, the tumor volume corresponds to the volume showing contrast enhancement on CT or MRI, and the limits of the tumor can thus be precisely estimated.[11,34,35] These tumors, comprising solid circumscribed tissue, can be entirely resected without a resultant deficit. Deep-seated tumors can also be treated by interstitial irradiation, which allows the destruction of a precise target volume.

In malignant structure type II gliomas, the extent of ITCs usually precludes complete surgical removal. Excision or selective radiosurgical destruction of the solid tumor tissue can theoretically be achieved in any location. Postoperative radiotherapy is the only available treatment for ITC components that cannot be removed. The microcirculation of ITC being that of the normal parenchyma, the intact blood-brain barrier in this element may explain, at least in part, the poor results reported for chemotherapy in high-grade structure type II gliomas.

In structure type III tumors, the extent of ITC infiltration also usually precludes complete surgical removal. Partial resection of these tumors, which occupy intact brain parenchyma, is of questionable benefit. On the other hand, the role of radiotherapy in low-grade infiltrative gliomas has not been clearly established.

PILOCYTIC ASTROCYTOMAS

Pilocytic astrocytomas are diagnosed mainly in children and show a distinct slow-growing behavior compared to ordinary astrocytomas. In these tumors, the histological criteria of

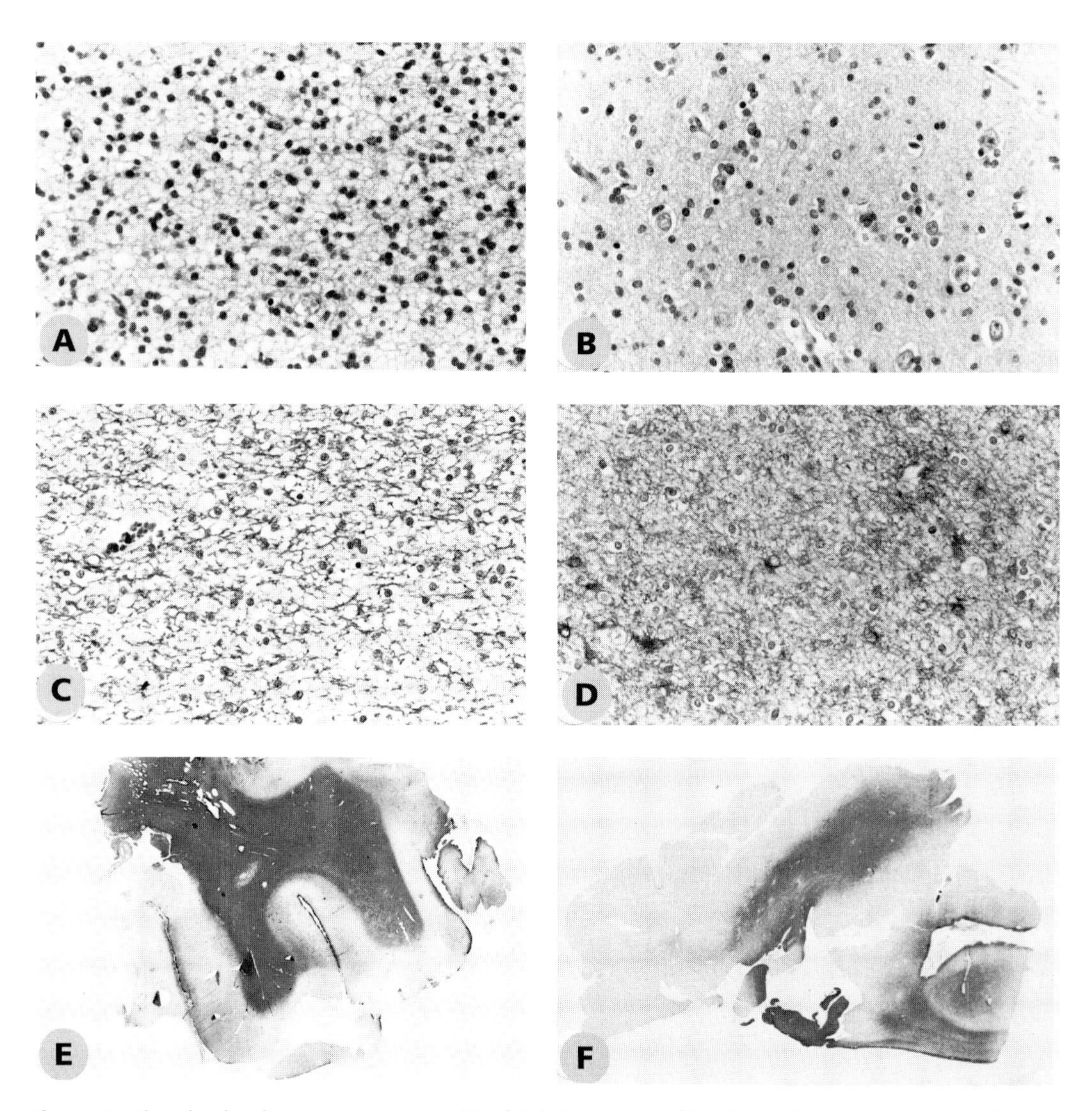

Figure 3: Oligodendroglioma structure type III. **A)** White matter infiltration with the appearance of "fibrillary astrocytoma." **B)** Cortex infiltrated by isolated tumoral oligodendrocytes. Note the absence of a fibrillary background. **(C** and **D)** As demonstrated by neurofilament (NF) (C) and GFAP (D) immunostaining, the fibrillary background in the white matter infiltrate is composed of axons and fibrillary reactive astrocytes. **E)** Area of GFAP positivity exactly delineates that of white matter. **F)** Changes in chronic epilepsy: GFAP demonstrates reactive gliosis of the white matter. Note that the pattern of GFAP positivity is identical to that of the oligodendroglioma structure type III under study. (hemalun-phloxine-safranin, original magnification × 170 [A and B]; NF immunostaining, original magnification × 170 [C]; GFAP immunostaining, original magnification × 170 [D], × 5 [E and F])

malignancy, such as the presence of nuclear atypia and endothelial proliferation, have no prognostic significance.[17,36,48,56] Accurate diagnosis and distinction of pilocytic astrocytomas from "ordinary" astrocytomas are thus of paramount importance in order to avoid over-grading these tumors and overtreatment of young patients.

Conventional histological classifications define pilocytic astrocytomas as tumors predominantly composed of bipolar fusiform piloid astrocytic cells.[36,49,56] However, malignant ordinary astrocytomas often contain fusiform astrocytes. Additionally, in certain structures (such as the brain stem and the corpus callosum) tumor cells of ordinary infiltrative astrocytomas, which are intermingled with parallel axons, may exhibit a bipolar pattern.[36] Cytological criteria are thus insufficient by themselves to establish the diagnosis of pilocytic astrocytoma. Together with cytological criteria, the pattern of tumor growth is important to consider in order to avoid misdiagnosis of these slow-growing neoplasms as ordinary astrocytomas. In fact, "true" pilocytic astrocytomas are of structure type I, being made up of a single solid tumor tissue element.[10,11]

Assessment of the pattern of growth is also useful in differentiating pilocytic astrocytomas from DNTs. The latter often contain pilocytic astrocytes (see below, Figures 6 and 7) but usually possess a distinct complex structure. Since DNTs are stable lesions whereas pilocytic astrocytomas are slow-growing tumors, it is obviously important from a therapeutic point of view to distinguish the two.

Being of structure type I, the volume of pilocytic astrocytomas can be accurately assessed on imaging, as it exactly corresponds to the area of contrast enhancement on CT or MRI.[11,34,36] These neoplasms, which contain only solid tumor tissue, can be entirely removed without a resultant deficit, even in eloquent brain structures.[34,40] When no residual contrast enhancement is seen on postoperative CT or MRI, radiotherapy is contraindicated.

OLIGODENDROGLIOMAS

Structural Types and Histological Diagnosis

Structure type III oligodendrogliomas (that is, oligodendrogliomas that consist only of ITCs infiltrating morphologically intact brain parenchyma) are traditionally misinterpreted as fibrillary astrocytomas for two reasons.[9,10] 1) Cytological criteria used for the diagnosis of oligodendrogliomas emphasize the characteristic fried-egg appearance of tumoral oligodendrocytes.[3,4,36,43] 2) Traditionally, in the histological assessment of gliomas, no consideration is given to identifying the pattern of tumor growth, whether solid or infiltrative.

As is apparent in Figure 2, which illustrates an example of oligodendroglioma structure type II, the tumor tissue and ITC components have a very different histological appearance. The solid tumor tissue (Figure 2A) shows the morphological features usually considered typical of oligodendrogliomas: on routine histological preparations (Figure 2A1), the tumor cells exhibit spherical nuclei surrounded by artifactually clear swollen cytoplasm; a well-defined plasma membrane gives a so-called "honeycomb" or "fried-egg" appearance. As seen in astrocytomas, the tumor tissue possesses newly formed microscopic blood vessels and contains no or only residual axons (Figure 2A3). In contrast, the infiltrative portion of the same tumor (Figure 2B1) exhibits the characteristic morphological appearance of the so-called "fibrillary astrocytoma": this tumoral element is described by the World Health Organization (WHO) classification of 1993[36] as showing "moderate density, the tumor cells have a scant and barely discernible cytoplasm and are scattered in a loose fibrillary matrix which consistently express GFAP" (glial fibrillary acidic protein). Accordingly, as the reader may see in Figure 35 of the WHO report, a tumor similar to this case of structure type II oligodendroglioma is given as an example of oligoastrocytoma.

As shown in Figure 2B, the fibrillary background seen in our example is in fact composed of axons and fibrillary astrogliosis of the white matter. Smear preparations, by distinguishing tumor cells from the background parenchyma, clearly demonstrate that the tumor cells, in fact, do not possess cell processes (Figure 2B2), and show that nuclei of the isolated tumor cells are identical to those seen in the solid tumor tissue: they are typically round and possess conspicuous dots of chromatin.

These observations concerning oligodendrogliomas with structure type II clearly explain why infiltrative oligodendrogliomas of structure type III are traditionally misinterpreted as fibrillary astrocytomas. In the example of a structure type III oligodendroglioma illustrated in Figure 3, the tumor infiltrated both the white matter (Figure 3A) and the cortex (Figure 3B). GFAP immunostaining shows that the area of GFAP positivity exactly delineates the white matter (Figure 3E), whereas the infiltrated cortex is GFAP-negative. This is because these slow-

TABLE 2
TUMOR STRUCTURAL TYPE AND HISTOLOGICAL GRADE IN 45 OLIGODENDROGLIOMAS EXPLORED BY SERIAL STEREOTACTIC BIOPSY*

	Tumor Structural Type		
Histological Grade	I	II	III
1	0	1	1
2	0	2	30
3	0	11	0
Totals	0	14 (31%)	31 (69%)

* Histological grade according to Daumas-Duport[9,10] (see text); for a definition of tumor structural type see text.

growing tumors induce a chronic fibrillary astrogliosis of the infiltrated white matter, whereas the protoplasmic astrocytes of the cortex do not show reactive changes. This pattern of gliosis is identical to that seen in other long-standing nontumoral disorders such as chronic epilepsy (see Figure 3F). In chronic astrogliosis, reactive fibrillary astrocytes lose the characteristic stellate appearance seen in acute reactive gliosis and form a continuous dense fibrillary network (Figure 3D).

Oligodendrogliomas are believed to be uncommon, accounting for 4% to 7% of intracranial gliomas.[3,22,42,43,49] Given that about two-thirds of oligodendrogliomas exhibit a structure type III (see Table 1) and are traditionally misinterpreted as fibrillary astrocytomas, and that structure type II oligodendrogliomas are often diagnosed as oligoastrocytomas, it is very likely that the actual incidence of these tumors is markedly underestimated. According to criteria in a recent series of 166 gliomas, oligodendrogliomas (45 cases) accounted for 27% of the total cases, ordinary astrocytomas for 57%, and oligoastrocytomas for 18%. At the time of diagnosis, the 45 patients harboring oligodendrogliomas ranged in age from 20 to 58 years, with one patient aged 70 years (mean 40 years).

Structural Types, Histological Grade, and Imaging Appearance

In Table 2, the 45 oligodendrogliomas in this study have been classified according to their structural type and histological grade of malignancy. The grading system currently used at our institution for grading oligodendrogliomas is based on recognition of three criteria: nuclear atypia, mitosis, and endothelial hyperplasia and/or endothelial proliferation. Similar to a system proposed for grading ordinary astrocytomas, the criteria are considered as present or absent. A summary of these criteria defines three grades as follows: no criterion, grade 1; one or two criteria (nuclear atypia and/or mitosis), grade 2; three criteria, grade 3.[9,10] In a preliminary study of 83 oligodendrogliomas, median survival times for each grade were estimated as follows: grade 2, 7.8 years; and grade 3, 2.2 years. The median survival time in nine patients with grade 1 oligodendrogliomas was more than 15 years (unpublished data).

Table 2 shows that, with few exceptions, oligodendrogliomas fell into two main categories, corresponding to grade 2 structure type III and grade 3 structure type II. As expected, these two categories have a distinct imaging appearance (see Table 3). Oligodendrogliomas grade 2 structure type III do not show contrast enhancement on CT or MRI. In oligodendrogliomas grade 3 structure type II contrast enhancement is seen in each patient undergoing MRI; however, in cases that show calcific hyperdensity, contrast enhancement may not be apparent on CT.

Slow-Growing Structure Type III Oligodendrogliomas

The median survival time of patients with oligodendroglioma grade 2 is about 8 years; thus, the oligodendroglioma grade 2 structure

TABLE 3

Imaging Appearance of Oligodendrogliomas Correlated with the Histological Grade and Structural Type*

Histological Grade & Structural Type	Calcific Hyperdensity	CT Contrast Enhancement	MRI Contrast Enhancement
Grade 2, III	10/30	0/30	0/11
Grade 3, II	5/11	5/11	6†/6

* For a definition of histological grade[9,10] and structural type see text.
† Two of these cases had calcific hyperdensity and no contrast enhancement on CT.

type III variant, defined by our system of classification, can be considered a slow-growing neoplasm. As will be detailed in a further publication, patients harboring infiltrative structure type III oligodendrogliomas have a similar clinical presentation, characterized by seizures with onset after 19 years of age and no neurological deficit. In addition, these slow-growing tumors have a characteristic appearance on imaging: they do not show contrast enhancement (Table 3) and, as best demonstrated on T2-weighted MRI, they involve both the cortex and the white matter and have a regular shape and sharply demarcated boundaries (see examples in Figure 4). Foci of calcific hyperdensity are seen inconstantly on CT scans, being encountered in one-third of the patients in this series (Table 3 and Figure 4B).

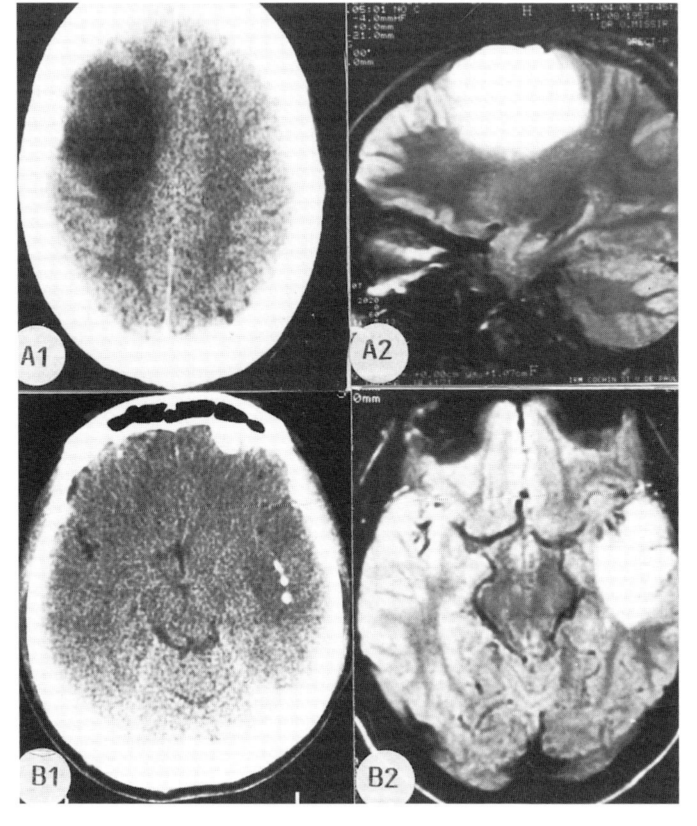

Figure 4: Imaging appearance of oligodendrogliomas grade 2 structure type III in two patients. **A)** In one patient, postcontrast CT (A1) of the tumor reveals an area of hypodensity . On T2-weighted MRI (A2) tumor involves the cortex and the white matter, and a well-demarcated hyperintensity signal is disclosed. **B)** In a second patient, CT without contrast enhancement (B1) shows calcific hyperdensity within an area of hypodensity. On T2-weighted MRI (B2), the appearance of the lesion is comparable to that seen in A2.

Does the area of hypersignal on T2-weighted MRI or hypodensity on CT depict the entire tumoral histological volume? This question is obviously of paramount importance from a therapeutic point of view. To investigate this problem, in patients who are explored by serial stereotactic biopsy at our institution biopsy tracks are chosen in order to obtain samples from both inside and outside the MRI lesional volume. Our preliminary results in five patients suggest that increased signal on T2-weighted MRI is equivalent to the histological volume; however, these results need confirmation in a larger series of patients.

Since the entire volume of structure type III oligodendrogliomas comprises morphologically and functionally intact brain parenchyma, the treatment of these slow-growing neoplasms is a challenging problem. In our experience, at time of first seizures, these tumors often occupy a large parenchymal volume and their location precludes complete surgical removal. This is likely explained by the fact that these slow-growing infiltrative lesions are well tolerated and remain asymptomatic for a long time.

The effectiveness of external beam irradiation in the treatment of these tumors has not yet been adequately investigated. Application of our criteria and comparison of survival times in retrospective series of patients who did or did not undergo external beam radiotherapy should determine if radiotherapy is effective in the treatment of low-grade structure type III oligodendrogliomas.

Dysembryoplastic Neuroepithelial Tumors

DNTs represent a recently defined category of brain tumors in young patients that histologically may resemble any form of benign or malignant gliomas, but, in fact, behave as stable lesions[7,8] Their distinction from a conventional form of glioma is thus of paramount importance in order to avoid undue aggressive radio- and/or chemotherapy in young patients with a normal life expectancy.

The different forms of DNT that we have identified to date were located in the supratentorial cortex. However, our ongoing studies indicate that DNTs may also originate in gray nuclei (in preparation). As discussed below, DNTs also arise in the subtentorial compartment.

The dysembryoplastic origin of DNTs has been inferred from the association of these tumors with foci of cortical dysplasia, the young age of patients at onset of first symptoms (as early as the first year of life), and the occurence of a bone deformity of the overlying skull. The generic term "dysembryoplastic neuroepithelial tumors" has been chosen in order that a large morphological spectrum of benign brain tumors of neuroepithelial derivation could be regrouped in this category.[15]

We have identified three different histological variants of DNTs: the "complex forms" and the "simple form": both possess specific histological features and nonspecific variants of DNT that cannot be histologically distinguished from conventional categories of gliomas.[7,8,15] These different morphological variants raise various problems in terms of histological diagnosis; it must be understood, however, that their distinction has no clinical or therapeutic implications. A summary of our previously published series of DNTs follows, which will show that the clinical presentation, tumor location, imaging appearance, and follow-up data are similar in each group.

These data will demonstrate that accurate diagnosis of supratentorial cortical DNTs requires that histological findings and clinical and imaging data be simultaneously considered. Independent of their histological appearance, glial tumors can be diagnosed as DNTs when all of the following criteria are present: 1) partial seizures with or without secondary generalization; 2) onset of seizures before 20 years of age; 3) no neurological deficit, or stable and likely congenital deficit such as quadrantanopsia; and 4) cortical location of the lesion on MRI.[7,8]

Complex Forms of DNTs

Definition of the complex forms of DNTs was prompted because, in the experience at our institution, conventional histological classifications were inadequate for the characterization of most glial tumors encountered among patients undergoing epilepsy surgery. It was observed that, despite a high polymorphism, certain tumors shared several features that clearly distinguished them from ordinary gliomas.[14,15] The features that characterize the "complex form" of DNTs are the following (Figures 5 and 6): 1) cortical location; 2) multinodular architecture with nodules being composed of multiple variants looking like astrocytomas, oligodendrogliomas, or oligo-astrocytomas (Figure 6D to I); 3) foci of dysplastic cortical disorganization (Figure 6C); and 4) presence of a particular element showing a columnar structure perpendicular to the cortical surface. This "specific glioneuronal element" of DNTs is composed of bundles of axons lined by small oligodendrocytes and of clearly visible neurons that seem to float within an interstitial fluid (Figure 6A and B).

A review of our histological files of epilepsy surgery performed between the years 1963 and 1984 has allowed us to identify 20 tumors that showed these morphological characteristics.[14] Nineteen further cases were collected on review of all supratentorial gliomas accumulated in the files of the Mayo Clinic.[15] In this series, clinical presentation and follow-up data were identical to those observed among Sainte-Anne Hospital cases, which allowed us to exclude the possibility that a clinical bias due to selection of patients for epilepsy surgery may be responsible for the uniform characteristics of these tumors.

In the revised WHO classification,[36] DNTs have been incorporated among the category of "neuronal and mixed neuronoglial tumors." However, this classification, which is based on our first restrictive histological criteria, permits recognition of only one of the multiple histological variants of DNTs.

Simple Form of DNTs with a Unique Glioneuronal Element

Identification of this morphological "simple" variant of DNT was further prompted by difficulties encountered in the diagnosis of DNTs explored by serial stereotactic biopsy. A series of 14 cases of simple DNTs treated at our institution between the years 1980 and 1989 were

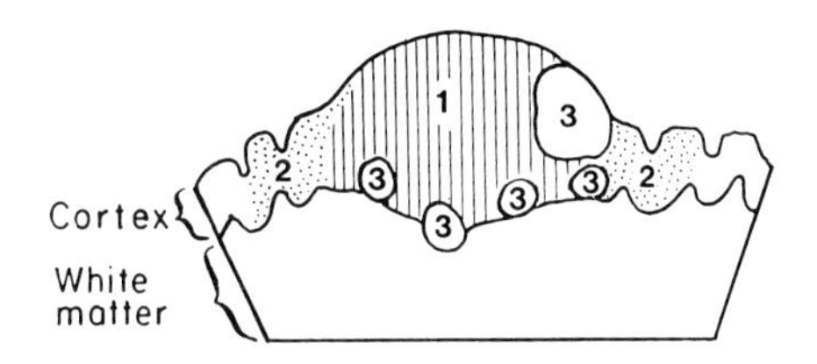

Figure 5: Schematic representation of complex forms of DNTs. 1 = a specific glioneuronal element; 2 = cortical dysplasia; and 3 = glial nodules.

studied. The presence of a unique glial element was confirmed in six of these patients who later benefited from epilepsy surgery. Clinical, imaging, and follow-up data in this series were similar to those found in the "complex forms." This study allowed demonstration that the spectrum of DNTs includes a simple form with a unique glioneuronal element.[7]

The following conclusions could be drawn: cortical tumors can be histologically diagnosed as DNTs and distinguished from conventional categories of gliomas if they possess a specific glioneuronal element (whether or not this element is related to glial nodules) or when glial nodules are associated with foci or cortical dysplasia.[7,8] Although the multinodular structure is a dominant characteristic of the complex forms of DNTs, a nodular pattern is occasionally encountered in ordinary gliomas. Nodules by themselves are thus insufficient for diagnosing DNTs.

Nonspecific Histological Forms of DNTs

In the series of patients surgically treated for long-standing seizures at our institution, the focus has been directed toward a remaining subset of glial tumors that did not show the morphological features that would allow for a diagnosis of complex or simple DNTs. Despite a strong feeling that conventional classifications were inadequate for characterization of the subset, it has not been possible to identify objective histological criteria to accurately distinguish them from ordinary gliomas. However, the study of a sample of 36 such cases again showed that clinical expression, tumor location, imag-

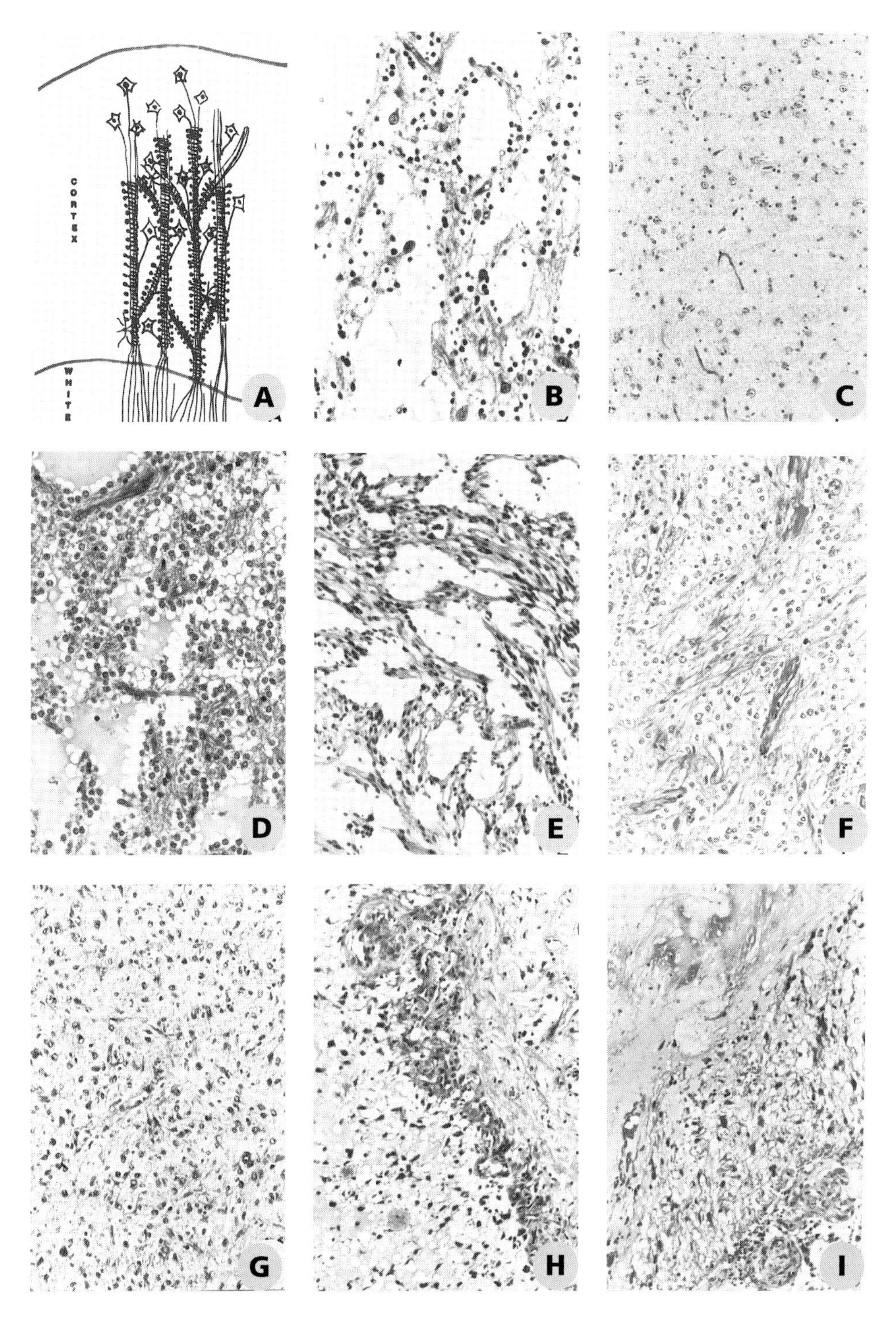

Figure 6: Histology of complex forms of DNTs. **A)** Schematic drawing of the glioneuronal element. Bundles of axons are attached by cell processes of small oligodendrocytes. At their proximal portion, neurons float within an interstitial fluid. This element contains scattered astrocytes. **B)** Specific glioneuronal element showing a columnar structure. **C)** Foci of cortical dysplasia with loss of lamination. **D-I)** Examples of some of the multiple glial components possibly seen in complex forms of DNTs: oligodendroglioma-like component (D); pilocytic astrocytoma-like element (E); oligoastrocytoma-like element (F); astrocytoma-like element (G); vascular arcades seen in a pilocytic element (H); foci of necrosis seen in a pilocytic component (I). (hemalun-phloxine-safranin, original magnification $\times$ 170 [B, F, and G], $\times$ 150 [C, E, H, and I], $\times$ 200 [D])

TABLE 4

SUPRATENTORIAL CORTICAL DNTs: CLINICAL PRESENTATION

Presentation	Complex Forms	Simple Form	Nonspecific Forms
No. of cases	39	14	36
Partial seizures	39	14	36
No neurological deficit	37	14	30
Quadrantanopsia	2	0	6
Age at onset of symptoms (yrs)	1-19 (mean 9)	2-17 (mean 9)	1-26* (mean 10)
Duration of seizures (yrs)	2-18 (mean 9)	2-19 (mean 9)	1-23 (mean 10)

*Only two patients were aged over 20 years.

ing appearance, and follow-up data were similar to those found in the "specific" forms of DNT.[8]

Tumors included in this group were histologically very heterogeneous. Their only common features were a more or less pronounced resemblance to conventional categories of gliomas and, when recognizable on surgical samples, a cortical location of the lesion. The following histological subdivisions only attempt to give an idea of the polymorphism of these lesions and of the range of misdiagnosis that may have resulted if histological criteria alone had been taken into consideration: the tumors resembled "ordinary astrocytomas" in 18 cases, pilocytic astrocytomas in seven cases, oligodendrogliomas in 10 cases, oligoastrocytomas in five cases; the remaining eight cases looked like atypical, unclassifiable gliomas (see examples in Figure 7). It is noteworthy that, just as in the complex form, nuclear abnormalities, mitosis, necrosis, and vascular proliferation could be seen in this group. By definition, these lesions did not show a specific glioneuronal element or an obvious multinodular pattern, but foci of cortical dysplasia were often observed. However, in the absence of other specific morphological features, foci of cortical dysplasia cannot be proposed as a diagnostic criterion of DNTs. Foci of cortical dysplasia may not be sampled or may be difficult to distinguish from secondary changes induced by the growth of ordinary gliomas.

In a recent review of our files of epilepsy surgery that included 93 cases of DNT, nearly half (48 cases) of the tumors were nonspecific variants.[8]

Supratentorial Cortical DNTs

Clinical Presentation

Table 4 summarizes clinical data in a previously published series of 39 complex, 14 simple, and 36 nonspecific forms of DNT, showing that clinical presentation in these different morphological variants are similar. All patients presented with partial seizures, with or without secondary generalization. In all but two patients, seizures occurred before the age of 20 years; the mean age at onset of symptoms was 9 or 10 years. In two patients harboring nonspecific forms of DNT, first seizures occurred at the age of 22 and 26 years. In a recent series of 12 complex forms of DNT used for imaging studies (see below), one patient had a late onset of seizures at age 38 years.[7] Thus, atypical clinical presentation may occasionally be encountered.

Patients harboring DNTs usually have no neurological deficit. A visual defect was found on neurological examination in seven (8%) of the 89 cases under study. Ignored by the patient, this neurological deficit was likely to be congenital. No patient and none of the families had stigmata of phacomatosis.

Tumor Location

Table 5 shows that DNTs may be encountered in any part of the supratentorial cortex. In the series under study, a majority of complex or nonspecific forms of DNT (51% and 72%, respectively) were located in the temporal lobe,

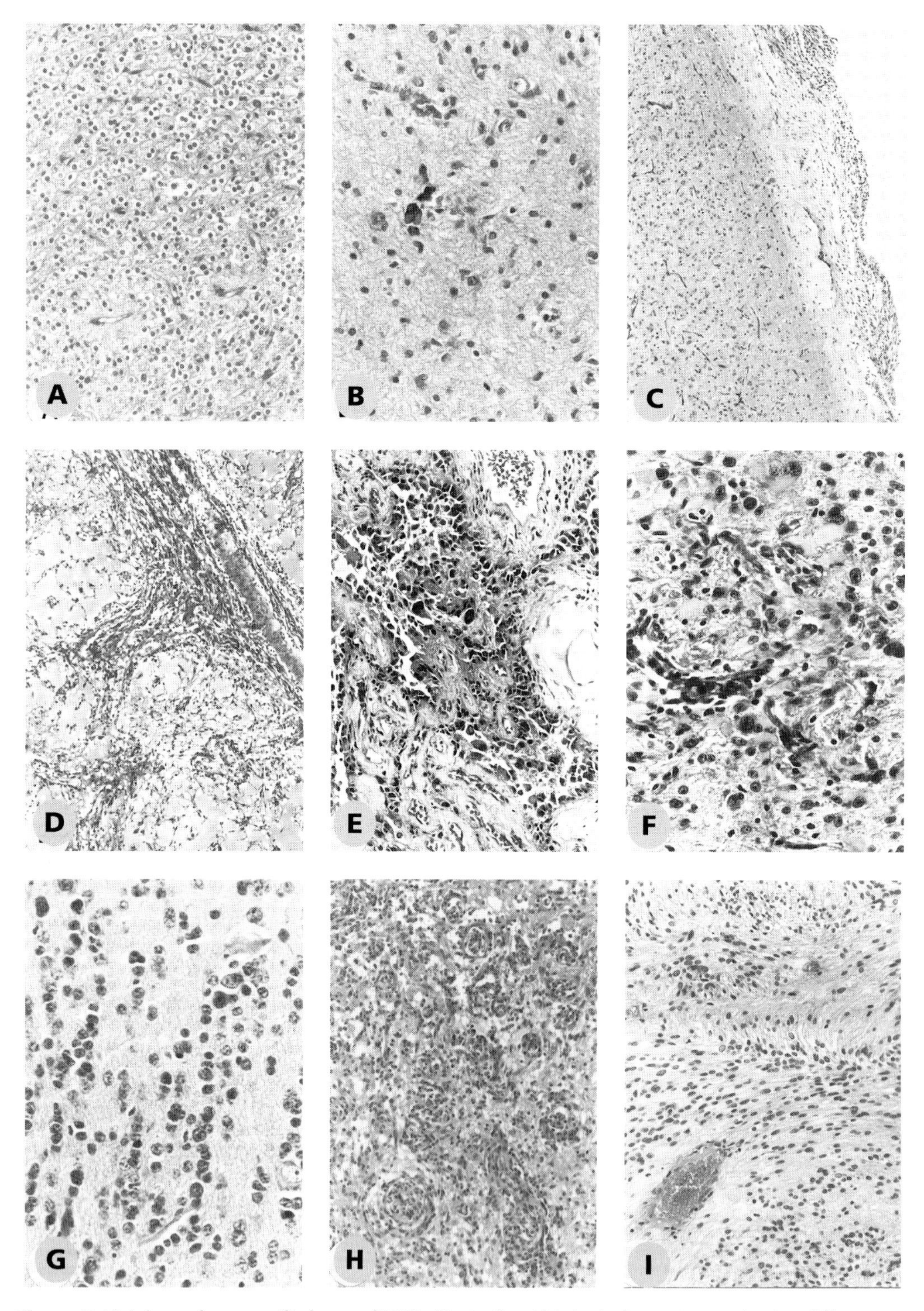

Figure 7: Histology of nonspecific forms of DNTs, illustrating histological aspects seen in nine different patients. The tumors resembled oligodendroglioma **(A)**, "fibrillary astrocytoma" **(B)**, infiltrative oligoastrocytoma with an exophytic part mimicking invasion of the leptomeninges **(C)**, "juvenile" pilocytic astrocytoma **(D)**, malignant astrocytoma **(E)**, atypical oligodendroglioma with pronounced nuclear atypia **(F)**, mixed oligoastrocytomas with nuclear abnormalities **(G)**, and atypical astrocytomas **(H** and **I)**. (hemalun-phloxine-safranin, original magnification × 150 [A, E, and I], × 200 [B, F, and G], × 80 [C and D], × 100 [H])

TABLE 5

LOCATION OF DIFFERENT FORMS OF DNT IN 89 PATIENTS

Presentation	Complex Forms	Simple Form	Nonspecific Forms
No. of cases	39	14	36
Temporal	20	5	26
Temporocentral or parietal	3	0	4
Temporoparieto-occipital	2	0	0
Frontal	9	1	3
Central, prerolandic, parietal	2	7	2
Occipital	1	0	0
Parieto-occipital	2	1	1

likely reflecting the selection of patients for epilepsy surgery. In the 14 cases of the simple form of DNT, all initially diagnosed by stereotactic biopsy, 50% of the lesions were located in the central, prerolandic, or parietal cortex.

Neuroimaging Appearance of DNTs

In all cases of either morphological form, neuroimaging demonstrated the cortical topography of the lesion. It is emphasized that MRI demonstrates the cortical location of these tumors better than CT (Figures 8, 9, and 10). Together with clinical presentation, the cortical site of a lesion is a paramount criterion for distinguishing DNTs from conventional categories of astrocytomas or oligodendrogliomas. Usually these latter tumors are not confined within the cortex, but also largely involve the white matter. It is, however, noteworthy that the area of the cortex involved by a DNT often largely encompasses that of normal cortical structures. Histologically, neurons are present even in the deeper part of DNTs, this being likely due to abnormal neuronal migration. In both morphological variants, when the lesions are superficially situated, CT often shows an overlying deformity of the skull (Figure 8A).

Results of imaging studies in 16 complex, 14 simple, and 21 nonspecific forms of DNT[7,8] are summarized in Table 6. Complex forms as well as nonspecific forms of DNT have a variable appearance on CT (Figures 9 and 10), the lesion being hypodense with or without calcific hyperdensity. Contrast enhancement, seen in about 40% of cases, is often ring-shaped (Figure 9A2). It is important to note that, even in cases showing contrast enhancement, the pattern of hypodensity on CT or hypersignal on T2-weighted MRI was in no patient suggestive of peritumoral edema.

The imaging pattern of the simple form of DNT is more uniform (Figure 8). These lesions do not show contrast enhancement on CT or MRI. Typically, the simple form of DNT appears as a hypodense pseudocystic lesion on CT or as a well-delineated increased signal on T2-weighted MRI, often looking like megagiry. In some instances, CT demonstrates hypercalcific density (in two of 14 cases in the analyzed series).

Follow-up Data

In our earlier studies of DNTs, which included 39 patients with complex forms and either complete or incomplete surgical removal, long-term follow-up (2 to 20 years, mean 9 years) showed neither clinical nor radiological evidence of recurrence in any patient.[15] In accordance with these data, our later studies of available preoperative imaging or follow-up imaging in patients who did not undergo surgery after

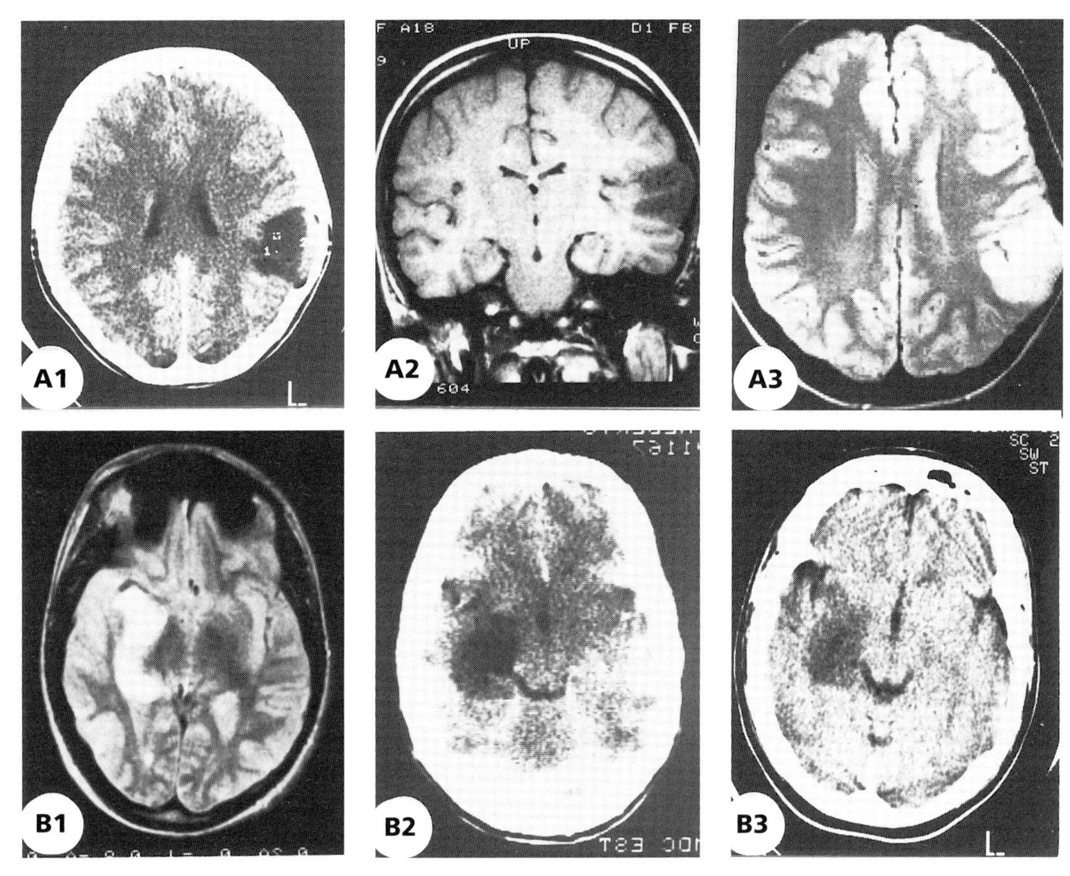

Figure 8: Imaging appearance of simple forms of DNTs in two patients. **A)** Left parietotemporal lesion in one patient. Postcontrast CT (A1) shows a well-demarcated low -attenuation area with a deformity of the overlying skull. T1- (A2) and T2-weighted (A3) MRI demonstrate the cortical topography of the lesion. **B)** Left mesial temporal lesion in a second patient. Well-demarcated hyperintense signal is seen on T2-weighted MRI (B1). CT scans of the same lesion obtained in 1981 (B2, postcontrast CT) and 1989 (B3, no contrast enhancement) demonstrate perfect stability of the lesion which appears as a well-demarcated low-attenuation area.

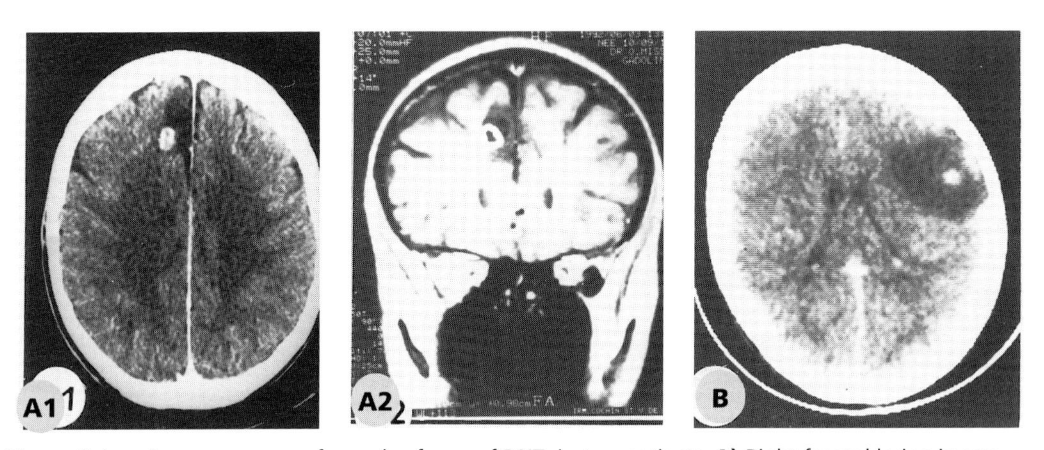

Figure 9: Imaging appearance of complex forms of DNTs in two patients. **A)** Right frontal lesion in one patient. A ring of contrast enhancement is seen in a low-attenuation area on postcontrast CT (A1) or within a hypointense T1-weighted signal on post-contrast MRI (A2). Note the absence of peritumoral edema. **B)** Left parietocentral lesion in a second patient. On CT, this is seen as a well-demarcated low-attenuation area with a calcific hyperdensity.

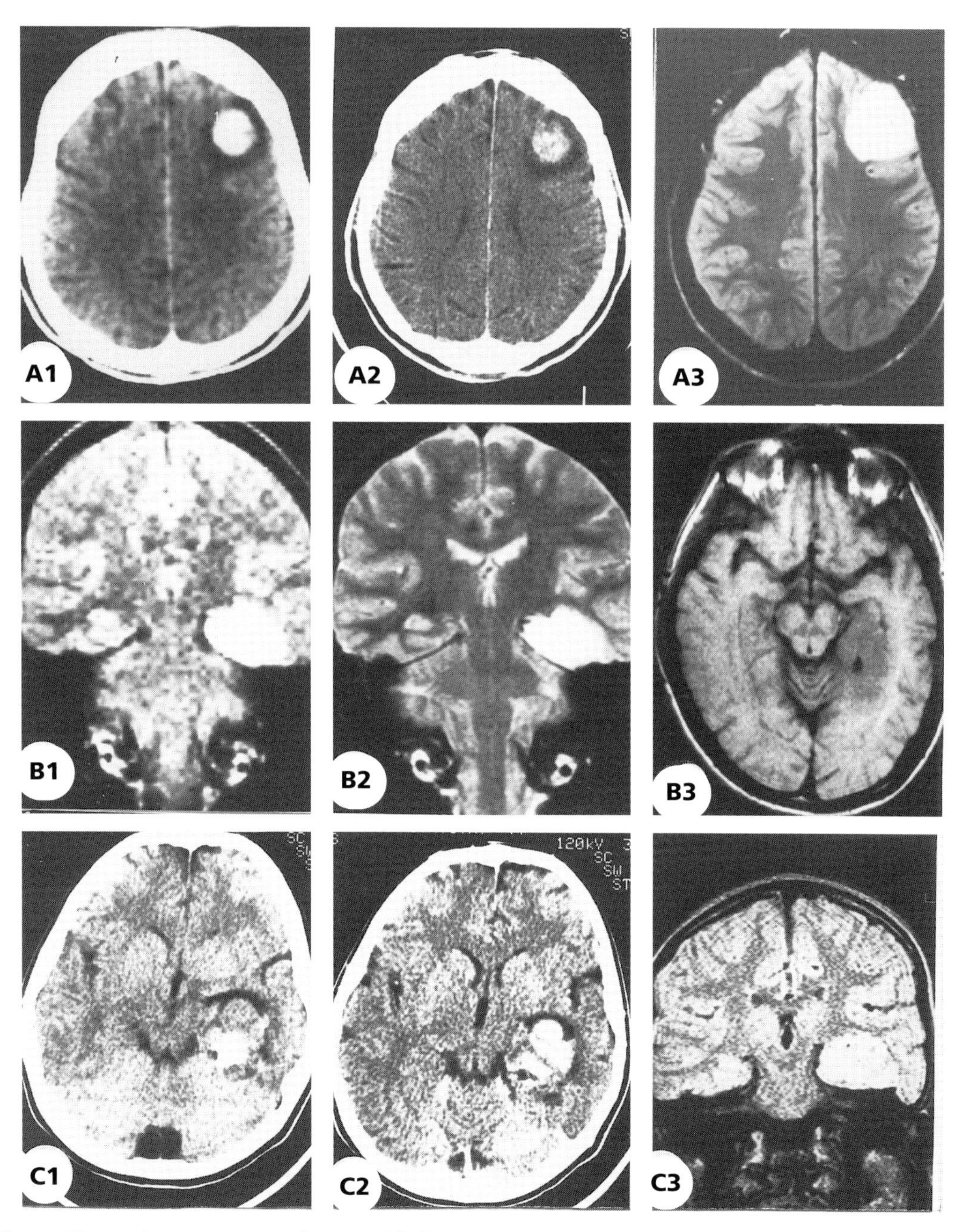

Figure 10: Imaging appearance of nonspecific forms of DNTs in three patients. **A)** Left frontal lesion in one patient. Comparative CT scans of the same lesion, one obtained in 1985 (A1) and one in 1989 (A2), demonstrate perfect stability of the lesion which appears as a well-demarcated area of contrast enhancement, surrounded by a zone of hypodensity. As seen preoperatively, the hypodense component reflects a cyst formation. T2-weighted MRI (A3) also demonstrates the cortical topography of the lesion. **B)** Right mesial temporal lesion in a second patient. Comparative MRIs of the same lesion, one obtained in 1987 (B1) and one in 1989 (B2), demonstrate perfect stability of the lesion which appears as a well-demarcated hyperintensity T2-weighted signal. The cortical topography of the lesion is also well seen on T1-weighted MRI (B3). **C)** Right mesial temporal lesion in a third patient. CT reveals calcific hyperdensity (C1) and contrast enhancement (C2). Note that this T2-weighted MRI (C3) better demonstrates the cortical topography of the lesion.

stereotactic biopsy exploration demonstrated that DNTs are perfectly stable lesions.[7,8] This important finding was confirmed without exception in 38 patients, including 11 cases of simple form (follow-up 2 to 10 years, mean 7 years), 12 cases of complex form (follow-up 2 to 7 years, mean 4.5 years), and 15 cases of nonspecific DNTs (follow-up 2 to 10 years, mean 5 years).

Kinetic Data

Using MIB-1 immunostaining, a marker that labels cycling cells (including G1, S, G2, and M phases), we have studied the growth fraction of 18 complex and simple forms of DNT.[7] In the complex form, a high labeling index comparable to that seen in high-grade ordinary astrocytomas was found; however, immunostaining for MIB-1 was negative in six of the seven simple forms. These findings indicate that kinetic markers which explore the tumor growth fraction cannot be used for differentiating DNTs from ordinary gliomas, and suggest that in these stable lesions the cell loss fraction is equivalent to that of the growth fraction.

The theory proposed by Pierce[45] is a tempting hypothesis for explaining the stability of DNTs. Based on experimental studies, this author has demonstrated the capacity of embryonic tissue to regulate or to induce maturation of its tumoral counterpart. If one admits that DNTs arise during embryogenesis, it becomes realistic to think that they may be regulated by or together with their normal embryonic environment.

Beyond the particular kinetics of DNTs, these findings raise important problems concerning the interpretation of current kinetic markers such as MIB-1, Ki-67, proliferating cell nuclear antigen, or bromodeoxyuridine. In well-defined histological tumor categories, a higher labeling index may correlate with higher potential for growth; however, the prognosis of neoplasms in general and of tumors that do not conform to conventional histological classification in particular cannot be deduced from their growth fractions. This is also true for the basic histological criteria of malignancy (cell density, mitosis, necrosis, etc.), which have no intrinsic significance, but may have a highly variable prognostic influence depending on the histological tumor type in which they are encountered.[9]

Diagnosis of DNTs: Therapeutic Implications

Accurate diagnosis of DNTs and their distinction from ordinary gliomas have important therapeutic implications. Aggressive radio- or chemotherapy must be avoided in order to spare these young patients with a normal life expectancy from the cohort of deleterious effects experienced from these aggressive treatments.[19] DNTs being carcinologically perfectly stable, in patients whose tumor is situated in functionally important brain structures, surgical removal as well as other aggressive treatment can be avoided. Therapeutic indications in patients harboring supratentorial cortical DNTs are, in fact, those of the treatment of epilepsy.

Application of the Concept of DNTs in the Interpretation of Glial Tumors in Children

Because DNTs were first identified among patients who underwent epilepsy surgery, this may wrongly suggest that such lesions are essentially encountered in specialized institutions. Since DNTs may easily be misdiagnosed as ordinary gliomas, we believe that the actual frequency of these lesions is underestimated. After the advent of modern imaging techniques, more systematic detection of supratentorial DNTs may account, at least in part, for the relative increase of supratentorial tumors in children shown by recent epidemiology studies.[50]

We believe with other authors[24,46] that conventional histological classification schemes and systems of grading gliomas, which are based on tumors in adults, are inadequate in a large proportion of glial tumors in children. Invariably, in the literature, survival curves are markedly better in childhood gliomas compared to those of adults.[26,30,31,37,38,41] This has long been considered as an "effect" of age; in fact, in most statistical studies, age appears as a major prognostic factor that supersedes other factors including the histological grade of malignancy.

TABLE 6

NEUROIMAGING APPEARANCE IN 51 PATIENTS WITH DNTs*

Presentation	Complex Forms	Simple Form	Nonspecific Forms
On CT			
Hypodensity only	8/16	12/14	6/21
Calcifications	2/16	2/14	11/21
Contrast enhancement	6/16	0/14	10/21
Normal	0/16	0/14	0/21
On MRI			
Hypointense on T1, hyperintense on T2	12/12	6/6	17/17
Contrast enhancement	2/2	0/4	7/17

*Results expressed as number of cases showing that appearance/number of cases studied.

A bias is likely to be introduced by misdiagnosis of distinct childhood tumoral entities that do not behave as "ordinary" astrocytomas. This is suggested by the usual plateau effect of survival curves of high-grade gliomas in children. For example, in a Surveillance, Epidemiology, and End Result (SEER) study of the National Cancer Institute,[20] the survival curve of high-grade astrocytomas in children showed a marked decrease in survival rates similar to that seen in adults until the second postoperative year; thereafter, the survival rate remained stable, showing that 40% of the children with "high-grade astrocytomas" are long-term survivors.

Obvious discordances are observed in survival curves of "low-grade astrocytomas" in children as well as in adults. For example, in the recent study of Westergaard et al[54] survival curves in patients with nonpilocytic supratentorial low-grade astrocytomas operated on before 20 years of age were markedly better and distinct from those of patients operated on after the age of 20 years.

Adherence to the concept of DNTs may provide better understanding of the distinct indolent behavior of a large proportion of glial tumors in children. From a practical point of view, we recommend that histological, clinical, and imaging data be considered together in the diagnosis of gliomas in children. Knowledge of the characteristic clinical presentation and imaging appearance helps with difficulties that may be encountered in the histological diagnosis of supratentorial cortical DNTs. However, for obvious reasons, the uniform criteria that we have proposed for the diagnosis of supratentorial cortical DNTs are inadequate for the identification of DNTs that may be encountered in other locations. In case of doubt, the growth potential of a tumor can nowadays be accurately estimated with the aid of successive postoperative or postbiopsy MRI. On the other hand, adjunctive radio- and/or chemotherapy are only palliative, whereas the long-term deleterious effects on children when these methods are used aggressively are well documented.[19] The risks of delaying adjunctive therapy are minor compared with the dangers of overtreating young patients with potentially long survival or a normal life expectancy. In our opinion, aggressive adjunctive therapy should not be considered in children without evidence of tumor growth on pre- or postoperative imaging follow-up.

DNTs vs. Benign Cerebellar Astrocytomas

Since the study of Cushing[6] in 1931, cerebellar astrocytomas in children and young patients are known to carry a favorable prognosis following surgery. He indiscriminately separated the cerebellar astrocytomas from the rest of the astrocytoma group. However, further studies have shown that the postoperative outcome of cerebellar astrocytomas is not uniform. It has been repeatedly observed that, after complete surgical removal, the tumor may recur and that, after partial surgical removal, the tumor may remain stable, or may behave as a slow-growing process.[1,23,27-29,44,52] The variable behavior of incompletely resected benign astrocytomas of the cerebellum in children has recently been well documented on postoperative CT.[49] Subcategorization of cerebellar astrocytomas has thus been attempted in order to better predict the postoperative prognosis of these tumors. It is now known that malignant ordinary astrocytomas may occur in the cerebellum and share the uniformly poor prognosis of their supratentorial equivalents. However, histological typing of benign gliomas of the cerebellum remains a subject of controversy.

Russell and Rubinstein[47] divided benign astrocytomas of the cerebellum into three groups: 1) a "typical juvenile form of pilocytic astrocytoma" indistinguishable from that encountered in the third ventricle; 2) closely allied to the former, a category of astrocytomas "showing an intimate and contiguous association of areas of compact pilocytic growth with other areas of loose-textured spongy character"; and 3) a "diffuse form" of astrocytomas, which is generally indistinguishable from the diffuse cerebral astrocytoma. Gjerris and Klinken[25] found that, in patients undergoing surgery in childhood, the 25-year cumulative survival rate for the diffuse form of the cerebellar astrocytomas was less than half as favorable as for the other forms. This was also confirmed by Davis and Joglekar.[18] However, the histoprognostic significance of such a subdivision has been denied by others.[44,52] These discrepances are likely to be explained by different definitions of "diffuse astrocytomas of the cerebellum" which, according to different authors, is exclusively applied to "fibrillary ordinary astrocytomas" or includes a morphological variant of pilocytic astrocytomas.[29] In fact, the description of the "diffuse form" given by Russell and Rubinstein[47,48] was ambiguous; it was said to be composed of fibrillated stellate or piloid cells and to be macroscopically cystic or solid. It is also important to note that these authors did not attribute a histoprognostic significance to their morphological classification of astrocytomas of the cerebellum.

Winston et al[55] and Gilles[24] proposed that cerebellar gliomas of children be assessed according to a cluster analysis of several histological features, and they classified the tumors as A, B, or C. The 10-year survival rates in these groups were 84%, 23%, and 68%, respectively. Probably because of its complexity and indiscriminate application to any type of gliomas including ependymomas, this system does not seem to have received a large acceptance.

Introduction of the concept of dysembryoplastic tumors may provide a better understanding of the variable behavior of gliomas of the cerebellum in children or young subjects, as well as a more accurate histoprognostication. In our opinion, a substantial proportion of tumors of the cerebellum, diagnosed as pilocytic astrocytomas according to conventional classifications,[36,56] and of the "diffuse" variant of cerebellar gliomas are in fact DNTs. If one admits that "true" pilocytic astrocytomas, DNTs, and the ordinary form of gliomas may all be encountered in this location, this may explain the variable postoperative outcome of cerebellar gliomas. "True" pilocytic astrocytomas, which are of structure type I, can be totally removed and cured by surgery, or will continue to behave as a slow-growing process after partial surgical removal. The occurrence of DNTs in the cerebellum may explain why, in other patients after incomplete removal or merely a biopsy and decompression of a cyst, the lesion may remain stable, and may be compatible with a normal lifespan.

As early as in 1937, Bergstrand[2] clearly voiced the opinion that cerebellar gliomas in childhood are congenital and are of dysembryoplastic origin. He accordingly proposed the term "gliocytoma embryonale"; however, his proposal was immediately rejected. The main argument leveled against the concept was that these tumors do recur in some patients.

Tumors of the cerebellum that we consider DNTs exhibit, like their supratentorial equivalent, several distinct features that allow their differentiation from pilocytic or ordinary gliomas. 1) Architectural disorganization of gyri adjacent to the tumor is often observed, evidenced by a more or less pronounced lack and/or abnormal disposition of neurons (Figure 11C). In agreement with Bergstrand,[2] we consider that these architectural abnormalities are of dysembryoplastic origin. These changes are, however,

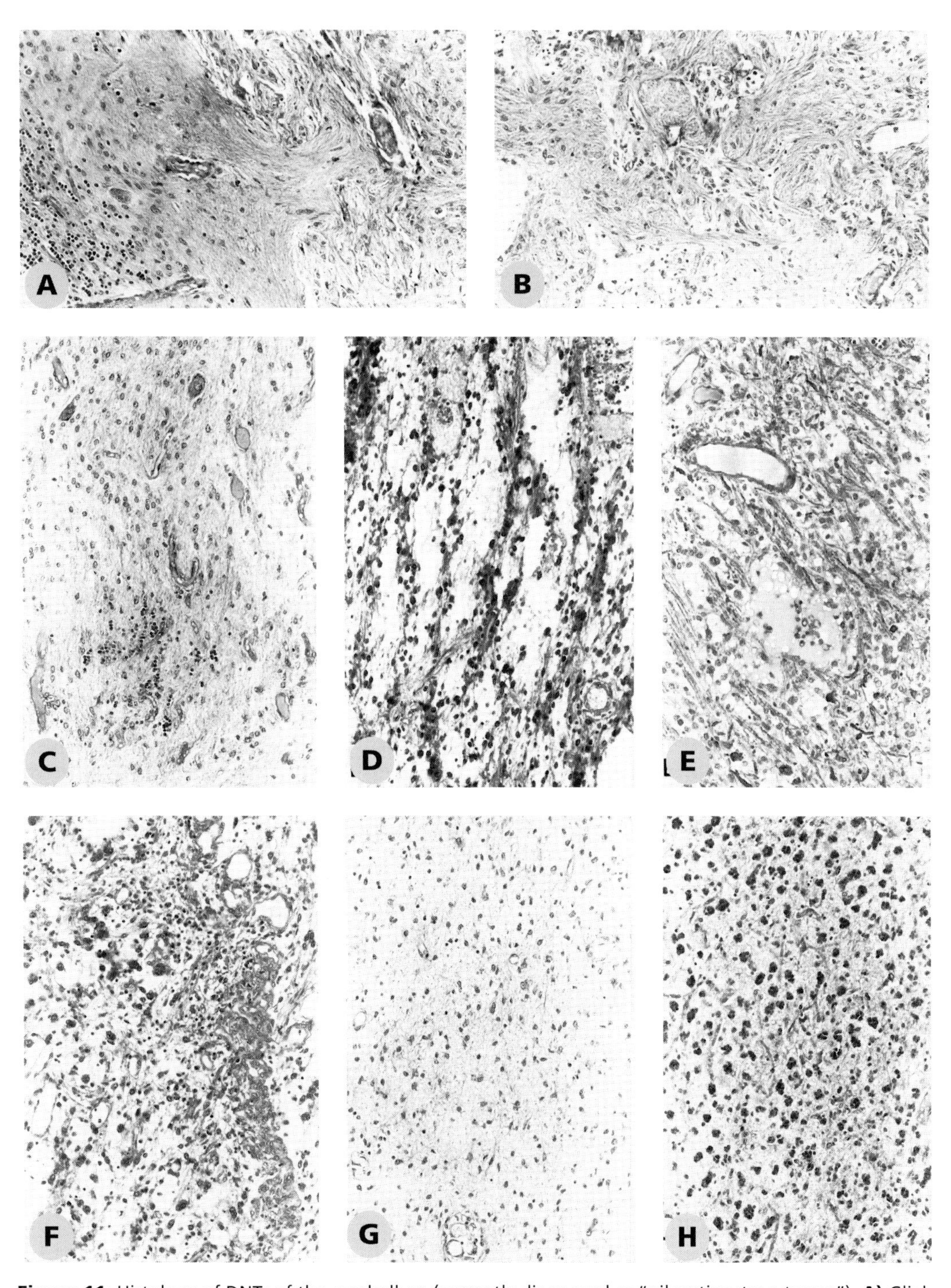

Figure 11: Histology of DNTs of the cerebellum (currently diagnosed as "pilocytic astrocytomas"). **A)** Glial bridge formations *(arrowheads)*: heterotopic tissue spreads from the molecular layer toward the exophytic part of the lesion. **B)** The so-called "tumoral invasion of the leptomeninge" shows a multinodular pattern made of intermingled elements issued from glial bridge formations. **C)** Zone of cortical dysplasia with abnormal disposition of granular and Purkinje neurons. **D** and **E)** Microcystic elements resembling "juvenile" pilocytic astrocytomas. **F)** Vascular arcades seen in a microcystic element. **G)** Astrocytic component with the appearance of "diffuse astrocytoma." **H)** Oligodendrocytic element with nuclei looking like "fleurettes." (hemalun-phloxine-safranin, original magnification × 100 [A and B], × 150 [C to H])

often interpreted as a result of chronic pressure induced by tumor growth (for a review, see Ilgren and Stiller[33]). 2) A so-called invasion of the pia is also commonly observed. With Bergstrand, we consider that this feature, which is well known to have no prognostic significance in "pilocytic astrocytomas" of the cerebellum, closely resembles the glial bridge formations encountered in various malformations of the cerebellum. As illustrated in Figure 11A and B, the multinodular pattern seen in the exophytic part of these tumors emanates from glial bridge formations and tends to reproduce these later. 3) As frequently seen in supratentorial DNTs, these lesions often show a complex structure, with juxtaposition of solid and pseudoinfiltrative patterns (Figure 11D-H). A nodular architecture may also be observed. Heterogeneous cell composition with an admixture of astrocytes and oligodendrocytes is also common.[2,18,33,48,55] This is, however, masked by conventional classifications based on the predominant cell type.

We believe that the recently identified "transependymal dorsally exophytic brain stem gliomas,"[32,51] "focal midbrain astrocytomas,"[53] and "intrinsic gliomas of the cervicomedullary junction"[21] are likely to be other topographic variants of DNTs. Encountered in children, these lesions show a favorable postoperative course and stability on imaging.[39] Previous indiscriminate inclusion of these benign stable lesions, which are still histologically interpreted as ordinary gliomas, probably explains the plateau effect that was seen in survival curves of astrocytomas of the brain stem in children.[5]

REFERENCES

1. Austin EJ, Alvord EC Jr: Recurrences of cerebellar astrocytomas: a violation of Collins' law. **J Neurosurg 68:**41-47, 1988
2. Bergstrand H: Weiteres über sog. Klein hern Astrocytome. **Virchows Arch [A] 229:**4-28, 1937
3. Bruner JM: Oligodendroglioma: diagnosis and prognosis. **Semin Diagn Pathol 4:**251-261, 1987
4. Burger PC, Rawlings CE, Cox EB, et al: Clinicopathological correlations in the oligodendroglioma. **Cancer 59:**1345-1352, 1987
5. Cohen ME, Duffner PK, Heffner RR, et al: Prognostic factors in brainstem gliomas. **Neurology 36:**602-605, 1986
6. Cushing H: Experiences with the cerebellar astrocytomas. A critical review of seventy-six cases. **Surg Gynecol Obstet 52:**129-204, 1931
7. Daumas-Duport C: Dysembryoplastic neuroepithelial tumours. **Brain Pathol 3:**283-295, 1993
8. Daumas-Duport C: Dysembryoplastic neuroepithelial tumours in epilepsy surgery, in Guerrini R (ed): **Dysplasia of Cerebral Cortex and Epilepsy.** New York, NY: Raven Press (In press)
9. Daumas-Duport C: Histological grading of gliomas. **Curr Opin Neurol Neurosurg 5:**924-931, 1992
10. Daumas-Duport C: Histoprognosis of gliomas. **Adv Tech Stand Neurosurg 21** (In press)
11. Daumas-Duport C, Monsaigneon V, Blond S, et al: Serial stereotactic biopsies and CT scan in gliomas: correlative study in 100 astrocytomas, oligo-astrocytomas and oligodendrocytomas. **J Neurooncol 4:** 317-328, 1986
12. Daumas-Duport C, Monsaigneon V, N'Guyen JP, et al: Some correlations between histological and CT aspects of cerebral gliomas contributing to the choice of significant trajectories for stereotaxic biopsies. **Acta Neurochir Suppl 33:**185-194, 1984
13. Daumas-Duport C, Monsaingeon V, Szenthe L, et al: Serial stereotactic biopsies: a double histological code of gliomas according to malignancy and 3-D configuration, as an aid to therapeutic decision and assessment of results. **Appl Neurophysiol 45:**431-437, 1982
14. Daumas-Duport C, Monsaingeon V, Vedrenne C, et al: Complex neuroepithelial tumours in epilepsy surgery. A series of 20 cases, in Broggi G (ed): **The Rational Basis of the Surgical Treatment of Epilepsies.** London: John Libbey, Ltd., 1988, pp 149-167
15. Daumas-Duport C, Scheithauer BW, Chodkiewicz JP, et al: Dysembryoplastic neuroepithelial tumor: a surgically curable tumor of young patients with intractable partial seizures. Report of thirty-nine cases. **Neurosurgery 23:**545-556, 1988
16. Daumas-Duport C, Scheithauer BW, Kelly PJ: A histologic and cytologic method for the spatial definition of gliomas. **Mayo Clin Proc 62:**435-449, 1987
17. Daumas-Duport C, Scheithauer BW, O'Fallon J, et al: Grading of astrocytomas. A simple and reproducible method. **Cancer 62:**2152-2165, 1988
18. Davis CH, Joglekar VM: Cerebellar astrocytomas in children and young adults. **J Neurol Neurosurg Psychiatry 44:**820-828, 1981
19. Duffner PK, Cohen ME: The long-term effects of central nervous system therapy on children with brain tumors. **Neurol Clin 9:**480-494, 1991
20. Duffner PK, Cohen ME, Myers MH, et al: Survival of children with brain tumors: SEER program, 1973-1980. **Neurology 36:**597-601, 1986
21. Epstein F, McCleary EL: Intrinsic brain-stem tumors of childhood: surgical indications. **J Neurosurg 64:**11-15, 1986
22. Favier J, Pizzolato GP, Berney J: Oligodendroglial tumors in childhood. **Childs Nerv Syst 1:**33-38, 1985
23. Garcia DM, Latifi HR, Simpson JR, et al: Astrocytomas of the cerebellum in children. **J Neurosurg 71:**661-664, 1989
24. Gilles FH: Classifications of childhood brain tumors. **Cancer 56:**1850-1857, 1985
25. Gjerris F, Klinken L: Long-term prognosis in children with benign cerebellar astrocytoma. **J Neurosurg**

49:179-184, 1978
26. Gol A: Cerebral astrocytomas in childhood. A clinical study. **J Neurosurg 19:**577-582, 1962
27. Gol A, McKissock W: The cerebellar astrocytomas. A report on 98 verified cases. **J Neurosurg 16:**287-296, 1959
28. Griffin TW, Beaufait D, Blasko JC: Cystic cerebellar astrocytomas in childhood. **Cancer 44:**276-280, 1979
29. Hayostek CJ, Shaw EG, Scheithauer B, et al: Astrocytomas of the cerebellum. A comparative clinicopathological study of pilocytic and diffuse astrocytomas. **Cancer 72:**856-869, 1993
30. Heiskanen O: Intracranial tumors of children. **Childs Brain 3:**69-78, 1977
31. Hirsch JF, Sainte Rose C, Pierre-Kahn A, et al: Benign astrocytic and oligodendrocytic tumors of the cerebral hemispheres in children. **J Neurosurg 70:**568-572, 1989
32. Hoffman HJ, Becker L, Craven MA: A clinically and pathologically distinct group of benign brain stem gliomas. **Neurosurgery 7:**243-248, 1980
33. Ilgren EB, Stiller CA: Cerebellar astrocytomas. Part I. Macroscopic and microscopic features. **Clin Neuropathol 6:**185-200, 1987
34. Kelly PJ: **Tumor Stereotaxis.** Philadelphia, Pa: WB Saunders, 1991, pp 296-357
35. Kelly PJ, Daumas-Duport C, Scheithauer BW, et al: Stereotactic histologic correlations of computed tomography- and magnetic resonance imaging-defined abnormalities in patients with glial neoplasm. **Mayo Clin Proc 62:**450-459, 1987
36. Kleihues P, Burger PC, Scheithauer BW: **Histological Typing of Tumours of the Central Nervous System. World Health Organization.** Berlin: Springer-Verlag, 1993
37. Laws ER Jr, Taylor WF, Clifton MB, et al: Neurosurgical management of low-grade astrocytoma of the cerebral hemispheres. **J Neurosurg 61:**665-673, 1984
38. Marchese MJ, Chang CH: Malignant astrocytic gliomas in children. **Cancer 65:**2771-2778, 1990
39. May PL, Blaser SI, Hoffman HJ, et al: Benign intrinsic tectal "tumors" in children. **J Neurosurg 74:**867-871, 1991
40. McGirr SJ, Kelly PJ, Scheithauer BW: Stereotactic resection of juvenile pilocytic astrocytomas of the thalamus and basal ganglia. **Neurosurgery 20:** 447-452, 1987
41. Mercuri S, Russo A, Palma L: Hemispheric supratentorial astrocytomas in children. Long-term results in 29 cases. **J Neurosurg 55:**170-173, 1981
42. Mørk SJ, Halvorsen TB, Lindegaard KF, et al: Oligodendroglioma. Histologic evaluation and prognosis. **J Neuropathol Exp Neurol 45:**65-78, 1986
43. Mørk SJ, Lindegaard KF, Halvorsen TB, et al: Oligodendroglioma: incidence and biological behavior in a defined population. **J Neurosurg 63:**881-889, 1985
44. Palma L, Russo A, Celli P: Prognosis of the so-called "diffuse" cerebellar astrocytoma. **Neurosurgery 15:**315-317, 1983
45. Pierce GB: The cancer cell and its control by the embryo. **Am J Pathol 113:**117-124, 1983
46. Rorke LB, Gilles FH, Davis RL, et al: Revision of the World Health Organization classification of brain tumors for childhood brain tumors. **Cancer 56:** 1869-1886, 1985
47. Russell DS, Rubinstein LJ: **Pathology of Tumours of the Nervous System, 4th ed.** London: Edward Arnold, 1977, pp 146-148
48. Russell DS, Rubinstein LJ: **Pathology of Tumours of the Nervous System, 5th ed.** London: Edward Arnold, 1989, pp 173-177
49. Schneider JH Jr, Raffel C, McComb JG: Benign cerebellar astrocytomas of childhood. **Neurosurgery 30:**58-63, 1992
50. Stevens MCG, Cameron AH, Muir KR, et al: Descriptive epidemiology of primary central nervous system tumours in children: a population-based study. **Clin Oncol 3:**323-329, 1991
51. Stroink AR, Hoffman HJ, Hendrick EB, et al: Transependymal benign dorsally exophytic brain stem gliomas in childhood: diagnosis and treatment recommendations. **Neurosurgery 20:**439-444, 1987
52. Szénásy J, Slowik F: Prognosis of benign cerebellar astrocytomas in children. **Childs Brain 10:**39-47, 1983
53. Vandertop WP, Hoffman HJ, Drake JM, et al: Focal midbrain tumors in children. **Neurosurgery 31:** 186-194, 1992
54. Westergaard L, Gjerris F, Klinken L: Prognostic parameters in benign astrocytomas. **Acta Neurochir 123:**1-7, 1993
55. Winston K, Gilles FH, Leviton A, et al: Cerebellar gliomas in children. **J Natl Cancer Inst 58:**833-838, 1977
56. Zülch KJ: **Histological Typing of Tumours of the Central Nervous System.** Geneva: World Health Organization, 1979, p 21

CHAPTER 8

GROWTH FACTORS AND PROLIFERATION POTENTIAL

DAVID R. HINTON, MD, FRCP(C)

The biological behavior of cerebral gliomas depends upon the age of the patient, the location of the tumor, the tendency of the tumor cells to infiltrate adjacent structures, the rate of tumor growth, and the response of the adjacent brain. In recent years, cerebral astrocytic tumors have been divided into two broad groups: the diffusely infiltrating fibrillary astrocytomas and the less common, more circumscribed "benign" gliomas encompassing pilocytic astrocytoma, pleomorphic xanthoastrocytoma, and subependymal giant cell astrocytoma.[19,39,40,43,47] The infiltrating tumors (astrocytoma, World Health Organization (WHO) grade II; anaplastic astrocytoma,WHO grade III; and glioblastoma multiforme,WHO grade IV) form a biological continuum in terms of their progressive genetic changes, histology, behavior, and tendency to transform into more malignant tumors with time.[31,39-41] The "benign" gliomas are well circumscribed, have a good prognosis, and rarely transform into malignant tumors.[35,62] The pathological characteristics of these tumors are described in detail in other chapters.

The growth in size of a tumor is based upon the rates of tumor cell proliferation, and cell death as well as the size of the tumor cells, their ability to invade, and the reactive changes of the adjacent brain tissues. While in fibrillary astrocytic tumors proliferation rates have correlated closely with tumor grade and prognosis, this has not proved to be true for the "benign" gliomas, suggesting that other factors, perhaps related to lack of invasiveness, are more critical for the behavior of these tumors. In this chapter, the literature concerning the proliferative potential of benign gliomas will be reviewed, particularly with respect to histology and biological behavior.

There has been an explosion of information in recent years about the factors controlling the growth and proliferation of normal and neoplastic cells, particularly cells of neuroectodermal origin. Much of this work has been done on malignant fibrillary astrocytomas because of the ease of cell culture and the clinical importance of developing therapeutic interventions. Little is known, however, about the factors controlling the growth of benign gliomas because of the difficulty in establishing in vitro models of tumor cell growth for these indolent tumors. Therefore, the review of the factors involved in glioma cell growth will draw from the literature on malignant fibrillary gliomas and extrapolate to the benign gliomas.

CELL CYCLE BIOLOGY

The cell cycle may be defined as the interval between the midpoint of mitosis and the midpoint of the subsequent mitosis in the daughter cells. There are four basic phases of the cell cycle. The S or deoxyribonucleic acid (DNA) synthesis phase is preceded by the G1 phase (gap 1) and followed by the G2 phase (gap 2). Mitosis is the culmination of the cell cycle and results in the creation of two daughter cells. Cells that are quiescent are in the G0 phase, a subphase of G1. The amount of time spent in the G1 phase is the most variable; slow-growing cells will have a longer G1 phase.

The relative proportions of DNA during the different phases of the cell cycle form the basis for understanding flow cytometry.[18] The normal diploid complement of DNA (2C) is found in the G1 phase. During DNA synthesis it increases to 4C or tetraploidy. Once the 4C level is reached, the cell enters G2 and subsequently mitosis. During the anaphase stage of mitosis the quantity of DNA per cell once again returns to 2C.

Cells move between G0 and G1 in response to changing environmental and growth conditions. Cells in G0 can also move into a permanent state of differentiation from which they cannot re-enter the cell cycle. The movement from G0 back to G1 requires the action of growth factors, many of which act through the *Ras* signaling pathway. This eventually results in phosphorylation and activation of a large number of factors including transcription factors (c-*myc*, c-*jun*) and cytoskeletal components (MAP-2, *tau*).[21]

The cell commits to progression through the cell cycle at a point in G1 termed the "restriction point." Once the cell cycle is initiated, there are specific checkpoints where the cycle can be halted if certain criteria are not met. These checkpoints occur in G1 and G2. The G1 checkpoint determines whether sufficient nutrients are available to proceed into S phase while the G2 checkpoint determines whether DNA replication is complete prior to entrance into mitosis.

Cell cycle regulation is achieved by activation of a family of protein kinases, the cyclin-dependent kinases (C_{dks}), which are activated at specific times in the cell cycle.[56] C_{dks} are activated after binding their regulatory cyclin partners. In general, the C_{dks} are present throughout the cell cycle while the cyclins are regulated and vary in different phases of the cycle. Many of the substrates for the C_{dks} have been identified and include a host of structural and regulatory proteins. For example, CDC2 (a cyclin-dependent kinase) is required for mitosis since its activation is involved in breakdown of the nuclear envelope and condensation of chromosomes. CDC2 complexes with, and is activated by, cyclin B late in the G2 phase, allowing initiation of mitosis.[28,51]

Cell Loss

Cell death is a fundamental property of the development and life of an organism and is a significant process in both benign and malignant neoplasms. Several lines of investigation have led to the concept that there are two fundamental types of cell death, apoptosis and necrosis (reviewed by Buja et al[4]).

Apoptosis is usually expressed as multifocal single-cell death and is typified by cell loss occurring during normal development of the nervous system. It is characterized by nuclear and cytoplasmic condensation of single cells, followed by loss of nuclear membrane and subsequent formation of multiple fragments of condensed nuclear material and cytoplasm. The resultant apoptotic bodies are phagocytosed by adjacent cells; however, an inflammatory reaction with leukocyte infiltration is absent. Apoptosis is associated with a perturbation of nuclear chromatin in which endonucleases are activated, resulting in cleavage of DNA at specific regions to form fragments of double-stranded DNA. In some situations, apoptosis is referred to as programmed cell death because the regulated activation of various genes produces or activates the endonucleases responsible for DNA cleavage. There is evidence that there are both repressors (bcl-2) and activators (*Fas* antigen, tumor necrosis factor (TNF)-α) of the genetic program for apoptosis.[66,71] The role of apoptosis in neoplasia is an area of active investigation. It has been hypothesized that suppression of apoptosis due to mutations in regulatory oncogenes may allow for clonal expansion. The promotion of apoptosis could be suggested as a potential therapy in patients with malignant gliomas.

Necrosis refers to the changes that accompany irreversible cell injury in living organisms and may be divided into coagulative, liquefactive, and fibrinoid forms. The evolution of

TABLE 1

PROLIFERATION-RELATED MARKERS USED ON TISSUE SECTIONS*

Marker	Description
MIB-1	Same antigen as Ki-67; used on formalin-fixed paraffin-embedded sections
^{3}H-thymidine	Incorporated in S phase; autoradiography performed with long exposures
BUdR	Incorporated in S phase; must be injected prior to surgery; used on ethanol-fixed paraffin-embedded sections
Ki-67	All cell cycles except G0; used on frozen sections
PCNA	Made in S phase, identified through remainder of cell cycle at low levels; used on formalin-fixed paraffin-embedded sections
AgNOR	Identifies nucleolar organizer regions in nuclei of formalin-fixed paraffin-embedded sections
Statin	Identifies cells in G0 phase; used on frozen sections

*For fuller description see text.

necrosis involves progressive damage to energy and substrate metabolism and is associated with progressive morphological changes. Early events include clumping of chromatin and intracellular edema and swelling, followed by advanced changes in chromatin, mitochondrial changes, and finally breaks in the plasma and organellar membranes, with cellular fragmentation. Necrosis is often accompanied by an inflammatory reaction, and may be focal or extensive.

METHODS TO MEASURE CELL PROLIFERATION AND CELL LOSS

Table 1 summarizes various proliferation-related markers used on tissue sections. These are described more fully below.

Mitotic Index

Pathologists have used a mitotic index to assess proliferation for many years; however, the method has proved to be unreproducible and inaccurate. Because of the rarity of mitotic figures in low-grade gliomas, there is a high rate of sampling error and sometimes ambiguity in what constitutes a mitotic figure histologically. For low- to intermediate-grade gliomas, a mitotic index (specified as number of mitotic figures per 10 or 20 microscopic fields) is likely to be 0 or 1; therefore, mitotic figures are usually indicated as rare or not observed.

^{3}H-Thymidine

Early studies employed autoradiographic analysis of tissue exposed to a pulse of [^{3}H]-thymidine to estimate proliferative potential of human brain tumors. Exogenous thymidine presented to a cell in S phase will be incorporated into nuclear DNA. When this thymidine contains [^{3}H]-thymidine, nuclei that incorporate it can be identified by autoradiography. Subjects are injected with [^{3}H]-thymidine shortly before craniotomy. The paraffin-embedded tissue sections are coated with photographic emulsion and exposed in light-tight boxes at 4°C for several months before developing.[24-26] This method is not currently employed in humans due to the necessity of injecting radionucleotides and the long tissue exposure time required.

Bromodeoxyuridine

Bromodeoxyuridine (BUdR), a thymidine analog, is incorporated specifically in the S phase of the cell cycle. It must be administered intravenously to the patient prior to surgery or incorporated in the tumor cells in vitro after establishment of a primary tumor culture. The nuclei incorporating BUdR are identified by use of an anti-BUdR antibody in paraffin-embedded ethanol-fixed tissue.[46] Sections are denatured with 2 N hydrochloric acid prior to incubation with monoclonal antibody. Pulse labeling with a second agent (iododeoxyuridine)

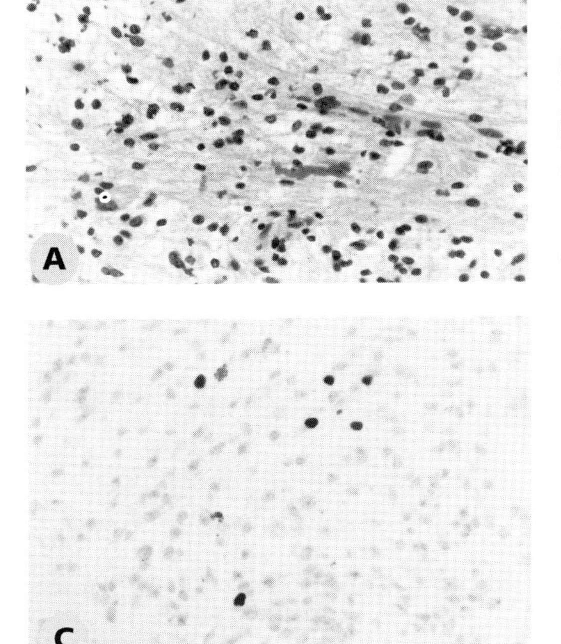

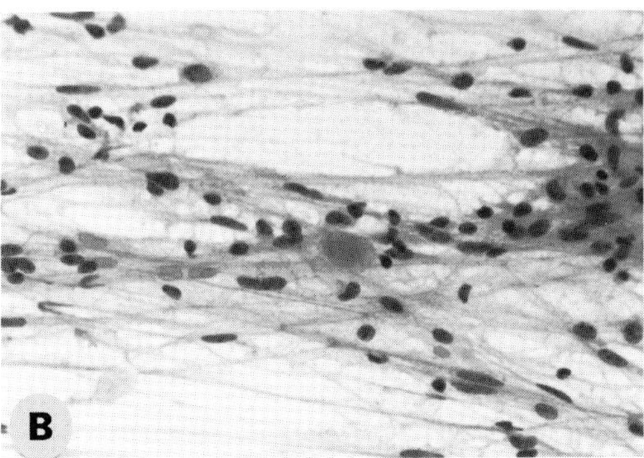

Figure 1: Ki-67 (MIB-1) immunoperoxidase staining of a supratentorial pilocytic astrocytoma. **A)** On this formalin-fixed paraffin-embedded section, note the interlacing bundles of tumor cells. **B)** The fine hair-like pilocytic processes can be seen. **C)** MIB-1 staining of an adjacent section, showing a significant proportion of positive cells.

can provide a sophisticated estimate of cell cycle duration.

Ki-67 Antibody

In 1983, Gerdes et al[14] reported the production of a mouse monoclonal antibody reactive with a human nuclear antigen associated with cellular proliferation. This antibody, designated Ki-67, was generated against the crude nuclear fraction of L428 cells, a Hodgkin's disease-derived cell line.

Extensive cell cycle analysis has determined that Ki-67-reactive antigen concentration increases with cell cycle progression and attains a maximum at the G2M phase in exponentially growing cells. Morphological studies have indicated that, in interphase nuclei, the antigen is present throughout the nucleus or in association predominantly with nucleoli, while in mitotic cells, it is associated with chromosomes.[13,14] Immunoblot analysis reveals that Ki-67 identifies a doublet of 395 and 345 kD.[60] The complementary DNA was recently cloned, and sequence analysis reveals that it encodes a nuclear and short-lived protein without any significant homology to known sequences. Ki-67 antigen-specific antisense oligonucleotides inhibit the proliferation of certain human cell lines, suggesting that Ki-67 may be required for cell proliferation.

Until recently, Ki-67 studies required fresh or snap-frozen tissue. The frozen tissue sections are air-dried, fixed with acetone, and stained by immunoperoxidase methods.[5] A new antibody directly against the Ki-67 antigen, MIB-1,[33] which is very effective in microwave-treated formalin-fixed paraffin-embedded sections, is now available (Figure 1), and has made possible the comprehensive analysis of archival material.

Proliferating Cell Nuclear Antigen

Proliferating cell nuclear antigen (PCNA) is a 36-kD nuclear protein which has been identified as the auxillary protein for DNA d-polymerase and may be important in cellular DNA replication and synthesis. PCNA is present throughout the cell cycle; however, it is synthesized in the S phase, resulting in the highest concentrations in the late G1 and S phases. Since the amount of PCNA in nonproliferating cells is low, the immunohistochemical labeling of cells may reflect proliferative activity. Several different clones of PCNA monoclonal antibodies are available for use and they vary in their reproducibility in frozen and permanent sections.[12,37] For some tumors PCNA labeling is out of proportion to proliferation indices obtained by other methods, suggesting that PCNA overexpression may be related to other than direct proliferative activity.[37] For example, one patient with a recurrent pilocytic astrocytoma had a PCNA labeling index of 6.7% while the Ki-67 labeling index was only 0.6%.[37]

Silver-Staining Nucleolar Organizer Regions

Nucleolar organizer regions (NORs) are segments of DNA that are associated with secondary constrictions of the five acrocentric chromosomes (chromosomes 13, 14, 15, 21, and 22), and represent the sites of the ribosomal ribonucleic acid (RNA) genes. In interphase nuclei, they are identified as fibrillar centers at the ultrastructural level. The argyrophilic method described by Smith and Crocker[65] detects proteins associated with the NORs (AgNORs), including RNA polymerase 1, C_{23} protein (nucleolin), and B_{23} protein. The specificity of the reaction has been confirmed ultrastructurally. The number of AgNORs within the cell nucleus reflects, in part, the level of ribosomal RNA transcription and should therefore provide important information about the nucleolus in benign and neoplastic conditions.

The reaction is easily performed on sections of paraffin-embedded formalin-fixed tissue and does not require special equipment. The number of dots/cell is counted at × 1,000 magnification and an average is determined. Factors affecting the AgNOR count include transcriptional activity of ribosomal genes, cell differentiation, and nucleolar association and dissociation.

Statin

Statin is a 57-kD protein with expression confined to the G0 phase of the cell cycle. It rapidly disappears on re-entry of the cell into G1 after stimulation with serum or growth factors such as platelet-derived growth factor (PDGF) or basic fibroblast growth factor (bFGF). It is localized to the nuclear envelope, resulting in a ring-like immunostaining pattern. Studies of lymphoid cells reveal that statin and Ki-67 antigen label distinct subsets of cells. Statin-positive cells in normal brain include neurons and some glia.[67]

Cell Loss Determination

Cell loss has been difficult to quantify in tumors. While zones of necrosis are often apparent on biopsy specimens and can be quantitated using image analysis, apoptosis can be very subtle. In situ nick translation methods to identify apoptosis in tissue sections have recently been developed and are now available commercially. Unfortunately, none of these methods has been applied to an analysis of specific grades of glioma.

Flow Cytometry

Proliferation data can be obtained based on knowledge of the DNA content in each phase of the cell cycle.[18] This has been facilitated by the development of automated flow cytometry, a method allowing for the rapid determination of the distribution of single-cell DNA content of large cell populations (Figure 2). Either fresh or paraffin-embedded material[20] may be studied. Single-cell suspensions are obtained by mechanical dissociation. DNA is labeled with propidium iodide in the presence of ribonuclease and detergent, and analyzed on a flow cytometer. Computer software designed for cell cycle analysis is utilized to evaluate the histograms. Proliferative activity is estimated by determining the S phase fraction.

Cell cycle analysis of human brain tumors is not restricted to cell kinetics evaluation alone. The analysis also characteristically includes

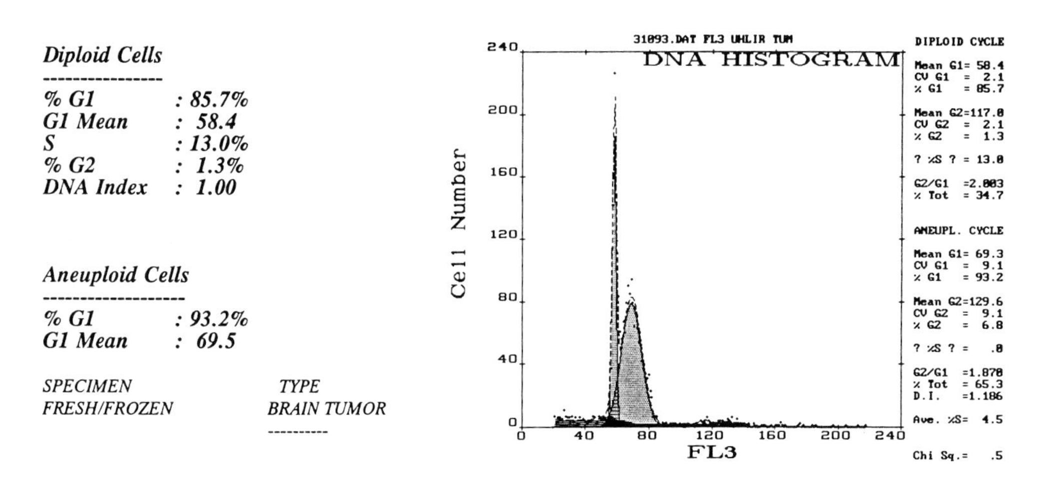

Figure 2: Flow cytometric analysis of a pilocytic astrocytoma. For description of the method see text.

ploidy determinations; aneuploid tumors demonstrate two or more G0-G1 phase peaks. Multivariate analysis of levels of critical cellular proteins such as c-*myc* can also be performed with respect to the different phases in the cell cycle.

Cell Kinetics Mathematics

The labeling index (LI) is a measure of the fraction of a cell population that incorporates a labeled precursor during a pulse exposure. Mathematically the observed LI (LI_{obs}) is expressed as:

$$LI_{obs} = \frac{\text{labeled cells}}{\text{labeled cells} + \text{unlabeled cells}}.$$

When labeled DNA precursors such as ^{3}H-thymidine or BUdR are used, the LI defines that population of cells actively involved in DNA synthesis (S phase): (cells in S)/(cells in G0 + G1 + S + G2 + M).

By following the percentage of labeled mitoses over time after the initial pulse, one can estimate the cell cycle time (T_c) and S phase time (T_s).

The LI cannot distinguish between unlabeled cells in a quiescent phase (G0) and a non-labeling proliferative phase (G1, G2, or M). Thus, the term "growth fraction" (GF) was introduced. It represents the number of cells actively cycling divided by the total number of cells (cycling and noncycling):

$$GF = \frac{\text{cells in G1} + \text{S} + \text{G2} + \text{M}}{\text{cells in G0} + \text{G1} + \text{S} + \text{G2} + \text{M}}.$$

Intuitively, the GF is 1 when there are no cells in the G0 phase. The GF is approximately measured by percentage Ki-67 labeling since this antibody binds only to cells that are actively cycling. Estimation of the GF is significant because it represents the population of cells most susceptible to chemotherapy.

Use of Proliferation Markers in the Biopsy Analysis of Benign Gliomas

A large body of data describing the cell kinetics of various central nervous system (CNS) tumors has accumulated in the last 15 years. When comparing the values between different studies, careful attention must be given to the method of labeling and the experimental protocol used. For instance, the BUdR LIs may vary because in vitro incubation with BUdR was used as opposed to in vivo infusion. Some recent studies have also analyzed the compatability of BUdR and Ki-67 antigen in evaluating similar tumors. Good correlation has been noted[58] and the following linear regression models have been proposed:

$$\text{BUdR} = 0.99 + (0.34)\ (\text{Ki-67}),\ r = 0.92$$
$$\text{Ki-67} = 1.15 + (1.59)\ (\text{BUdR}),\ r = 0.89.$$

TABLE 2

SUMMARY OF PROLIFERATION-RELATED MARKERS IN PILOCYTIC ASTROCYTOMAS

- Presence of mitoses does not correlate with prognosis
- No association between S phase by flow cytometry and prognosis
- BUdR labeling index ranges from 0.22% to 4.3% (higher in younger patients and in recurrent subtotally resected tumors)
- Ki-67 labeling index varies from <0.05% to 5.6%
- PCNA labeling varies from 0.6% to 6.7%

Pilocytic Astrocytomas

Table 2 presents a summary of proliferation-related markers used in pilocytic astrocytomas. The presence of even a single mitotic figure in a biopsy from a fibrillary astrocytoma is associated with a poorer prognosis; however, in pilocytic astrocytomas this has proved not to be true. Clinicopathological analysis of 51 patients with supratentorial pilocytic astrocytoma revealed no association between histological grade and patient survival time.[10] In particular, the presence of mitoses, which were identified in small numbers in 35%, readily found in 6%, and common in 2%, did not correlate with prognosis.

In an attempt to determine if more quantitative analysis of proliferation could show prognostic significance, the authors performed flow cytometry on 34 of the 51 patients. No association between S phase fraction or ploidy pattern and specific histological features or prognosis could be found.

The most extensive analysis of proliferation in pilocytic astrocytomas has been performed using BudR labeling. Several small series[15,25] showed a median LI of less than 1%; however, a wide range of values were present with LI as high as 7.9% in occasional patients (it should be noted that this LI is in the range reported for anaplastic astrocytomas). A large series of 50 juvenile pilocytic astrocytomas reported from the University of California at San Francisco[29] showed BUdR LIs ranging from 0.22% to 4.3% (<1% in 34 and >1% in 16; mean ± standard error of the mean: 1.05% ± 0.13%). Tumors from male patients exhibited a higher LI than those from female patients, and tumors in the cerebellum had a higher LI than those in the hypothalamus. Cerebral tumors had a low LI similar to hypothalamic tumors (0.73% ± 0.52%). The LI did not correlate with the gross appearance of the tumor. Of great interest, tumors from younger patients often had a higher LI than those from older patients, suggesting that as tumors aged they lost their proliferative activity. Among tumors that were subtotally resected, those that recurred had a higher LI (2.6% ± 0.7% versus 0.74% ± 0.09%, $P<.005$). Overall, including both incompletely and completely excised tumors, there was no relationship between LI and recurrence. The authors concluded that, although most juvenile pilocytic astrocytomas have a low LI, some tumors have a high LI, particularly in young patients; however, if mass effect is controlled the growth rate is likely to slow with a subsequent favorable clinical course.

Labeling indices for Ki-67 antigen have also been quite variable. Tsanaclis et al[68] reported a single pilocytic tumor with an LI of 5.6%, while Giangaspero et al[16] described a single patient with an LI of 1%. A larger series of 13 patients reported by Shibata et al[63] revealed a 0.3% to 1.6% range of LIs (mean 0.9%), while Jay et al,[30] in a series of 20 patients, showed a range from 0% to 2.23% (mean 0.93%). The recent development of an antibody (MIB-1) identifying Ki-67 antigen in paraffin-embedded sections should allow for more complete studies of proliferative potential. A recent study of brain tumors by Karamitopoulou et al[33] provided a survey of LIs, but in the results of their astrocytoma groups they did not distinguish between fibrillary and pilocytic tumors.

Small numbers of pilocytic astrocytomas have been studied by labeling for PCNA. In one patient the PCNA LI was high (6.7%) while an adjacent area showed a Ki-67 LI of only 0.6%, suggesting a falsely elevated PCNA.[37]

Desmoplastic Cerebral Astrocytomas of Infancy

VandenBerg[70] described a series of 22 desmoplastic infantile gangliogliomas and cerebral astrocytomas of infancy. He suggested that, although these patients have a long postoperative survival, their prognosis depends in part on gross total removal of the tumor. These tumors may have a significant proliferative potential if incompletely excised.

Aydin et al[2] reported proliferation data in a single patient with desmoplastic cerebral astrocytoma of infancy. Using flow cytometry, they found that 11.7% of the cells in this tumor were in the S phase, indicating high proliferative activity. AgNOR counting also revealed a high number of AgNORs/nucleus in the astrocytic population (6.07/nucleus) while smaller numbers were present in fibroblasts and endothelial cells. PCNA labeling was variable but ranged from 10% to 30% with an average of 20%.

A second single patient was reported by Paulus et al.[50] In that patient less than1% of cells were positive, indicating a very low growth fraction.

Pleomorphic Xanthoastrocytomas

The benign nature of pleomorphic xanthoastrocytoma is implied by its long clinical course, rarity of mitotic figures, and absence of necrosis.[34,36] Only a small number of these tumors have been assessed for their proliferative potential. Analysis of AgNORs by Sawada et al[59] revealed an average of 2.34/nucleus in pleomorphic xanthoastrocytomas, a level similar to that found in low-grade fibrillary astrocytomas. Ki-67 immunoreactivity in one case revealed an LI of less than 1%. DNA flow cytometry in another single case revealed an S phase fraction of less than 0.25%.[27]

Dysembryoplastic Neuroepithelial Tumors

Dysembryoplastic neuroepithelial tumors comprise a group of benign supratentorial cortical neoplasms of mixed neuronal-glial histology. A recent study of 18 tumors included LIs for MIB-1. Most cases were negative or showed small numbers of labeled nuclei; however, in three cases the LI was high and in the range found for anaplastic astrocytomas. It was suggested that the Ki-67 antigen LI is unreliable in these tumors as a prognostic indicator, possibly because of increased cell loss.[8]

Low-Grade Fibrillary Astrocytomas

The differentiation of low-grade fibrillary astrocytomas from reactive gliosis may be difficult in some cases. This difficulty suggested to neuropathologists that proliferation-related markers may be useful in distinguishing gliosis from glioma. Unfortunately, reactive astrocytes may be labeled with markers such as Ki-67 antigen at a level similar to that found in gliomas so that this marker may not be used on its own as an independent indicator of tumorgenicity. Recently, Louis et al[44] described using the AgNOR technique to differentiate between gliosis and low-grade fibrillary astrocytomas. In gliosis, AgNOR counts averaged 1.18 ± 0.11/nucleus while low-grade fibrillary astrocytomas averaged 2.22 ± 0.39. Although compound AgNORs were frequent in grade II astrocytomas, they were extremely rare in reactive gliosis. The authors concluded that this technique is a useful adjunct in the diagnosis of CNS neoplasia.

There has been a good correlation between histological grade of fibrillary astrocytomas and proliferation indices. Hoshino et al[25] found a significant correlation between survival times and BUdR LIs in both malignant gliomas and low-grade astrocytomas. Patients with low-grade astrocytomas with an LI greater than 1% had more recurrences and poorer survival times when compared to patients with a tumor LI less than 1%. In higher-grade tumors, there was better patient survival when the LI was greater than 5% as compared to less than 5%. Similar results had been demonstrated earlier using ^{3}H-thymidine.[26]

A larger number of studies have been performed showing a correlation between histological grade and Ki-67 LI for fibrillary gliomas.[7,15,16,30,48,49,54,55,68,73] They reveal that, on average, astrocytomas range from 0.3% to 1.8%, anaplastic astrocytomas from 4.1% to 8.6%, and glioblastomas multiforme from 6.4% to 13.5%. A recent study using MIB-1 revealed that astrocytomas had an LI of 2.03 ± 2.03, anaplastic astrocytomas 12.8 ± 6.29, and glioblastomas multiforme 14.57 ± 6.77.[33]

PCNA labeling has also been utilized in the analysis of fibrillary astrocytic tumors.[3,38] In one recent study, Kim et al[38] graded tumors based on the percentage of positive nuclei (grade 0, no positive nuclei; grade 1, ≤10% positive; grade 2, 11% to 50% positive; grade 3, >50% positive). The mean PCNA grade score for glioblastoma was 1.8 ± 0.18, for anaplastic astrocytoma 1.2 ± 0.11, and for astrocytoma 0.63 ± 0.24.

A recent study of 230 fibrillary astrocytomas by Coons et al[7] examined the prognostic significance of flow cytometric analysis of proliferative activity. Multivariate analysis revealed that S phase fraction showed significant independent prognostic importance (*P*<.01). On the basis of S phase fraction, patients could be divided into three groups with significantly different survival rates (<3%, 3% to 5.9%, and >6%).

Expression of Growth Factors

Table 3 summarizes growth factors implicated in glioma growth, some of which are angiogenic factors.

TABLE 3

GROWTH FACTORS IMPLICATED IN GLIOMA GROWTH

- Transforming growth factor-β*
- Vascular endothelial growth factor*
- Platelet-derived growth factor (PDGF)/PDGF receptor
- Basic fibroblast growth factor*
- Epidermal growth factor (EGF)/EGF receptor
- Cytokines: TNF-α,* IL-1, IL-6*

*Angiogenic factor.

Angiogenic Factors

Angiogenesis describes the collective events involved in the formation of new vessels from pre-existing vessels and is critical to the development of many tumors. Angiogenesis involves proteolytic digestion of extracellular matrix, migration of endothelial cells, proliferation of these cells, extracellular matrix production, vascular tube formation, and anastomosis of newly formed channels. A variety of angiogenic factors have been elucidated in both reactive and neoplastic conditions. Factors with significant angiogenic potential include: transforming growth factor-beta (TGF-β), vascular endothelial growth factor (VEGF), PDGF, and basic fibroblast growth factor (bFGF); others are TNF-α, urokinase plasminogen activator (uPA), and interleukins (IL). For tumors of the CNS, angiogenesis research has centered around the neovascular proliferation characteristic of glioblastoma multiforme. For example, VEGF, a factor whose the receptors are limited to endothelial cells, has been shown to be expressed in malignant gliomas in association with the presence of vascular proliferation.[53] Neovascularization is also characteristic of the pilocytic astrocytoma; however, there is no specific information on the presence of angiogenic factors in benign gliomas although it is implied that some angiogenic factor(s) must be expressed.

Transforming Growth Factor-Beta

TGF-β comprises a family of closely related peptides with pleiotropic effects involving growth regulation, wound healing, and morphogenesis. In general, TGF-β promotes growth of mesenchyme and inhibits epithelial cells. It promotes deposition of extracellular matrix and suppresses immune function during inflammation. Three isoforms of TGF-β (TGF-β1, -2, and -3) have been characterized in human glial tumors. TGF-β2 was first purified and cloned from a human glioblastoma cell line and found to inhibit the generation of allogeneic cytotoxic T cells and T cell growth induced by IL-2. A study by Constam et al[6] compared glioblastoma with primary cultured astrocyes and brain macrophages. They found that astrocytes secrete latent TGF-β1 and -2 and, although they have the messenger RNA (mRNA) for TGF-β3, they do not secrete it. Brain macrophages, however, have the mRNA for and secrete only TGF-β1. Glioblastoma cell lines release both latent and active TGF-β1 and -2 ; however, they share with astrocytes the inability to secrete TGF-β3. Schneider et al[61] reported the immunohistochemical presence of TGF-β in a series of malignant gliomas; benign (grade I) astrocytic tumors were not studied.

TGF-β is a potent growth inhibitor of many malignant cell lines and also appears to inhibit growth of certain glioblastoma cells in soft agar.[22] However, it also appears to be mitogenic to hyperdiploid glioblastoma cells. In contrast, near-diploid low-grade astrocytoma cells are growth inhibited by TGF-β1 and -2 in vitro. These results have suggested an autocrine hypothesis for the action of TGF-β in malignant gliomas.[32] Specific studies on the role of TGF-β in benign (grade I) gliomas have not been performed.

Vascular Endothelial Growth Factor

VEGF is a potent angiogenic factor and vascular permeability factor with receptors limited to endothelial cells. Its mRNA is markedly elevated in glioblastoma multiforme when compared to astrocytoma. It is significantly up-regulated adjacent to areas of necrosis, suggesting that it is induced by localized hypoxia. The presence of abundant VEGF receptors on tumor vascular endothelial cells suggests that VEGF may mediate angiogenesis through paracrine loops involving secretion of VEGF by tumor cells with resultant stimulation of adjacent endothelial cells.[53,64] There have been no studies concerning the presence of VEGF in bengin (grade I) gliomas.

Platelet-Derived Growth Factor

PDGF has a molecular weight of 30 kD and consists of two peptide chains (A and B) which may associate in three isoforms (AA, BB, and AB) and bind with different affinities to two types of cell surface receptors (α and β). It is a potent growth factor for glial cells and, when injected into the brains of marmoset monkeys with simian sarcoma virus, may form malignant glial tumors. It is of interest that the v-*sis* oncogene of simian sacrcoma virus is the retroviral homolog of the PDGF-B chain. Glioblastoma tumor cells have been shown to express both PDGF-A and -B chains as well as PDGF-α receptor, suggesting the possibility of an autocrine growth loop. The presence of up-regulated PDGF-β receptor on endothelial cells in malignant gliomas provides support for a paracrine angiogenesis mechanism. Gene amplification of the PDGF-α receptor has been reported in about 8% of glioblastoma tumors.[9,23,52] The specific role of PDGF in benign gliomas has not been investigated.

Basic Fibroblast Growth Factor

Basic FGF was originally purified from normal bovine brain and pituitary. It is a heparin-binding protein mitogenic toward a variety of mesodermal and neuroectodermal-derived cells and is a potent angiogenic factor. Immunohistochemical studies show that glioblastoma multiforme specimens exhibit prominent reactivity in both neoplastic astrocytes and endothelial cells. In low-grade astrocytomas, astrocytic cells are weakly and inconsistently stained. Reactive astroglial cells show variable reactivity. FGF-receptor-1 is expressed on both tumor cells and endothelial cells and the level of expression correlates with the level of FGF. Antisense oligonucleotides against bFGF inhibit colony formation by glioma cells in soft agar. The results suggest that bFGF is involved as a potential autocrine/paracrine growth factor in malignant gliomas. The expression pattern in benign gliomas has not been explored; however, the relatively low expression in low-grade fibrillary astrocytomas and reactive gliosis suggest that this is an unlikely mechanism.[45,69,72]

Epidermal Growth Factor Receptor

EGF is a 6-kD protein that stimulates growth of astrocytes and proliferation, migration, and invasiveness of glioma cells in vitro. The EGF receptor gene is the commonest amplified gene in glioblastoma (c-*erb*B1). The EGF receptor contains an intracellular domain with tyrosine kinase activity and an extracellular domain that binds EGF and TGF-α. Since malignant gliomas express both EGF and its receptor, an EGF autocrine loop has been suggested as a potential growth mechanism in these tumors. It has also been shown that EGF stimulation of EGF receptor on glioma cells may lead to increased production of VEGF, leading to increased angiogenesis.[17] Recent studies of large numbers of glial tumors have shown that EGF receptor expression is essentially limited to malignant gliomas, particularly glioblastoma multiforme. Approximately 50% of glioblastomas multiforme showed evidence of EGF receptor expression; however, none of the 25 grade I pilocytic astrocytomas studied showed evidence of EGF receptor expression, suggesting that this is an unlikely mechanism of growth control in these benign gliomas.[1,57]

Cytokines

Cytokines are important regulatory proteins controlling growth and differentiation, often in an autocrine or paracrine manner. Although originally described as products of lymphocytes and macrophages, cells of the CNS including astrocytes have been shown to be effective sources and targets for cytokines. Cytokines, acting through their specific cell-surface receptors, have been implicated as potential growth factors for a variety of tumors including malignant gliomas. The action of cytokines is pleiotropic, however, and thus the specific nature of the complex interactions between producing (tumor cells, leukocytes) and target cells (tumor cells, reactive astrocytes, endothelial cells, leukocytes) are not clear. Glioblastoma multiforme cell lines have been shown to produce and respond to several cytokines, including IL-1, TNF-α, and IL-6. TNF-α may result in either stimulation or inhibition of tumor cell growth, depending on the cell line studied, suggesting possible regulation at the level of the TNF receptor. Both TNF-α and IL-6 may also have angiogenic actions and have been implicated in tumor-associated angiogenesis. Analysis of a group of 15 malignant gliomas revealed prominent reactivity of infiltrating macrophages in five of 15 tumors for TNF-α and IL-6, while the tumor cells were only weakly positive.[60] Although it would seem illogical that the host would produce tumor-promoting factors, one could speculate that cytokine production by leukocytes is an attempt to inhibit tumor growth. Certain cytokines (TGF-β, IL-6) target specific nuclear downstream genes (c-*myc*, Rb, cyclin A) in vitro with resultant G0/G1 arrest and growth suppression. This study emphasizes the importance of understanding the complexities of the interrelationships between the tumor and its host in the analysis of growth factor action. There have been no specific studies of the localization or effects of cytokines in benign gliomas.

CONCLUSION

There is extensive literature concerning the assessment of proliferative potential and role of growth factors in progression of malignant gliomas. While there is, in general, a good correlation between grade and proliferative potential for fibrillary gliomas, benign (WHO grade I) gliomas show considerable variability in proliferative potential as we measure it, which does not appear to correlate with prognosis. This is important to recognize, since the finding of a high labeling index for a proliferation-related marker in a small fragment of biopsy material could result in inappropriately aggressive therapy. Potential reasons for this lack of correlation could include the necessity of correlating cell death with proliferation and the importance of other factors, such as invasiveness.

Several growth factors have been implicated for their role as autocrine/paracrine factors for glioma growth or neovascularizaton; however, there is very limited information about these factors in benign (grade I) gliomas. The apparently paradoxical presence of features associated with a poor prognosis for fibrillary tumors in benign pilocytic astrocytomas, including high metabolic rate as shown by proton emission tomography, contrast enhancement on computed tomography,[11,42] and vascular proliferation, suggest that similar growth factors may be active in these tumors. Future studies of the biology of benign gliomas will need to address the reasons for their more indolent behavior, including analyses of cell death, decreased invasiveness, and growth factor production and responsiveness.

REFERENCES

1. Agosti RM, Leuthold M, Gullick WJ, et al: Expression of the epidermal growth factor receptor in astrocytic tumours is specifically associated with glioblastoma multiforme. **Virchows Arch** [A] **420**:321-325, 1992
2. Aydin F, Ghatak NR, Salvant J et al: Desmoplastic cerebral astrocytoma of infancy. A case report with immunohistochemical, intrastructural and proliferation studies. **Acta Neuropathol 86**:666-670, 1993
3. Beppu T, Arai H, Kanaya H, et al: [Measurement of PCNA labeling index in astrocytic tumors.] **No Shinkei Geka 20**:1255-1259, 1992 (Jpn)
4. Buja LM, Eigenbrodt ML, Eigenbrodt EH: Apoptosis and necrosis. Basic types and mechanisms of cell death. **Arch Pathol Lab Med 117**:1208-1214, 1993
5. Burger PC, Shibata T, Kleihues P: The use of the monoclonal antibody Ki-67 in the identification of proliferating cells: application to surgical neuropathology. **Am J Surg Pathol 10**:611-617, 1986
6. Constam DB, Phillipp J, Malipiero UV, et al: Differential expression of transforming growth factor-β1, -β2, and -β3 by glioblastoma cells, astrocytes, and microglia. **J Immunol 148**: 1404-1410, 1992
7. Coons SW, Johnson PC, Pearl DK: Prognostic significance of flow cytometry DNA analysis of human astrocytomas. **Neurosurgery 35**:114-126, 1994
8. Daumas-Duport C: Dysembryoplastic neuroepithelial tumours. **Brain Pathol 3**:283-295, 1993
9. Fleming TP, Saxena A, Clark WC, et al: Amplification and/or overexpression of platelet-derived growth factor receptors and epidermal growth factor receptor in human glial tumors. **Cancer Res 52**:4550-4553, 1992
10. Forsyth PA, Shaw EG, Scheithauer BW, et al: Supratentorial pilocytic astrocytomas. A clinicopathologic, prognostic, and flow cytometric study of 51 patients. **Cancer 72**:1335-1342, 1993
11. Fulham MJ, Melisi JW, Nishimiya J, et al: Neuroimaging of juvenile pilocytic astrocytomas: an enigma. **Radiology 189**:221-225, 1993
12. Garcia RL, Coltrera MD, Gown AM: Analysis of proliferative grade using anti-PCNA/Cyclin monoclonal antibodies in fixed, embedded tissues. **Am J Pathol 134**:733-739, 1989
13. Gerdes J, Lemke H, Baisch H, et al: Cell cycle analysis of a cell proliferation-associated human nuclear antigen defined by the monoclonal antibody Ki-67. **J Immunol 133**:1710-1715, 1984
14. Gerdes J, Schwab U, Lemke H, et al: Production of a mouse monoclonal antibody reactive with a human nuclear antigen associated with cell proliferation. **Int J Cancer 31**:13-20, 1983
15. Germano IM, Ito M, Cho KG, et al: Correlation of histopathological features and proliferative potential of gliomas. **J Neurosurg 70**:701-706, 1989
16. Giangaspero F, Doglioni C, Rivano MT, et al: Growth fraction in human brain tumors defined by the monoclonal antibody Ki-67. **Acta Neuropathol 74**:179-182, 1987
17. Goldman CK, Kim J, Wong WL, et al: Epidermal growth factor stimulates vascular endothelial growth factor production by human malignant glioma cells: a model of glioblastoma multiforme pathophysiology. **Mol Biol Cell 4**:121-133, 1993
18. Gray JW, Dolbeare F, Pallavicini MG, et al: Cell cycle analysis using flow cytometry. **Int J Radiat Biol 49**:237-255, 1986
19. Hayostek CJ, Shaw EG, Scheithauer B, et al: Astrocytomas of the cerebellum. A comparative clinicopathological study of pilocytic and diffuse astrocytomas. **Cancer 72**:856-869, 1993
20. Hedley DW, Friedlander ML, Tayler IW: Application of DNA flow cytometry to paraffin-embedded archival material for the study of aneuploidy and its clinical significance. **Cytometry 6**:327-333, 1985
21. Heintz N: Temporal regulation of gene expression during the mammalian cell cycle. **Curr Opin Cell Biol 1**:275-278, 1989
22. Helseth E, Unsgaard G, Dalen A, et al: The effects of type beta transforming growth factor on proliferation and epidermal growth factor receptor expression in a human glioblastoma cell line. **J Neurooncol 6**:269-276, 1988
23. Hermanson M, Funa K, Hartman M, et al: Platelet-derived growth factor and its receptors in human glioma tissue: expression of messenger RNA and protein suggests the presence of autocrine and paracrine loops. **Cancer Res 52**:3213-3219, 1992
24. Hoshino T: A commentary on the biology and growth kinetics of low-grade and high-grade gliomas. **J Neurosurg 61**:895-900, 1984
25. Hoshino T, Nagashima T, Murovic JA, et al: *In situ* cell kinetics studies on human neuroectodermal tumors with bromodeoxyuridine labeling. **J Neurosurg 64**:453-459, 1986
26. Hoshino T, Townsend JJ, Muraoka I, et al: An autoradiographic study of human gliomas: growth kinetics of anaplastic astrocytoma and glioblastoma multiforme. **Brain 103**:967-984, 1980
27. Hosokawa Y, Tsuchihashi Y, Okabe H, et al: Pleomorphic xanthoastrocytoma. Ultrastructural, immunohistochemical, and DNA cytofluorometric study of a case. **Cancer 68**:853-859, 1991
28. Hunt T: Maturation promoting factor, cyclin and the control of M-phase. **Curr Opin Cell Biol 1**: 268-274, 1989
29. Ito S, Hoshino T, Shibuya M, et al: Proliferative characteristics of juvenile pilocytic astrocytomas determined by bromodeoxyuridine labeling. **Neurosurgery 31**:413-419, 1992
30. Jay V, Parkinson D, Becker L, et al: Cell kinetic analysis in pediatric brain and spinal tumors: a study of 117 cases with Ki-67 quantitation and flow cytometry. **Pediatric Pathol 14**:253-276, 1994
31. Jenkins RB, Kimmel DW, Moertel CA, et al: A cytogenetic study of 53 human gliomas. **Cancer Genet**

Cytogenet 39:253-279, 1989
32. Jennings MT, Maciunas RJ, Carver R, et al: TGF-B1 and TGF-B2 are potential growth regulators for low-grade and malignant gliomas *in vitro*: evidence in support of an autocrine hypothesis. **Int J Cancer** 49:129-139, 1991
33. Karamitopoulou E, Perentes E, Diamantis I, et al: Ki-67 immunoreactivity in human central nervous system tumors: a study with MIB1 monoclonal antibody on archival material. **Acta Neuropathol** 87:47-54, 1994
34. Kawano N: Pleomorphic xanthoastrocytoma: some new observations. **Clin Neuropathol** 11:323-328, 1992
35. Kehler U, Arnold H, Müller H: Long-term follow-up of infratentorial pilocytic astrocytomas. **Neurosurg Rev** 13:315-320, 1990
36. Kepes JJ: Pleomorphic xanthoastrocytoma: the birth of a diagnosis and a concept. **Brain Pathol** 3: 269-273, 1993
37. Khoshyomn S, Maier H, Morimura T, et al: Immunostaining for proliferating cell nuclear antigen: its role in determination of proliferation in routinely processed human brain tumor specimens. **Acta Neuropathol** 86:582-589, 1993
38. Kim DK, Hoyt J, Bacchi C, et al: Detection of proliferating cell nuclear antigen (PCNA) in gliomas and adjacent resection margin. **Neurosurgery** 33: 619-626, 1993
39. Kleihues P, Burger PC, Scheithauer BW: **Histological Typing of Tumors of the Central Nervous System. World Health Organization.** Berlin: Springer-Verlag, 1993
40. Kleihues P, Burger PC, Scheithauer BW: The new WHO classification of brain tumours. **Brain Pathol** 3:255-268, 1993
41. Kleinman GM, Schoene WC, Walshe TM III, et al: Malignant transformation in benign cerebellar astrocytoma. Case report. **J Neurosurg** 49:111-118, 1978
42. Lee YY, Van Tassel P, Bruner JM, et al: Juvenile pilocytic astrocytomas: CT and MR characteristics. **AJR** 152:1263-1270, 1989
43. Lewis RA, Gerson LP, Axelson KA, et al: von Recklinghausen neurofibromatosis. II. Incidence of optic gliomata. **Ophthalmology** 91:929-935, 1984
44. Louis DN, Meehan SM, Ferrante RJ, et al: Use of the silver nucleolar organizer region (AgNOR) technique in the differential diagnosis of central nervous system neoplasia. **J Neuropathol Exp Neurol** 51:150-157, 1992
45. Morrison RS, Giordano S, Yamaguchi F, et al: Basic fibroblast growth factor expression is required for clonogenic growth of human glioma cells. **J Neurosci Res** 34:502-509, 1993
46. Nagashima P, DeArmond SJ, Murovic J, et al: Immuncytohistochemical demonstration of S-phase cells by anti-bromodeoxyuridine monoclonal antibody in human brain tumor tissues. **Acta Neuropathol** 67:155-159, 1985
47. Nishizaki T, Orita T, Abibo S, et al: Subependymal giant cell astrocytoma associated with tuberous sclerosis: with special reference to cell kinetic studies—a case report. **Neurol Med Chir** 30:695-697, 1990
48. Nishizaki T, Orita T, Furutani Y, et al: Flow-cytometric DNA analysis and immunohistochemical measurement of Ki-67 and BUdR labeling indices in human brain tumors. **J Neurosurg** 70:379-384, 1989
49. Ostertag CB, Volk B, Shibata T, et al: The monoclonal antibody Ki-67 as a marker for proliferating cells in stereotactic biopsies of brain tumors. **Acta Neurochir** 89:117-121, 1987
50. Paulus W, Schlote W, Perentes E, et al: Desmoplastic supratentorial neuroepithelial tumours of infancy. **Histopathology** 21:43-49, 1992
51. Pines J, Hunter T: Isolation of a human cyclin cDNA: evidence for cyclin mRNA and protein regulation in the cell cycle and for interaction with $p34_{cdc2}$. **Cell** 58:833-846, 1989
52. Plate KH, Breier G, Farrell CL, et al: Platelet-derived growth factor receptor-β is induced during tumor development and upregulated during tumor progression in endothelial cells in human gliomas. **Lab Invest** 67:529-534, 1992
53. Plate KH, Breier G, Welch HA, et al: Vascular endothelial growth factor is a potential tumor angiogenesis factor in human gliomas in vivo. **Nature** 359:845-848, 1992
54. Prados MD, Krouwer HGJ, Edwards MSB, et al: Proliferative potential and outcome in pediatric astrocytic tumors. **J Neurooncol** 13:277-282, 1992
55. Raghavan R, Steart PV, Weller RD: Cell proliferation patterns in the diagnosis of astrocytomas, anaplastic astrocytomas, and glioblastoma multiforme: a Ki-67 study. **Neuropathol Appl Neurobiol** 16:123-133, 1990
56. Reddy GPV: Cell cycle: regulatory events in $G_1 \rightarrow S$ transition of mammalian cells. **J Cell Biochem** 54: 379-386, 1994
57. Reifenberger G, Prior R, Deckert M, et al: Epidermal growth factor receptor expression and growth fraction in human tumours of the nervous system. Virchows **Arch** [A] 414:147-155, 1989
58. Sasaki K, Matsumura K, Tsuji T, et al: Relationship between labeling indices of Ki-67 and BrdUrd in human malignant tumors. **Cancer** 62:989-993, 1988
59. Sawada T, Oinuma T, Katada H, et al: [Argyrophilic nucleolar organizer region proteins in human central nervous tumors.] **Rinsho Byori** 40:1179-1184, 1992 (Jpn)
60. Schlüter C, Duchrow M, Wohlenberg C, et al: The cell proliferation-associated antigen of antibody Ki-67: a very large, ubiquitous nuclear protein with numerous repeated elements, representing a new kind of cell cycle-maintaining protein. **J Cell Biol** 123:513-522, 1993
61. Schneider J, Hofman FM, Apuzzo MLJ, et al: Cytokines and immunoregulatory molecules in malignant glial neoplasms. **J Neurosurg** 77:

265-273, 1992

62. Schwartz AM, Ghatak NR: Malignant transformation of benign cerebellar astrocytoma. **Cancer 65:**333-336, 1990
63. Shibata T, Burger PC, Kleihues P: Ki-67 immunoperoxidase stain as marker for the histological grading of nervous system tumours. **Acta Neurochir Suppl 43:**103-106, 1988
64. Shweiki D, Itin A, Soffer D, et al: Vascular endothelial growth factor induced by hypoxia may mediate hypoxia-initiated angiogenesis. **Nature 359:** 843-845, 1992
65. Smith R, Crocker J: Evaluation of nucleolar organizer region-associated proteins in breast malignancy. **Histopathology 12:**113-25, 1988
66. Stewart BW: Mechanisms of apoptosis: integration of genetic, biochemical and cellular indicators. **JNCI 86:**1286-1246, 1994
67. Trudel MA, Oligny L, Caplan S, et al: Statin—a novel marker of nonproliferation. **Am J Clin Pathol 101:**421-425, 1994
68. Tsanaclis AM, Robert F, Michaud J, et al: The cycling pool of cells within human brain tumors: *in situ* cytokinetics using the monoclonal antibody Ki-67. **Can J Neurol Sci 18:**12-17, 1991
69. Ueba T, Takahashi JA, Fukumoto M, et al: Expression of fibroblast growth factor receptor-1 in human glioma and meningioma tissues. **Neurosurgery 34:**221-226, 1994
70. VandenBerg SR: Desmoplastic infantile ganglioglioma and desmoplastic cerebral astrocytoma of infancy. **Brain Pathol 3:**275-281, 1993
71. Wong GHW, Goeddel DV: Fas antigen and p55 TNF receptor signal apoptosis through distinct pathways. **J Immunol 152:**1751-1755, 1994
72. Zagzag D, Miller DC, Sato Y, et al: Immunohistochemical localization of basic fibroblast growth factor in astrocytomas. **Cancer Res 22:**7393-7398, 1990
73. Zuber P, Hamou MF, de Tribolet N: Identification of proliferating cells in human gliomas using the monoclonal antibody Ki-67. **Neurosurgery 22:** 364-268, 1988

CHAPTER 9

Molecular Genetic Basis of Cerebral Gliomas

David N. Louis, MD, Bernd R. Seizinger, MD, PhD, and Webster K. Cavenee, PhD

The past few years have witnessed the emergence of a considerable body of knowledge concerning the molecular genetic alterations that characterize glial tumors. Together with investigations into the molecular basis of other common human tumors (such as colon and breast carcinoma), clinical and basic scientists have begun to trace the genetic pathways that lead to glial tumorigenesis. This chapter reviews current knowledge concerning the molecular genetic basis of cerebral gliomas. The discussion begins by highlighting the basic principles of molecular genetics of human tumors and the unique insights afforded by the neurological tumor syndromes, such as the neurofibromatoses. The majority of the review will focus on the diffuse fibrillary astrocytomas that affect the cerebral hemispheres of adults, since these are the most common and the most extensively studied of human gliomas. Finally, the genetic characteristics of the less common and less well-studied gliomas, such as pilocytic astrocytomas, oligodendrogliomas, and ependymomas, will be discussed.

Oncogenes and Tumor Suppressor Genes

The evolving era of molecular genetics has resulted in significant insights into the fundamental mechanisms of tumor development. Neoplastic transformation appears to be a multistep process in which the normal controls of cell proliferation and cell-cell interaction are lost, thus transforming a benign into a malignant phenotype. Studies of numerous different human and experimental tumors have shown that this tumorigenic process involves an interplay between two classes of genes: oncogenes and tumor suppressor genes[16] (see Glossary).

An oncogene is an abnormally activated version of a cellular gene, which is known as a "proto-oncogene" and which promotes normal cell proliferation and growth.[4] Proto-oncogenes typically code for growth-promoting proteins, such as growth factors, cell-surface receptors, or nuclear regulatory proteins. Abnormal activation of the proto-oncogene results in an exaggerated impulse for the cell to grow and divide. A proto-oncogene can be converted to an oncogene by a variety of genetic mechanisms, including point mutation, translocation, and amplification. In gliomas, most oncogene abnormalities identified to date have been gene amplifications, in which there is an increased copy number of a particular gene (Figure 1). In addition to structural changes such as point mutation, translocation, and amplification (see Glossary) growth factors may be abnormally overexpressed in tumor cells because of altered gene regulation (Figure 1). This mechanism also appears to be important in primary gliomas.

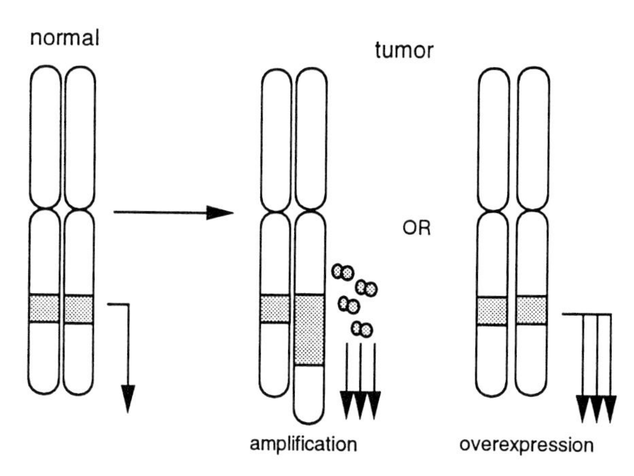

Figure 1: The *left* panel illustrates normal tissues. In this panel a proto-oncogene produces a growth signal (*single downward arrow*). In gliomas, a proto-oncogene can be converted into an oncogene by two common mechanisms. The *middle* panel shows gene amplification with overexpression (*multiple arrows*), as in the case of the EGFR gene in GBMs. The *right* panel illustrates overexpression (*multiple arrows*) by other mechanisms, as in the case of the PDGF ligands and receptors in astrocytomas.

Tumor suppressor genes are normal genes that act to inhibit cell proliferation and growth.[58] Thus, the loss or inactivation of these genes may result in tumor formation or progression. As opposed to oncogenes, which require activation of just one allelic copy of a proto-oncogene and therefore act in a genetically "dominant" manner, both allelic copies of a tumor suppressor gene must be inactivated to provide an oncogenic stimulus. Tumor suppressor genes are therefore genetically "recessive" and have been alternatively termed "recessive oncogenes." In some situations, however, a single mutant tumor suppressor allele may have an oncogenic effect and is said to act in a "dominant negative" manner. The most common scenario for inactivation of both copies of a tumor suppressor gene is mutation of one allelic copy, followed by loss of all or part of the chromosome bearing the second allelic copy, either by nondysjunction, deletion, or mitotic recombination (Figure 2). Consequently, the identification of consistent regions of chromosomal loss in specific tumor types is evidence that a tumor suppressor gene resides in that chromosomal region. Allelic chromosomal loss also provides a convenient means for identifying potential tumor suppressor genes: loss of heterozygosity (LOH) studies (see Glossary).[76] These studies employ genetic polymorphisms, such as restriction fragment length polymorphisms (RFLP) or microsatellite polymorphisms, to distinguish the patient's normal maternal and paternal alleles in normal (usually blood) deoxyribonucleic acid (DNA). If a particular polymorphism identifies two alleles in a patient, the patient is said to be "heterozygous" or "informative" at that locus. Comparison of the polymorphism in normal and tumor DNA will show allelic loss if either the maternal or paternal allele is absent in the tumor. This LOH implies allelic loss at the chromosomal region of interest (Figure 2). In many cases, these LOH studies provide the only means of searching for tumor suppressor gene inactivation, since the number of well-characterized tumor suppressor genes remains quite limited. These analyses are now robust in many tumor types[76] and, as discussed below, they have been integral to the identification of putative tumor suppressor loci in human gliomas. In addition, the loss or inactivation of tumor suppressor genes also plays a role in many of the inherited tumor syndromes, including a host of neurological tumor syndromes, which are discussed in greater detail below.

In most non-nervous system tumors, multiple genetic events appear necessary before a tumor is formed. Furthermore, certain genetic

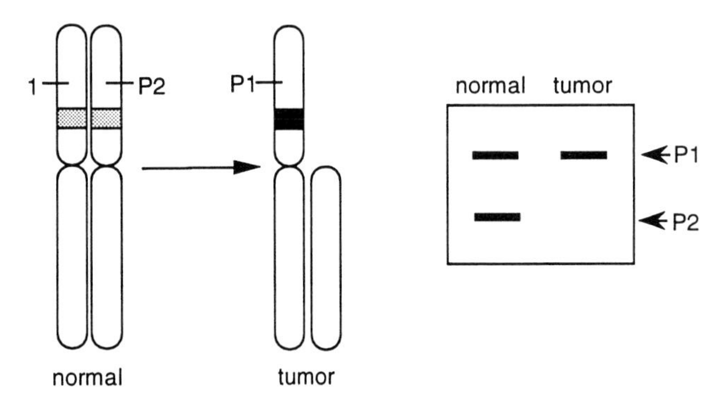

Figure 2: In normal tissues, tumor suppressor genes *(shaded boxes)* suppress cell growth *(left)*. In tumors, both tumor suppressor gene alleles become inactivated, one by mutation *(black box)* and one by loss of the second allele. Loss of a chromosomal arm can be detected by studying a polymorphism (P), which is different in a patient's paternal and maternal alleles (P1 and P2). Comparison of normal and tumor DNA on a Southern blot study *(right)* will then demonstrate loss of one allele (P2) in the tumor.

events are characteristic of specific stages in tumor development. In colon carcinoma, for instance, specific genetic alterations are associated with precursor polyps, while other genetic changes characterize the transition to carcinoma.[16] Such detailed knowledge of the specific genetic events that are involved in the formation of specific tumors is also beginning to provide important clinical information. Oncogene activation has been correlated with clinical course in some tumors, such as N-*myc* gene amplification in neuroblastoma,[5] while tumor suppressor gene alterations have been correlated with the clinical course in other tumors, such as p53 abnormalities in breast carcinoma.[76] Such studies provide a background for recent investigations suggesting that analysis of genetic events in gliomas may also result in useful clinical and pathogenetic information.

Neurological Tumor Syndromes

Hereditary neurological tumor syndromes, in which patients have a high incidence of multiple nervous system tumors, have provided important clues to the genetic basis of gliomas and other brain tumors. The neurological tumor syndromes in which gliomas are common include the so-called "neurocutaneous syndromes," such as neurofibromatosis (NF) 1, NF2, tuberous sclerosis (TS), and other tumor conditions such as Li-Fraumeni cancer syndrome, Turcot's syndrome, and isolated glioma families. Each syndrome is accompanied by a characteristic panoply of tumors, both neurological and non-neurological. A catalog of only the gliomas would feature optic nerve gliomas and other astrocytomas in NF1; ependymomas and astrocytomas in NF2; subependymal giant cell astrocytomas in TS; and various malignant gliomas in Li-Fraumeni cancer syndrome, Turcot's syndrome, and the hereditary glioma pedigrees.

Linkage studies (see Glossary) have provided powerful means for tracking down the genes associated with these tumor syndromes, and have assigned the NF1 gene to chromosome 17q11.2 (see Glossary),[77] the NF2 gene to chromosome 22q11.2-q12,[70] and the TS gene or genes to chromosomes 9q32-34 and 16p13.3.[32,45] The NF1 gene codes for a guanosine triphosphatase-activating protein (GAP) are termed "neurofibromin."[10,91,96] Neurofibromin interacts with the p21 product of the *ras* oncogene and is most likely important in growth factor-mediated signal transduction.[31] The NF2 gene codes for a protein, termed "merlin" (that is homologous with moesin, ezrin, and radixin), suggesting that the protein functions to link the cytoskeleton and cell surface.[69,80] One of the TS genes, TSC2 on chromosome 16p, has also recently been identified.[15] Like NF1, TSC2 encodes a GAP. While TSC2 GAP is not homologous with neurofibromin, these proteins may nonetheless be involved in similar cellular pathways. For the Li-Fraumeni cancer syndrome, mutational analyses have implicated the p53 gene on chromosome 17p13.1;[57] this is perhaps the most studied of all tumor genes. This nuclear phosphoprotein has been implicated in many cell functions, including cell cycle arrest, differentiation, DNA damage and repair, and apoptosis.[52] The other neurological tumor syndrome genes await identification and characterization.

These tumor syndromes provide unique insights into tumor suppressor genes. For instance, the hereditary retinoblastoma syndrome, which provided much of the impetus for current tumor suppressor gene research, results from a mutation in the retinoblastoma (Rb) tumor suppressor gene on chromosome 13q14. The retinoblastoma story revealed that both copies of this gene must be inactivated to overcome its tumor suppressor function.[8] In the case of familial retinoblastoma, the patient inherits one mutant, inactive copy of the Rb gene and thus carries a "germline" mutation in every cell.[9] A tumorigenic process begins in a cell when the second copy of the gene is inactivated, either by mutation or by loss of a portion of chromosome 13q. A patient with sporadic retinoblastomas does not carry the germline mutation and must acquire both inactivating "hits" in the same cell during his or her life. Therefore, a familial retinoblastoma patient, in whom every cell contains a mutation, is much more likely to develop a second retinoblastoma than a sporadic retinoblastoma patient.[21] In addition, sporadic retinoblastomas occur later in life than their familial counterparts. Consequently, in the case of glial tumors, patients with the above neurological tumor syndromes, who already have germline mutations, have a greatly increased incidence of gliomas, may develop multiple gliomas, and usually acquire these tumors at an earlier age than patients with sporadic gliomas.

Molecular Genetics of Diffuse Fibrillary Astrocytoma

Over the past few years, a number of investigators have applied molecular genetic techniques to astrocytomas in order to understand the molecular basis of astrocytoma formation and progression. The work from our laboratories and from other investigators has focused on the common diffuse fibrillary astrocytomas that affect adults, since these are by far the most common of cerebral gliomas. These studies have implicated the epidermal growth factor receptor (EFGR), the platelet-derived growth factor (PDGF) and its receptors, and the tumor suppressor genes on chromosomes 9p, 10, 11p, 13q, 17p, 19q, and 22q in astrocytoma tumorigenesis. These genetic alterations are diagrammed in Figure 3. The following discussion outlines the genetic alterations that characterize each stage of astrocytoma progression and presents data suggesting the existence of genetic subsets of glioblastoma multiforme (GBM).

The Formation of Low-Grade Astrocytoma

The p53 Gene and Chromosome 17p

The p53 gene, a tumor suppressor gene located on chromosome 17p, is the most frequently mutated gene in a number of common human cancers and has been the subject of intensive investigation over the past few years. It appears to have an integral role in a number of cellular processes, including cell cycle arrest, response to DNA damage, differentiation, and apoptosis. These protective roles have given p53 the nickname "guardian of the genome." Since the details of p53 alterations in brain tumors are beyond the scope of this chapter, we will only summarize some of the salient features and refer the reader to a recent review for further information.[52]

Our studies, as well as those of others, have clearly implicated the p53 gene in astrocytoma

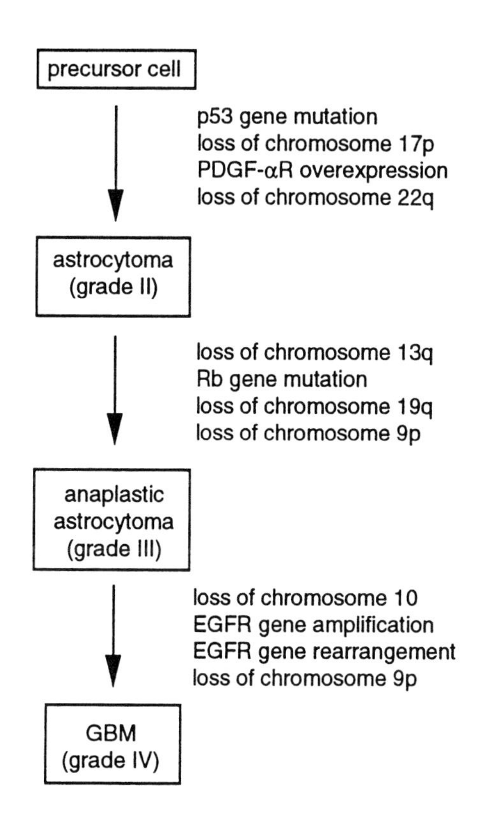

Figure 3: Molecular genetic alterations characteristic of different stages of astrocytoma progression. Grading according to the World Health Organization classification.[49]

tumorigenesis.[11,20,24,27,40,54,75,78,85] Mutations of p53 and allelic loss of chromosome 17p are observed in approximately one-third of all three grades of adult astrocytomas, suggesting that inactivation of p53 is important in the formation of low-grade astrocytomas (grade II on the World Health Organization (WHO) classification system[49]). These mutations are primarily missense (that is, leading to a change in an amino acid) and preferentially affect the evolutionally conserved domains in exons 5, 7, and 8. Particular hot-spots for mutations include codons 175, 248, and 273, in which spontaneous deamination of 5-methylcytosine residues most likely leads to C to T transition mutations.[52]

Mutations of p53 are closely correlated with allelic loss of chromosome 17p.[52,85] In this regard, p53 conforms to the classic paradigm of tumor suppressor gene inactivation, with mutation inactivating one allele and chromosomal loss inactivating the second. A remaining question, however, has been whether chromosome 17p harbors a second, more distal astrocytoma tumor suppressor gene. Such a gene has been implicated in other human tumors, including medulloblastomas.[2] The close correlation of p53 mutation and 17p loss, however, suggests that p53 is the target of allelic loss on chromosome 17p. We have studied astrocytomas at multiple 17p loci, in the area of the p53 gene and telomeric to the gene,[85] but have been unable to detect any cases with allelic loss telomeric to p53 that maintained heterozygosity at the p53 locus itself. While two astrocytomas have been reported to have strictly telomeric 17p loss, both cases also exhibited mutations in the p53 gene.[75] Therefore, there is as yet no firm evidence to suggest a second astrocytoma tumor suppressor gene on 17p.

A number of studies have also examined p53 protein expression in astrocytomas.[54] Most human tumors with p53 mutations have p53 protein stabilization, which enables the protein to be detected by immunohistochemistry. While many astrocytomas showed protein accumulation in the presence of gene mutation, we have demonstrated that tumors with frameshift p53 mutations are immunohistochemically negative. More problematic, however, has been the observation that some astrocytomas have elevated levels of wild-type p53 protein.[73] Although the product of the MDM2 oncogene binds wild-type p53 and could account for p53 accumulation, analysis of astrocytomas with accumulated wild-type p53 has not revealed MDM2 gene amplification.[73] MDM2 amplification has been noted in 8% to 10% of only one series of astrocytomas,[67] but was not detected in three other series.[61,73,75] Thus, evidence suggests that some astrocytomas may accumulate wild-type p53 protein, but probably not as a result of MDM2 gene amplification. The functional relevance of accumulation of a tumor suppressor in a neoplasm seems counterintuitive, but this phenomenon may reflect a physiological response by p53 to such stimuli as DNA damage in the tumor cells.

Platelet-Derived Growth Factor-Alpha Receptor Overexpression

While a number of growth factors are overexpressed in astrocytomas, PDGF has been the best studied and the most clearly implicated. PDGF exists as a homo- or heterodimer of two chains, A and B, while the PDGF receptor is a homo- or heterodimer of transmembrane receptor tyrosine kinases, α and β.[33] Studies of astrocytomas have shown overexpression of cognate ligands and receptors and have thus strongly suggested the presence of autocrine stimulatory loops.[35,62] Interestingly, it has been demonstrated that PDGF-AA and PDGF-α receptors are primarily overexpressed in astrocytoma cells, while the PDGF-BB and PDGF-β receptors are overexpressed in proliferating endothelial cells.[36] The mechanisms for overexpression in most cases, however, have not been elucidated, although rare astrocytomas do display amplification of the PDGF-α receptor gene.[18]

A recent analysis of PDGF ligand and receptor expression in a series of astrocytomas has shown PDGF-α receptor overexpression in 60% to 80% of all grades of diffuse fibrillary astrocytoma, suggesting that such overexpression is important in the initial stages of astrocytoma formation (M. Hermanson and D. N. Louis, unpublished data). Furthermore, there is a tight correlation between the loss of chromosome 17p and PDGF-α receptor overexpression, in that 17p loss is only seen in astrocytomas with PDGF-α receptor overexpression. These observations may imply that p53 mutations have an oncogenic effect only in the presence of PDGF α-receptor overexpression. Alternatively, PDGF α-receptor overexpression, perhaps through enhanced mitogenesis and thereby increased numbers of susceptible mitoses, may predispose to p53 mutation and 17p loss. These relationships are discussed below with regard to putative genetic subsets of GBM.

Chromosome 22q

Allelic loss of chromosome 22q is found in approximately 20% to 30% of astrocytomas.[26,39] Because allelic loss of 22q is found in low-grade as well as high-grade astrocytomas, the tumor suppressor gene on 22q may be important in the early stages of astrocytoma tumorigenesis. The NF2 gene is a tumor suppressor gene on chromosome 22q that is responsible for NF2, a hereditary tumor syndrome in which patients develop multiple schwannomas and meningiomas. Since NF2 patients also have a higher incidence of gliomas (particularly ependymomas but astrocytomas as well) the NF2 gene is a good candidate for the astrocytoma tumor suppressor on chromosome 22q.

The recent cloning of the NF2 gene[80] has enabled us to examine the entire coding sequence of the NF2 gene in 25 astrocytomas of different grades. We did not detect any NF2 mutations in astrocytomas,[71] making it unlikely that the NF2 gene is the astrocytoma tumor suppressor gene on chromosome 22q. Furthermore, deletion mapping (see Glossary) of 22q in astrocytomas (see bracketed region on the chromosome 22q map, Figure 4) has revealed three cases with 22q loss telomeric to NF2, but with maintenance of both NF2 alleles.[65] Coupled with our data, this suggests that the astrocytoma tumor suppressor gene on chromosome 22q is distal to NF2.

The Progression to Anaplastic Astrocytoma

The Rb Susceptibility Gene and Chromosome 13q

Loss of chromosome 13q occurs in up to 50% of human astrocytomas,[82] suggesting the presence of an astrocytoma tumor suppressor gene on that chromosome. To determine if the Rb gene on 13q14 contributes to the formation of astrocytomas, we examined 77 tumors for LOH at the intragenic Rb 1.20 locus.[34] LOH was detected in 16 (30%) of 53 informative high-grade astrocytomas, but was not detected in low-grade gliomas. Deletion mapping with flanking markers on 13q revealed that the 13q14 region containing Rb was preferentially targeted by the deletions. Sixteen tumors with LOH at Rb 1.20 were examined for mutations in the remaining Rb allele, and mutations were detected in four cases. These were primarily deletions that resulted in frameshifts or altered splice junction sites. Rb protein (pRb) expression, as assessed by immunohistochemistry, was altered in some of the cases with LOH. In the only previous study to specifically analyze the Rb locus,[82] LOH was detected at a variable-number tandem repeat polymorphism within the Rb gene in four of nine glioblastomas, and one of the four tumors contained an interstitial deletion in the remaining allele.[78]

The data suggest that Rb gene inactivation is restricted to high-grade tumors, since no low-grade tumor had LOH at Rb 1.20. Furthermore, LOH at Rb 1.20 was detected more frequently in GBMs than in anaplastic astrocytomas in our series, lending credence to the notion that Rb inactivation also occurs during progression to GBM. Similarly, LOH at Rb was not detected in any of four low-grade astrocytomas but it was found in four of nine GBMs in a previous study,[82] and an analysis of pRb expression revealed the absence of detectable pRb in four of 10 high-grade astrocytomas, whereas all seven low-grade tumors expressed pRb.[1] These data are all consistent with the hypothesis that Rb inactivation occurs in astrocytoma progression, and thereby implicate Rb as the second known tumor suppressor gene (after p53) to be involved in astrocytoma formation.

Chromosome 19q

Allelic losses on chromosome 19q have been observed in up to 40% of medium- and high-grade astrocytomas, and in the majority of oligodendrogliomas and mixed oligodendroglioma-astrocytomas, indicating the presence of a glial tumor suppressor gene on chromosome 19q.[88] Furthermore, such data demonstrate genetic similarities between astrocytomas, oligodendrogliomas, and mixed glial tumors. To narrow the location of the 19q tumor suppressor gene, we have recently studied astrocytomas with numerous closely spaced microsatellite polymorphisms on chromosome 19q. Analysis of cases with partial or interstitial deletions suggests that the common region of overlap localizes to 19q13.2-13.4, between markers D19S178 and D19S180 (see bracketed region on the chromosome 19q map, Figure 4).[72,89]

The chromosome 19q tumor suppressor gene is of particular interest for a number of reasons. The first is that, while allelic loss of chromosomes such as 17p and 10 are common in other human tumors, loss of chromosome 19q appears to be unique to glial tumors.[76] This may suggest the presence of a glial-specific tumor suppressor gene on this chromosome. The second reason for the importance of chromosome 19q is that it harbors a handful of DNA repair genes, such as ERCC1, ERCC2, XRCC, and DNA ligase I. Given the emerging relationship between DNA repair and tumor suppressor pathways,[47,50] these may prove promising candidate tumor suppressor genes.

Chromosome 9p

Initial studies of chromosome 9p showed that approximately 50% of anaplastic astrocytomas and GBMs have 9p deletions in the region of the interferon (IFN) gene cluster, including some GBMs with homozygous deletions.[41] Although the probes from this study were restricted to the IFN region, they suggested that allelic losses may be centered in the centromeric end of the region. Subsequent studies found 9p loss in approximately one-third of primary astrocytomas, predominantly in GBMs.[64] In glioma cell lines, 9p loss was noted in two-thirds of cases, which most likely represented the high number of cell lines that were derived from higher-grade tumors.[64] Interestingly, in our experience, the frequency of 9p loss increases not only at the transition from astrocytoma to anaplastic astrocytoma, but also at the transition from anaplastic astrocytoma to GBM, implying that the 9p tumor suppressor plays a role in astrocytoma progression at different stages.[84] It has been suggested that loss of one 9p allele is usually seen in anaplastic astrocytoma, while loss of both alleles is seen only in GBM.[12] One explanation for such a phenomenon would be a dosage effect, whereby a cell with one allele is hampered in its ability to suppress the next oncogenic step, but not as impaired as a cell lacking both copies.

Genomic deletion mapping and studies of methylthioadenosine phosphorylase (MTAP) protein expression suggested that the chromo-

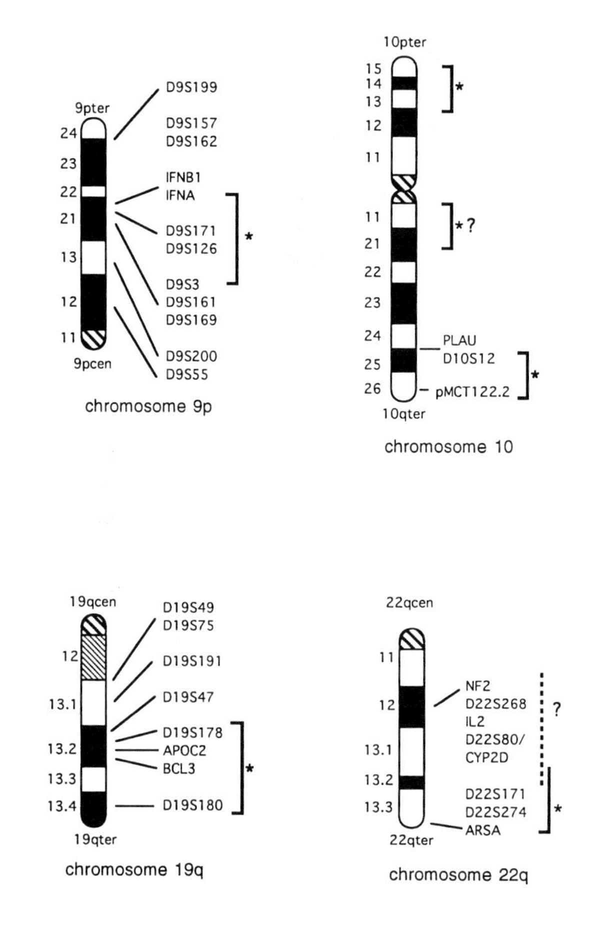

Figure 4: Maps of chromosomes 9p, 10, 19q, and 22q, with locations (*bracketed regions with asterisks*) of putative astrocytoma tumor suppressor genes.

some 9p region of interest lay between the centromeric end of the IFN gene cluster and the MTAP gene locus.[64] Recent Southern blotting deletion mapping studies in glioma cell lines have narrowed the region of interest to a portion of 9p21-p22, which includes the centromeric portions of IFN and extends to the next centromeric marker, D9S126 (Figure 4).[43] We have studied primary high-grade astrocytomas (including GBMs) for chromosome 9p loss with multiple polymorphic microsatellite loci on chromosome 9p and have shown that the common region of deletion in primary high-grade astrocytomas conforms to that shown in glioma cell lines: in the approximately 7 to 8 centiMorgans (cM) of 9p21 proximal to IFNA but distal to D9S3 region.[81] While such studies implicate a gene on 9p in the region of the centromeric end of the IFN gene cluster, the IFN genes themselves are probably not the targets. One study of IFN function in gliomas showed no correlation between IFN region deletions and sensitivity to IFN,[60] and deletion studies in other human tumors, such as malignant melanoma, have suggested a slightly more centromeric locus, involving only D9S126, but not extending to the telomeric IFN or to the centromeric D9S3 (see bracketed region on the chromosome 9p map, Figure 4).[19]

The Progression to Glioblastoma Multiforme

Chromosomes 10q and 10p

Chromosome 10 loss is a frequent finding in high-grade gliomas, both at the cytogenetic and molecular genetic level. Studies have found allelic loss of chromosome 10 in 60% to 95% of GBMs, but in only occasional cases of anaplastic astrocytoma.[22,26,39,83,87] In our series of 106 gliomas, allelic loss of chromosome 10 was restricted to GBMs, and was not seen in any low- or medium-grade gliomas.[87] These findings strongly suggest the presence of at least one tumor suppressor gene on chromosome 10 that is involved in the transition to GBM. Attempts to identify this chromosome 10 tumor suppressor gene by deletion mapping, however, have been hampered by the observation that, in most cases, the entire chromosome is lost. However, a number of recent deletion mapping studies have demonstrated telomeric losses restricted to band q25[25,46,66] (see lowest bracketed region on the chromosome 10 map, Figure 4). In addition, a number of studies have detected cases with loss of only the short arm of chromosome 10, suggesting the presence of a second tumor suppressor gene on the short arm[46,87] and one study has postulated that a third locus may exist on the long arm, near the centromere[46] (see other bracketed region on chromosome 10 map, Figure 4). Attempts to isolate these genes are underway, and will no doubt shed light on these putative tumor suppressor genes. The relationship of chromosome 10 loss to EGFR gene amplification is discussed below.

The Epidermal Growth Factor Receptor Gene

EGFR is a transmembrane receptor tyrosine kinase, with ligands including EGF and transforming growth factor-α. The EGFR gene is the most frequently amplified oncogene in astrocytic tumors,[23] and is amplified in approximately 40% of all GBMs.[87] (Less commonly amplified oncogenes include N-*myc*, *gli*, PDGF-α receptor, c-*myc*, *myb*, K-*ras*, and MDM2.) In our series of 106 gliomas, EGFR gene amplification was restricted to GBMs and was not seen in a variety of astrocytic and non-astrocytic low- or medium-grade gliomas.[87] Other authors have reported occasional cases of anaplastic astrocytoma with EGFR gene amplification.[14,37] GBMs with EGFR gene amplification display overexpression of EGFR at both the messenger ribonucleic acid (mRNA) and protein levels, suggesting that activation of this growth signal pathway is integral to malignant progression in astrocytomas.[14,94] Approximately one-third of those GBMs with EGFR gene amplification also have EGFR gene rearrangements, some of which produce truncated molecules similar to the v-*erb* B oncogene.

We[87] and others[14] have also examined EGFR amplification in patients from whom we obtained both primary and recurrent GBMs. Only those recurrent tumors with EGFR amplification in the initial GBMs exhibited EGFR amplification in the recurrent tumors, with no change in the gene copy number. The findings are similar to those reported in neuroblastoma, in which N-*myc* amplification remains stable between primary and recurrent tumors.[5]

Those GBMs that exhibit EGFR gene amplification have almost always lost genetic material on chromosome 10.[87] This close association suggested a relationship between these two genetic events, and is akin to other tumors, such as neuroblastoma[5] and Wilms tumor,[13] in which interactions occur between oncogenes and tumor suppressor genes. Moreover, we suggested that loss of a tumor suppressor gene on chromosome 10 most likely precedes EGFR gene amplification in the temporal sequence of GBM formation (Figure 3). It is possible that loss of function of a chromosome 10 tumor suppressor gene allows the cell to acquire a growth advantage or leads to genomic instability,[51] which in turn may enable the cell to undergo amplification of the EGFR gene. Alternatively, EGFR gene amplification may exert an oncogenic effect only if there has been previous loss of the chromosome 10 tumor suppressor, and therefore clones with EGFR gene amplification would only arise from cells with prior loss of chromosome 10.

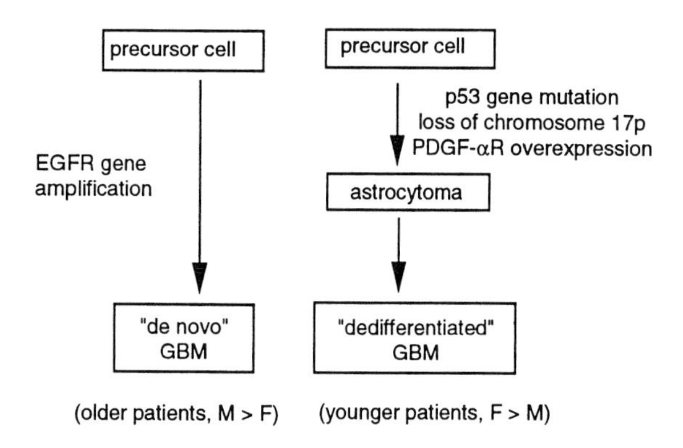

Figure 5: Molecular genetic subsets of GBM. M = male; F = female. See text for details.

Subsets of Glioblastoma Multiforme

The assumption that all astrocytomas progress through distinct genetic stages in a linear fashion, as depicted in Figure 3, is most likely an oversimplification. Indeed, it appears as if there are biological subsets of astrocytomas that may reflect the clinical heterogeneity observed in these tumors. For instance, we have shown that GBMs can be divided on the basis of molecular genetic analysis. As stated above, loss of chromosome 17p and associated p53 gene mutation occur in tumors with PDGF-α receptor overexpression (M. Hermanson and D.N. Louis, unpublished data), and EGFR gene amplification is seen in tumors with loss of chromosome 10.[87] However, EGFR gene amplification almost never occurs in GBMs with loss of chromosome 17p.[90] We examined GBMs from 67 patients and found only one patient with both EGFR gene amplification and 17p loss. We therefore explored the possibility that genetic analysis of 17p loss and the EGFR gene amplification could be used to subdivide GBMs into distinct clinical groups. Glioblastomas with loss of chromosome 17p occurred in patients significantly younger (mean age 40.5 years) and more frequently in women than glioblastomas characterized by EGFR gene amplification (mean age 56.3 years) (P=.001).[90] These subsets are corroborated by data comparing PDGF-α receptor overexpression and gene amplification with EGFR gene amplification, since tumors with PDGF-α receptor overexpression or gene amplification do not show EGFR gene amplification.

These findings allow the separation of GBMs into at least two subsets: GBMs with EGFR gene amplification and GBMs with loss of chromosome 17p, p53 mutations, and PDGF-α receptor overexpression[90] (M. Hermanson and D.N. Louis, unpublished data). This is illustrated in Figure 5. The former occur more commonly in older patients, while the latter are more common in younger adults. This finding offers preliminary evidence that genetic analysis can provide clinical information not available using traditional methods of tissue analysis.

We have postulated that the genetic pathway involving chromosome 17p loss may involve progression from a lower-grade astrocytic lesion, since loss of chromosome 17p, p53 gene mutation, and PDGF-α receptor overexpression occur as commonly in lower-grade as in higher-grade astrocytomas (see above). This is exemplified by one of our patients, who exhibited LOH on 17p in an initial low-grade astrocytoma and additional loss of chromosome 10 in the subsequent GBM. On the other hand, it is tempting to speculate that those GBMs with EGFR amplification arise either *de novo* or rapidly from a pre-existing tumor, without a clinically evident preceding lower-grade astrocytoma. None of the patients in our study with EGFR gene amplification had a history of an earlier lower-grade astrocytoma.

Younger age at initial diagnosis has been an important prognostic parameter among patients with GBM, with younger patients faring better than older patients.[6,7,48] The predominance of tumors with 17p loss in a younger population of astrocytoma patients may therefore reflect the age-based difference in prognosis. Indeed, in our earlier study, patients with p53 gene mutations had somewhat better prognoses than those without p53 mutations.[11] In addition, it is possible that those patients with anaplastic gliomas and a previous history of lower-grade glioma who do better clinically ("dedifferentiated GBM")[93] are the same subset as our GBM patients with 17p loss. The data suggest that genetic analysis may begin to explain the clinical observations concerning patient age and sex differences in astrocytic tumors.

MOLECULAR GENETICS OF OTHER GLIOMAS

Other Astrocytomas

Pilocytic Astrocytomas

Pilocytic astrocytoma is the most common astrocytic tumor of childhood and differs clinically and histopathologically from the diffuse fibrillary astrocytoma that affects adults. We have examined pilocytic astrocytomas for allelic losses on chromosomes 10, 17p, and 19q and for amplification of the EGFR gene, but have not detected genomic alterations at these loci. Because pilocytic astrocytomas frequently affect patients with NF1 and the NF1 gene has been mapped to 17q11.2, we have also examined pilocytic astrocytomas for allelic loss at multiple loci on the long arm of chromosome 17.[86] Allelic loss was observed on chromosome 17q in one-quarter of cases, including one tumor with an interstitial deletion that included the NF1 gene. These data suggest the presence of a tumor suppressor gene on 17q that is associated with pilocytic astrocytomas. A potential candidate for this gene is the NF1 tumor suppressor gene. However, no detailed mutational analysis of the NF1 gene in pilocytic tumors has yet been performed.

Pediatric Brain Stem Gliomas

We have also studied brain stem gliomas, a form of pediatric diffuse fibrillary astrocytoma, for p53 gene mutations and chromosome 17p loss.[53] Brain stem gliomas had not been studied previously since biopsies of these tumors are rare and biopsy fragments extremely small. We investigated the molecular genetic composition of brain stem gliomas using polymerase chain reaction assays[56] and showed that chromosome 17p loss and p53 gene mutations are common in these tumors.[53] Interestingly, none of the cases showed amplification of the EGFR gene.

These data suggest that pediatric brain stem GBMs share genetic features with those adult GBMs that affect younger patients: p53 gene and chromosome 17p alterations without EGFR gene amplification. Since brain stem gliomas are predominantly tumors of childhood, this may suggest a common oncogenic pathway for those diffuse fibrillary astrocytic tumors that affect younger patients, regardless of their anatomical location. On the other hand, it has been shown that there are regional differences in the astrocytes that populate different brain areas.[17] For instance, there is considerable variation in the transcription levels of particular growth factors and proto-oncogenes in different normal glial cell populations.[28] It is therefore possible that at different ages there are distinct susceptibilities of certain astrocytes to the same genetic alterations.

Pleomorphic Xanthoastrocytomas

Pleomorphic xanthoastrocytoma is a superficial low-grade astrocytic tumor that predominantly affects young adults. While these tumors have a bizarre histological appearance, they are typically slow-growing tumors that may be amenable to surgical cure. In our series, we examined three pleomorphic xanthoastrocytomas for allelic losses on chromosomes 10 and 17, and for EGFR gene amplification. No genetic alterations were detected in these tumors (A. von Deimling and D.N. Louis, unpublished data).

Subependymal Giant Cell Astrocytomas

Subependymal giant cell astrocytoma (SEGA) is a periventricular, low-grade astrocytic tumor usually associated with TS, and is histologically identical to the so-called "candle-gutterings" that line the ventricles of TS patients. Similar to the other tumorous lesions in TS, these are slow-growing and may be more akin to hamartomas than true neoplasms. The association of SEGA with TS predicts the involvement of a tumor suppressor gene; TS patients would inherit one mutant copy, which would predispose them to the panoply of TS tumors, while sporadic SEGA would arise in those rare instances in which both tumor suppressor alleles were somatically altered in the same periventricular cell. Linkage studies have identified the location of a number of TS genes, with one gene on chromosome 9q and another on 16p. As discussed above, the 16p gene, designated TSC2, has recently been cloned.[15] Loss of heterozygosity studies have shown allelic loss of chromosome 16p loci in one SEGA, again suggesting that the TS gene is a tumor suppressor.[29] However, the 9q loci have not been studied. Confirmation of the role of the TS genes in glial tumorigenesis must await analysis of TSC2 on 16q, and eventually of the 9q TSC1 gene in cases of SEGA.

Desmoplastic Infantile Gliomas

Desmoplastic cerebral astrocytoma of infancy and desmoplastic infantile ganglioglioma are large, superficial, usually cystic, benign astrocytomas that affect children in the first year or two of life. Both variants have conspicuous collagen-rich stroma, with the desmoplastic infantile gliomas having an additional ganglion cell component. We have studied allelic chromosomal loss in two cases of desmoplastic cerebral astrocytoma of infancy, and did not detect loss of chromosomes 17 or 10 in either case.[55]

Gangliogliomas

Our series included eight cases of gangliogliomas in adults. Analysis of EGFR gene amplification and of allelic loss on chromosomes 10, 13q, 17p, 19q, and 22q did not reveal genetic alterations (A. von Deimling and D.N. Louis, unpublished data).

Oligodendrogliomas and Mixed Gliomas (Oligoastrocytomas)

There have been relatively few cytogenetic analyses of oligodendrogliomas and mixed gliomas, and these have produced varied results. In oligodendrogliomas, loss of the Y chromosome and chromosomes 1p and 6q, and structural alterations of 9p have been reported,[3,44,65] while other studies have revealed no karyotypic abnormalities.[30] Cytogenetic studies of mixed gliomas have not revealed characteristic alterations.[44]

Molecular genetic studies of oligodendrogliomas and mixed gliomas have also been few in number. A study of seven oligodendrogliomas using Southern blotting for at least one polymorphic marker on each chromosome arm showed four tumors with chromosome 19q loss, two cases with allelic loss of chromosome 1p, and one case with loss of the Y chromosome.[65] To evaluate whether loss of chromosome 19q alleles is common in oligodendrogliomas and mixed gliomas, we performed LOH analysis of chromosome 19 loci in oligodendrogliomas, anaplastic oligodendrogliomas, low-grade mixed gliomas, and anaplastic mixed gliomas. Allelic loss was noted in two of five oligodendrogliomas (both anaplastic oligodendrogliomas), five of eight mixed gliomas, and five of seven anaplastic mixed gliomas, confirming that 19q loss is very common in gliomas that have an oligodendroglial component.[88] Because of the frequent loss of this locus in low-grade oligodendrogliomas and mixed gliomas, it is likely that this tumor suppressor gene is important early in oligodendroglial tumorigenesis. Deletion mapping of this locus has suggested that it is the same as the astrocytoma gene on chromosome 19q.

The p53 tumor suppressor gene is not involved in human oligodendrogliomas.[63] Most other studies have included very few oligodendroglial tumors, but it has been suggested that allelic loss of chromosome 10 may be a common finding in high-grade malignant gliomas, whether they are astrocytic or oligodendroglial in original lineage.[39] This may be supported by a reported case of an aggressive oligodendroglioma with allelic loss of chromosome 10 that rapidly recurred as a GBM.[95] Finally, it is important to note that oncogene amplification has only rarely been noted in oligodendroglial tumors.[23]

Ependymomas

Molecular genetic and cytogenetic studies have demonstrated that chromosome 22q loss is common in ependymomas.[42,65,92] While such analyses have suggested that chromosome 22q harbors an ependymoma tumor suppressor gene, they have not narrowed down the location of this putative tumor suppressor gene. A candidate glioma tumor suppressor gene on chromosome 22q is the neurofibromatosis NF2 gene.[80] Patients with NF2 develop bilateral vestibular schwannomas (acoustic neuromas), schwannomas in other sites, and multiple meningiomas. In addition, NF2 patients have a higher incidence of gliomas, particularly ependymomas.[59] We therefore evaluated the NF2 gene in eight sporadic ependymomas and 30 sporadic astrocytomas to determine whether the NF2 gene is the glioma tumor suppressor gene on chromosome 22q.[71] Screening of the NF2 gene in eight ependymomas revealed a single migration shift, which occurred in exon 7 of an ependymoma that had lost the remaining wild-type allele. DNA sequencing of this exon revealed a deletion of a single thymidine (base 840) in codon 207. The frameshift mutation resulted in a stop in codon 208, thus leading to a severely truncated protein product. The mutation was not in the patient's constitutional DNA. The combination of mutation of one NF2 allele and chromosomal loss of the second allele thus fulfills the classic paradigm of NF2 as a tumor suppressor gene in ependymomas.

Thus, the NF2 gene appears to be the target of 22q allelic loss in at least some ependymomas. It is tempting to speculate that NF2 mutations may be particular to intramedullary spinal ependymomas, since these are the types of ependymomas characteristically associated with NF2[74] and we did not detect NF2 mutations in any of the six intracranial ependymomas. To evaluate this possibility, we screened six intraspinal and six myxopapillary ependymomas of the cauda equina for NF2 mutations, but did not detect alterations (S. Cortez and D.N. Louis, unpublished data). Alternatively, the lack of mutations in the remainder of cases may imply the presence of a second chromosome 22q ependymoma tumor suppressor gene, or that NF2 mutations may be larger deletions or occur in non-exonic portions of the gene, such as in promoters or introns. Our recent screening of the NF2 gene in NF2 patients has revealed some cases without detectable mutations in the same regions assayed in the present study,[38] supporting the possibility that mutations may occur in other regions of the gene.

The p53 gene does not appear to be involved in ependymomas.[63] We have also excluded a role for mutations of the p53 gene in the malignant transformation of ependymomas to anaplastic ependymoma (S. Cortez and D.N. Louis, unpublished data).

Conclusion

Molecular genetic studies of human astrocytomas have identified genetic alterations that are characteristic of each stage of astrocytoma progression. For instance, the formation of grade II astrocytoma involves inactivation of the p53 tumor suppressor gene on chromosome 17p, as well as overexpression of the PDGF-α receptor and loss of a putative tumor suppressor gene on chromosome 22q. The transition from astrocytoma to anaplastic astrocytoma is associated with inactivation of the Rb gene on chromosome 13q and putative tumor suppressor genes on chromosomes 9p and 19q. Finally, progression to GBM involves loss of at least one putative tumor suppressor gene on chromosome 10 and amplification of the EGFR gene. Furthermore, molecular genetic analysis has been used to distinguish subsets of astrocytomas. For instance, one type of GBM, characterized by p53 gene mutations, is more common in younger patients and may be associated with slower progression from lower-grade astrocytoma, while another type of GBM, characterized by EGFR gene amplification, is more common in older patients and may be associated with more rapid progression or de novo growth. For the less common gliomas, molecular genetic studies have defined only isolated genetic alterations. At the present time, such genetic schemata remain quite preliminary and it is clear that these glimpses are merely visions of the tip of a genetic iceberg.

REFERENCES

1. Anker L, Hamel W, Laas R, et al: Immunodetection of tumor suppressor gene products in primary brain tumors and glioma cell lines. **Clin Neuropathol 10:**10, 1991 (Abstract)
2. Biegel JA, Burk CD, Barr FG, et al: Evidence for a 17p tumor related locus distinct from p53 in pediatric primitive neuroectodermal tumors. **Cancer Res 52:**3391-3395, 1992
3. Bigner SH, Mark J, Bigner DD: Cytogenetics of human brain tumors. **Cancer Genet Cytogenet 47:**141-154, 1990
4. Bishop JM: Molecular themes in oncogenesis. **Cell 64:**235-248, 1991
5. Brodeur GM: Neuroblastoma—clinical applications of molecular parameters. **Brain Pathol 1:**47-54, 1990
6. Burger PC, Green SB: Patient age, histologic features, and length of survival in patients with glioblastoma multiforme. **Cancer 59:**1617-1625, 1987
7. Burger PC, Vogel FS, Green SB, et al: Glioblastoma multiforme and anaplastic astrocytoma. Pathologic criteria and prognostic implications. **Cancer 56:**1106-1111, 1985
8. Cavenee WK, Dryja TP, Phillips RA, et al: Expression of recessive alleles by chromosomal mechanisms in retinoblastoma. **Nature 305:**779-784, 1983
9. Cavenee WK, Murphree AL, Shull MM, et al: Prediction of familial predisposition to retinoblastoma. **N Engl J Med 314:**1201-1207, 1986
10. Cawthon RM, Weiss R, Xu G, et al: A major segment of the neurofibromatosis type 1 gene: cDNA sequence, genomic structure, and point mutations. **Cell 62:**193-201, 1990
11. Chung R, Whaley J, Kley N, et al: TP53 mutation and 17p deletions in human astrocytomas. **Genes Chromosom Cancer 3:**323-331, 1991
12. Collins VP, James CD: Gene and chromosomal alterations associated with the development of human gliomas. **FASEB J 7:**926-930, 1993
13. Drummond IA, Madden SL, Rohwer-Nutter P, et al: Repression of the insulin-like growth factor II gene by the Wilms tumor suppressor WT1. **Science 257:**674-678, 1992
14. Ekstrand AJ, James CD, Cavenee WK, et al: Genes for epidermal growth factor receptor, transforming growth factor a, and epidermal growth factor and their expression in human gliomas *in vivo.* **Cancer Res 51:**2164-2172, 1991
15. European Chromosome 16 Tuberous Sclerosis Consortium: Identification and characterization of the tuberous sclerosis gene on chromosome 16. **Cell 75:**1305-1315, 1993
16. Fearon ER, Vogelstein B: A genetic model for colorectal tumorigenesis. **Cell 61:**759-767, 1990
17. Federoff S, Vernadakis A: **Astrocytes.** Orlando, Fla: Academic Press, 1986
18. Fleming TP, Saxena A, Clark WC, et al: Amplification and/or overexpression of platelet-derived growth factor receptors and epidermal growth factor receptor in human glial tumors. **Cancer Res 52:**4550-4553, 1992
19. Fountain JW, Karayiorgou M, Ernstoff MS, et al: Homozygous deletions within human chromosome band 9p21 in melanoma. **Proc Natl Acad Sci USA 89:**10557-10561, 1992
20. Frankel RH, Bayona W, Koslow M, et al: p53 mutations in human malignant gliomas: comparison of loss of heterozygosity with mutation frequency. **Cancer Res 52:**1427-1433, 1992
21. Friend SH, Dryja TP, Weinberg RA: Oncogenes and tumor-suppressing genes. **N Engl J Med 318:** 618-622, 1988
22. Fujimoto M, Fults DW, Thomas GA, et al: Loss of heterozygosity on chromosome 10 in human glioblastoma multiforme. **Genomics 4:**210-214, 1989
23. Fuller GN, Bigner SH: Amplified cellular oncogenes in neoplasms of the human central nervous system. **Mutat Res 276:**299-306, 1992
24. Fults D, Brockmeyer D, Tullous MW, et al: p53 mutation and loss of heterozygosity on chromosome 17 and 10 during human astrocytoma progression. **Cancer Res 52:**674-679, 1992
25. Fults D, Pedone C: Deletion mapping of the long arm of chromosome 10 in glioblastoma multiforme. **Genes Chromosom Cancer 7:**173-7, 1993
26. Fults D, Pedone CA, Thomas GA, et al: Allelotype of human malignant astrocytoma. **Cancer Res 50:**5784-5789, 1990
27. Fults D, Tippets RH, Thomas GA, et al: Loss of heterozygosity for loci on chromosome 17p in human malignant astrocytoma. **Cancer Res 49:**6572-6577, 1989
28. Gillaspy GE, Mapstone TB, Samols D, et al: Transcriptional patterns of growth factors and protooncogenes in human glioblastomas and normal glial cells. **Cancer Lett 65:**55-60, 1992
29. Green AJ, Yates JRW: Loss of heterozygosity on chromosome 16p in hamartomata from patients with tuberous sclerosis. **Am J Hum Genet 53 (Suppl):**244, 1993 (Abstract)
30. Griffin CA, Long PP, Carson BS, et al: Chromosome abnormalities in low-grade central nervous system tumors. **Cancer Genet Cytogenet 60:**67-73, 1992
31. Gutmann DH, Collins FS: Recent progress toward understanding the molecular biology of von Recklinghausen neurofibromatosis. **Ann Neurol 31:** 555-561, 1992
32. Haines JL, Short MP, Kwiatkowski DJ, et al: Localization of one gene for tuberous sclerosis within

9q32-9q34, and further evidence for heterogeneity. **Am J Hum Genet 49:**764-772, 1991

33. Heldin CH: Structural and functional studies on platelet-derived growth factor. **EMBO J 11:** 4251-4259, 1992
34. Henson JW, Schnitker BL, Correa K, et al: The retinoblastoma gene is involved in the malignant progression of astrocytomas. **Ann Neurol** (In press)
35. Hermansson M, Funa K, Hartman M, et al: Platelet-derived growth factor and its receptors in human glioma tissue: expression of messenger RNA and protein suggests the presence of autocrine and paracrine loops. **Cancer Res 52:**3213-3219, 1992
36. Hermansson M, Nistér M, Betsholtz C, et al: Endothelial cell hyperplasia in human glioblastoma: coexpression of mRNA for platelet-derived growth factor (PDGF) B chain and PDGF receptor suggests autocrine growth stimulation. **Proc Natl Acad Sci USA 85:**7748-7752, 1988
37. Hurtt MR, Moossy J, Donovan-Peluso M, et al: Amplification of epidermal growth factor receptor gene in gliomas: histopathology and prognosis. **J Neuropathol Exp Neurol 51:**84-90, 1992
38. Jacoby LB, MacCollin M, Louis DN, et al: Exon scanning for mutation in the NF2 gene in schwannomas. **Hum Molec Genet 3:**413-419, 1994
39. James CD, Carlblom E, Dumanski JP, et al: Clonal genomic alterations in glioma malignancy stages. **Cancer Res 48:**5546-5551, 1988
40. James CD, Carlbom E, Nordenskjold M, et al: Mitotic recombination of chromosome 17 in astrocytomas. **Proc Natl Acad Sci USA 86:**2858-2862, 1989
41. James CD, He J, Carlbom E, et al: Chromosome 9 deletion mapping reveals IFN α and IFN β-1 gene deletions in human glial tumors. **Cancer Res 51:**1684-1688, 1991
42. James CD, He J, Carlbom E, et al: Loss of genetic information in central nervous system tumors common to children and young adults. **Genes Chromosom Cancer 2:**94-102, 1990
43. James CD, He J, Collins VP, et al: Localization of chromosome 9p homozygous deletions in glioma cell lines with markers constituting a continuous linkage group. **Cancer Res 53:**3674-3676, 1993
44. Jenkins RB, Kimmel DW, Moertel CA, et al: A cytogenetic study of 53 human gliomas. **Cancer Genet Cytogenet 39:**253-279, 1989
45. Kandt RS, Haines JL, Smith M, et al: Linkage of an important gene locus for tuberous sclerosis to a chromosome 16 marker for polycystic kidney disease. **Natl Genet 2:**37-41, 1992
46. Karlbom AE, James CD, Boethius J, et al: Loss of heterozygosity in malignant gliomas involves at least three distinct regions on chromosome 10. **Hum Genet 92:**169-174, 1993
47. Kastan MB, Onyekwere O, Sidransky D, et al: Participation of p53 protein in the cellular response to DNA damage. **Cancer Res 51:**6304-6311, 1991
48. Kim TS, Halliday AL, Hedley-Whyte ET, et al: Correlates of survival and the Daumas-Duport grading system for astrocytomas. **J Neurosurg 74:**27-37, 1991
49. Kleihues P, Burger PC, Scheithauer BW: **Histological Typing of Tumors of the Central Nervous System.** World Health Organization. Berlin: Springer-Verlag, 1993
50. Kuerbitz SJ, Plunkett BS, Walsh WV, et al: Wild-type p53 is a cell cycle checkpoint determinant following irradiation. **Proc Natl Acad Sci USA 89:**7491-7495, 1992
51. Livingstone LR, White A, Sprouse J, et al: Altered cell cycle arrest and gene amplification potential accompany loss of wild-type p53. **Cell 70:**923-935, 1992
52. Louis DN: The p53 gene and protein in human brain tumors. **J Neuropathol Exp Neurol 53:** 11-21, 1994
53. Louis DN, Rubio MP, Correa K, et al: Molecular genetics of pediatric brain stem gliomas. Application of PCR techniques to small and archival brain tumor specimens. **J Neuropathol Exp Neurol 52:**507-515, 1993
54. Louis DN, von Deimling A, Chung RY, et al: Comparative study of p53 gene and protein alterations in human astrocytomas. **J Neuropathol Exp Neurol 52:**31-38, 1993
55. Louis DN, von Deimling A, Dickersin GR, et al: Desmoplastic cerebral astrocytomas of infancy. A histopathologic, immunohistochemical, ultrastructural, and molecular genetic study. **Hum Pathol 23:**1402-1409, 1992
56. Louis DN, von Deimling A, Seizinger BR: A $(CA)_n$ dinucleotide repeat assay for evaluating loss of allelic heterozygosity in small and archival human brain tumor specimens. **Am J Pathol 141:** 777-782, 1992
57. Malkin D, Li FP, Strong LC, et al: Germ line p53 mutations in a familial syndrome of breast cancer, sarcomas, and other neoplasms. **Science 250:** 1233-1238, 1990
58. Marshall CJ: Tumor suppressor genes. **Cell 64:** 313-326, 1991
59. Martuza RL, Eldridge R: Neurofibromatosis 2 (bilateral acoustic neurofibromatosis). **N Engl J Med 318:**684-688, 1988
60. Miyakoshi J, Dobler KD, Allalunis-Turner J, et al: Absence of IFNA and IFNB genes from human malignant glioma cell lines and lack of correlation with cellular sensitivity to IFNs. **Cancer Res 50:** 278-283, 1990
61. Newcomb EW, Madonia WJ, Pisharody S, et al: A correlative study of p53 protein alteration and p53 gene mutation in glioblastoma multiforme. **Brain Pathol 3:**229-235, 1993
62. Nistér M, Claesson-Welsh L, Eriksson A, et al: Differential expression of platelet-derived growth factor receptors in human malignant glioma cell lines. **J Biol Chem 266:**16755-16763, 1991
63. Ohgaki H, Eibl RH, Wiestler OD, et al: p53 mutations in nonastrocytic human brain tumors. **Cancer Res 51:**6202-5, 1991
64. Olopade OI, Jenkins RB, Ransom DT, et al: Molecular analysis of deletions of the short arm of chromosome 9 in human gliomas. **Cancer Res 52:** 2523-2529, 1992

65. Ransom DT, Ritland SR, Kimmel DW, et al: Cytogenetic and loss of heterozygosity studies in ependymomas, pilocytic astrocytomas, and oligodendrogliomas. **Genes Chromosom Cancer 5**:348-356, 1992
66. Rasheed BKA, Fuller GN, Friedman AH, et al: Loss of heterozygosity for 10q loci in human gliomas. **Genes Chromosom Cancer 5**:75-82, 1992
67. Reifenberger G, Liu L, Ichimura K, et al: Amplification and overexpression of the *MDM2* gene in a subset of human malignant gliomas without p53 mutations. **Cancer Res 53**:2736-2739, 1993
68. Rey JA, Bello MJ, Jiménez-Lara AM, et al: Loss of heterozygosity for distal markers on 22q in human gliomas. **Int J Cancer 51**:703-706, 1992
69. Rouleau GA, Merel P, Lutchman M, et al: Alteration in a new gene encoding a putative membrane-organizing protein causes neuro-fibromatosis type 2. **Nature 363**:515-21, 1993
70. Rouleau GA, Wertelecki W, Haines JL, et al: Genetic linkage of bilateral acoustic neurofibromatosis to a DNA marker on chromosome 22. **Nature 329**: 246-248, 1987
71. Rubio MP, Correa KM, Ramesh V, et al: Analysis of the neurofibromatosis 2 gene in human ependymomas and astrocytomas. **Cancer Res 54**:45-47, 1994
72. Rubio MP, Correa KM, Ueki K, et al: The putative glioma tumor suppressor gene on chromosome 19q maps between APOC2 and HRC. **Cancer Res 54**:4760-4763, 1994
73. Rubio MP, von Deimling A, Yandell DW, et al: Accumulation of wild type p53 protein in human astrocytomas. **Cancer Res 53**:3465-3467, 1993
74. Russell DS, Rubinstein LJ: **Pathology of Tumours of the Nervous System, 5th ed.** Baltimore: Williams & Wilkins, 1989
75. Saxena A, Clark WC, Robertson JT, et al: Evidence for the involvement of a potential second tumor suppressor gene on chromosome 17 distinct from p53 in malignant astrocytomas. **Cancer Res 52**:6716-6721, 1992
76. Seizinger BR, Klinger HP, Junien C, et al: Report of the committee on chromosome and gene loss in human neoplasia. **Cytogenet Cell Genet 58**: 1080-1096, 1991
77. Seizinger BR, Rouleau GA, Ozelius LJ, et al: Genetic linkage of von Recklinghausen neurofibromatosis to the nerve growth factor receptor gene. **Cell 49**:589-594, 1987
78. Sidransky D, Mikkelsen T, Schwechheimer K, et al: Clonal expansion of p53 mutant cells is associated with brain tumor progression. **Nature 355**:846-847, 1992
79. Thor AD, Moore DH, Edgerton SM, et al: Accumulation of p53 tumor suppressor gene protein: an independent marker of prognosis in breast cancers. **J Natl Cancer Inst 84**:845-855, 1992
80. Trofatter JA, MacCollin MM, Rutter JL, et al: A novel moesin-, ezrin-, radixin-like gene is a candidate for the neurofibromatosis 2 tumor suppressor. **Cell 72**:791-800, 1993
81. Ueki K, Rubio MP, Ramesh V, et al: MTS1/CDKN2 gene mutations are rare in primary human astrocytomas with allelic loss of chromosome 9p. **Hum Molec Genet 3**:1841-1845, 1994
82. Venter DJ, Bevan KL, Ludwig RL, et al: Retinoblastoma gene deletions in human glioblastomas. **Oncogene 6**:445-448, 1991
83. Venter DJ, Thomas DGT: Multiple sequential molecular abnormalities in the evolution of human gliomas. **Br J Cancer 63**:753-757, 1991
84. von Deimling A, Bender B, Jahnke R, et al: Loci associated with malignant progression in astrocytomas: a candidate on chromosome 19q. **Cancer Res 54**:1397-1401, 1994
85. von Deimling A, Eibl RH, Ohgaki H, et al: P53 mutations are associated with 17p allelic loss in grade II and grade III astrocytoma. **Cancer Res 52**:2987-2990, 1992
86. von Deimling A, Louis DN, Menon AG, et al: Deletions on the long arm of chromosome 17 in pilocytic astrocytoma. **Acta Neuropathol 86**:81-85, 1993
87. von Deimling A, Louis DN, von Ammon K, et al: Association of epidermal growth factor receptor gene amplification with loss of chromosome 10 in human glioblastoma multiforme. **J Neurosurg 77**:295-301, 1992
88. von Deimling A, Louis DN, von Ammon K, et al: Evidence for a tumor suppressor gene on chromosome 19q associated with human astrocytomas, oligodendrogliomas and mixed gliomas. **Cancer Res 52**:4277-4279, 1992
89. von Deimling A, Nagel J, Bender B, et al: Deletion mapping of a putative tumor suppressor gene on chromosome 19q associated with human gliomas. **Int J Cancer 57**:676-680, 1994
90. von Deimling A, von Ammon K, Schoenfeld D, et al: Subsets of glioblastoma multiforme defined by molecular genetic analysis. **Brain Pathol 3**:19-26, 1993
91. Wallace MR, Marchuk DA, Andersen LB, et al: Type 1 neurofibromatosis gene: identification of a large transcript disrupted in three NF1 patients. **Science 249**:181-186, 1990
92. Weremowicz S, Kupsky WJ, Morton CC, et al: Cytogenetic evidence for a chromosome 22 tumor suppressor gene in ependymoma. **Cancer Genet Cytogenet 61**:193-196, 1992
93. Winger MJ, Macdonald DR, Cairncross JG: Supratentorial anaplastic gliomas in adults. The prognostic importance of extent of resection and prior low-grade glioma. **J Neurosurg 71**:487-493, 1989
94. Wong AJ, Bigner SH, Bigner DD, et al: Increased expression of the epidermal growth factor receptor gene in malignant gliomas is invariably associated with gene amplification. **Proc Natl Acad Sci USA 84**:6899-6903, 1987
95. Wu JK, Folkerth RD, Ye Z, et al: Aggressive oligodendroglioma predicted by chromosome 10 restriction fragment length polymorphism analysis. Case study. **J Neurooncol 15**:29-35, 1993
96. Xu G, O'Connell P, Viskochil D, et al: The neurofibromatosis type 1 gene encodes a protein related to GAP. **Cell 62**:599-608, 1990

Glossary of Cancer Genetics

Cancer Genes

The two major classes of genes involved in oncogenesis are:

1. *Oncogenes:* Oncogenes are abnormally activated versions of normal growth-promoting genes known as *proto-oncogenes.* These genes encode proteins that function in signal transduction pathways from the cell surface to the nucleus, and include cell surface receptors and their ligands, cytoplasmic "second messengers," and nuclear transcription factors.
2. *Tumor suppressor genes:* Tumor suppressor genes are normal genes that inhibit cell growth and division. It is the inactivation of such genes that leads to tumor formation. Tumor suppressor genes encode proteins with a wide variety of functions. The most studied tumor suppressor genes, Rb and p53, are nuclear proteins that regulate the cell cycle.

Oncogenic Alterations in Cancer Genes

Normal cellular genes can be converted to oncogenic genes by a number of genetic mechanisms. In the case of proto-oncogenes, such generic alterations are activating, and result in abnormally mitogenic proteins. In the case of tumor suppressor genes, on the other hand, these genetic alterations are inactivating, and destroy the normal suppressive function of the protein. These genetic mechanisms include:

1. *Gene mutation:* A mutation is an alteration of the nucleotide sequence in a gene. Some types of mutations include:
   a. *Point mutations,* in which one nucleotide is substituted for another. These can be further divided into *missense mutations,* in which the nucleotide change results in an amino acid alteration, and *nonsense mutations,* which the nucleotide change results in a stop codon and a truncated protein. Missense mutations may activate proto-oncogenes or inactivate tumor suppressor genes, while nonsense mutations are typically inactivating.
   b. *Frameshift mutations,* in which one or more nucleotides (but not a multiple of three) are either inserted or deleted from the gene, resulting in a "shift" of the normal reading frame and an abnormal, truncated protein. Such frameshift mutations are usually inactivating changes.
2. *Gene amplification:* Gene amplification is a process whereby a cell develops an increased number of copies of a particular gene, either a structurally normal proto-oncogene or an abnormal oncogene. This is depicted in Figure 1. The increased number of genes and, consequently, gene products, results in an excessive growth signal.
3. *Translocation:* Translocation refers to the transfer of genetic material from one chromosome to another. If this transfer interrupts the middle of a gene, such as a tumor suppressor gene, that gene may be inactivated. On the other hand, translocation may activate an oncogene, by placing a proto-oncogene near a highly active gene or by abnormally fusing part of an oncogene with another active gene.

Polymorphisms, Alleles, Linkage, and Loss of Heterozygosity

1. *Polymorphisms* are natural variations in nucleotide sequence that occur throughout a population and that do not usually alter the amino acid sequence. These polymorphisms include:
   a. *Restriction fragment length polymorphisms* (RFLP), in which a single nucleotide change alters the recognition site of highly specific restriction endonucleases.
   b. *Repeat polymorphisms*, in which there are variable numbers of short, repeated nucleotide sequences (e.g. CACACACACA).
2. *Alleles* are alternate copies of the same gene or chromosome that are inherited from different parents. In diploid cells, such as in humans, there are therefore two alleles for each gene and chromosome, one maternal and one paternal. Some polymorphisms, such as the repeat polymorphisms, may have many different forms; thus, while each individual can have only two alleles, many more alleles may exist in the whole population. *Polymorphisms* enable the distinction of different *alleles*, since polymorphic sites are often different between the maternal and paternal allele. For instance, in the case of repeat polymorphisms, the maternal allele may have five repeats, while the paternal allele has ten repeats. If a given polymorphism can distinguish two alleles in a given patient, the patient is *heterozygous* or *informative* at that polymorphism.
3. *Linkage* studies rely on polymorphisms to determine whether a disease phenotype is associated with or "linked" to a certain chromosomal region. For example, if all affected members of a family with a hereditary syndrome have a particular allele, while the unaffected members have other alleles, the syndrome phenotype would be "linked" to that polymorphism and, consequently, "linked" to the chromosomal region containing that polymorphism.
4. *Loss of heterozygosity* studies (see Figure 2) use polymorphisms to compare the maternal and paternal alleles in normal tissue with these alleles in tumor tissue. If a patient's normal tissue is *heterozygous* for a particular polymorphism, and the patient's tumor shows only one of the two alleles, the one allele has been lost in the tumor. This is termed "*loss of heterozygosity*," and implies tumor-specific loss of one chromosomal allele. As depicted in Figure 2, this often reflects the presence of a nearby tumor suppressor gene.
5. *Deletion mapping* studies are loss of heterozygosity studies that use multiple polymorphisms on a given chromosome. The common area of deletion represents the most likely site for a tumor suppressor gene. The results of some of these studies are depicted in Figure 4.

Chromosomes and Chromosomal Loci

1. Each *chromosome* can be divided into a *short arm*, designated *p*, and a long arm, designated *q*. The end (*telomere*) of the short arm is known as *pter*, for p-terminus, and the end (*telomere*) of the long arm as *qter*, for q-terminus, while the *centromere* defines the proximal ends of the two arms (*pcen* and *qcen*). Each arm is divided into regions and subregions, designated by numbers and as black and white regions on chromosome maps (see Figure 4).
2. *Chromosomal loci* are sites on the chromosomes that are either known genes or polymorphisms. Known genes are given abbreviated names, e.g., NF2 (for the neurofibromatosis 2 gene) on the chromosome 22q map in Figure 4. Polymorphisms are given working designations which state the chromosome after a "D" and the polymorphism number (indicating only the order of discovery) after an "S", e.g., D22S274 on the chromosome 22q map in Figure 4.

CHAPTER 10

MALIGNANT PROGRESSION IN GLIOMAS

THOMAS C. CHEN, MD, DAVID R. HINTON, MD, FRCP(C) AND
MICHAEL L. J. APUZZO, MD

Astrocytomas comprise 10% to 15% of all brain tumors and 25% to 35% of all gliomas.[35] While most patients with glioblastoma multiforme (GBM) present with this lesion at the time of initial diagnosis, many GBMs have been documented to increase in malignancy from an astrocytoma or anaplastic astrocytoma at initial diagnosis to a GBM at the time of recurrence.[22,30,33,37,45,52,53,57] This phenomenon whereby tumors become more aggressive and acquire greater malignant potential over a period of time is termed "tumor progression." This chapter attempts to define the scientific basis for progression by: 1) defining the pathological basis for malignant progression and the clonal hypothesis; 2) presenting the clinical evidence for dedifferentiation in astrocytomas; and 3) providing an update on current genetic findings supporting a clonal origin for gliomas and a molecular basis for progression.

PROGRESSION AND THE CLONAL HYPOTHESIS

The concept of malignant progression in neoplasms is not new and has been well documented in various carcinomas.[58] Neoplasia represents some degree of escape from normal growth control. In the 1950s, Foulds[10,11] defined progression as the "development of a neoplasm by way of permanent irreversible qualitative change in one or more of its characters." These changes occur in several steps, and multiple factors (e.g., host immune system, local environment, therapeutic interventions) may be involved. The first step, "initiation," represents an acquired genetic instability in the original transformed cell, resulting in an alteration in the cell's reactivity to certain stimuli, which are normally noncarcinogenic. Continued exposure to these growth factors may result in expansion of the cell population and tumor growth, leading to tumor progression. Subsequent dedifferentiation of the tumor may occur by advancement either along a predetermined path to a predictable endpoint or along an erratic and unpredictable route to a carcinoma. Whatever the pathway to dedifferentiation, the outcome is the same: a more malignant stage of the tumor with well-defined histological features.

To explain the concept of progression at the cellular level, the clonal hypothesis was advanced in 1976 by Nowell.[40] According to Nowell's model, neoplasms arise from a single cell of origin. Tumor progression results from an acquired genetic alteration within the original clone, allowing sequential selection of more aggressive sublines. These genetic alterations may result

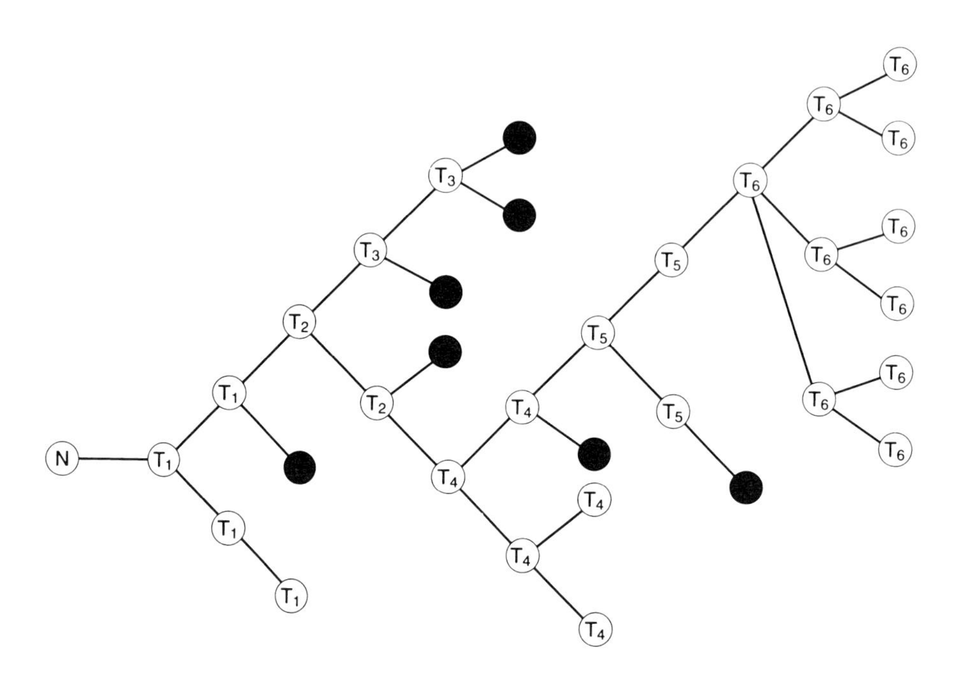

Figure 1: Clonal hypothesis. Tumor initiation results in a genetic alteration in a normal (N) cell that confers a growth advantage to an affected daughter cell (T1). Subsequent tumor progression results in a number of daughter clones with genetic variability (T2 to T6). Most of the clones die; however, a certain number survive with enhanced growth potential and genetic variability. These alterations, associated with tumor progression, result in tumor genetic heterogeneity. The relative proportion of tumor cell subpopulations is dependent upon the growth advantage conferred by the cumulative genetic changes in the individual clone over time. The *blackened circles* represent lethal mutations.

from development of oncogenes, loss of tumor suppressor genes, or both. A cancer-causing oncogene is an abnormally activated form of a cellular gene called a "proto-oncogene," which normally codes for growth-promoting proteins. On the other hand, tumor suppressor genes are normal genes that inhibit cell proliferation and growth.[12] Volpe[59] proposed that three types of genetic events may lead to neoplastic initiation and progression: 1) errors resulting in accumulation of one or several oncogenes may lead to the occurrence of benign tumors; 2) loss of a tumor suppressor gene may increase the chance of gaining future mutations; and 3) both oncogene overexpression and mutation occurring together in tumor suppressor gene lead to a much greater chance of forming a malignant tumor. As a result of genetic instability, mutant daughter clones are selected. The majority of these daughter cells will die; however, a Darwinian genetic selection process ensures that an occasional mutant will have a growth advantage with respect to the original tumor or to normal cells. This newly selected mutant will then become a precursor for a new predominant subpopulation. Thus, despite the fact that most malignant tumors are monoclonal in origin, by the time they become clinically evident their constituent cells are extremely heterogeneous. Ultimately, the fully developed malignancy with its unique karyotype, associated aberrant metabolic behavior, and specific antigenic properties

TABLE 1
INCIDENCE OF PROGRESSION IN MAJOR SERIES OF GLIOMAS

Authors & Year	Reference No.	No. of Cases	Initial Diagnosis by Biopsy Alone	No. Cases Examined (autopsy, repeat surgery)	Documented Progression	Median Time to Recurrence
Marsa et al, 1975	30	256	0%	31	33%	—
Müller et al, 1977	37	137	0%	72	86%	2.6 yrs
Laws et al, 1984	22	461	—	79	49%	—
Piepmeier, 1987	45	60	25%	8	13%	4.75 yrs
Soffietti et al, 1989	52	85	0%	24	79%	5 yrs
Steiger et al, 1990	53	50	28%	10	20%	—
Vertosick et al, 1991	57	25	80%	8	87%	—
McCormack et al, 1992	33	53	17%	7	86%	4.5 yrs

will have the capability of continued growth and variation as long as the tumor persists (Figure 1).

Heim et al[14] expanded on Nowell's clonal hypothesis[39-41] by postulating four tumor progression scenarios. In the first model, the original clone is stable until the patient dies. The second model is similar to Nowell's original hypothesis: clonal stability may be followed by divergence, leading to massive genetic heterogeneity. Third, an initially heterogeneous neoplastic population is converted to a state of pseudomonoclonality by genetic convergence that eliminates all but one or a few clones, which subsequently expand to form a neoplasm. Last, the initial convergence may give rise to later divergence during disease progression.[14]

The implications of Nowell's clonal hypothesis[39-41] and subsequent modifications are as follows. 1) Advanced human malignancies have highly individual karyotypes and biological behavior. 2) Over time, there is an increased risk of dedifferentiation, with the neoplasm becoming more aggressive and "malignant" during its life history. The rate of dedifferentiation will depend not only on tumor genotypic instability but also on its microenvironment. Therefore, the age of the patient, his or her nutritional status, and therapeutic interventions by physicians will have an impact on the tumor's progression.[38] 3) The heterogeneous histological appearance of malignant gliomas may represent accumulation of genetic alterations in individual clones in various stages of dedifferentiation.[61]

TUMOR PROGRESSION IN GLIOMAS: CLINICAL SERIES

What is the evidence for progression and dedifferentiation in astrocytomas to form an anaplastic astrocytoma or GBM? Table 1 summarizes the results of large published series of patients with tumor progression in astrocytomas. Diagnosis of the initial tumor was usually obtained from specimens acquired at subtotal or total resection, not from biopsy material alone. Therefore, the incidence of sampling error often associated with biopsy alone is low in these series. In the recurrent tumors obtained at autopsy or reoperation, the incidence of progressive malignancy was >50%. The series with the lowest incidence of progression was that of Piepmeier,[45] with progression in 13% of cases. This low rate may be secondary to the short length of follow-up (5 years). The average interval to recurrence in the series was approximately 4 years (Table 1).

CLONAL ORIGIN OF MALIGNANT GLIOMAS

Do malignant gliomas arise from a single clone? To answer this question, molecular genetic analysis employing two techniques, X chromosome inactivation or somatic mutations, may be utilized.[15] X chromosome inactivation works on the principle that one X chromosome is inactivated early in the embryonic development. This X chromosome inactivation is maintained in a stable fashion in all progeny cells, including tumor cells. Therefore, in monoclonal cell populations, the same X chromosome will be inactive in all tumors.

Glucose-6-phosphate dehydrogenase (GPD) and restriction fragment length polymorphisms (RFLP) have been used as markers to determine which X chromosome has been inactivated. In these studies, clonality is determined by the existence of identical GPD isozyme or methylation patterns (resulting in differential endonuclease digestion) in both the parent and daughter cells. Specific somatic mutations may be identified by cytogenetics, loss of heterozygosity, deoxyribonucleic acid (DNA) fingerprinting, or point mutations so that clonality may be determined independent of sex. In all cases, an abnormality in a chromosome is determined in a tumor cell, and the same DNA mutation is identified in the recurrent tumor.[15] A detailed discussion of RFLP, loss of heterozygosity, and point mutations is presented in the preceding chapter by Louis et al.[27]

Several studies have been performed to determine the clonality of gliomas. Sidransky et al[51] used somatic mutation analysis with point mutations in the p53 gene as a tumor cell marker in 10 primary brain tumor pairs; p53 is a tumor suppressor gene located on chromosome 17 that appears to have an important role in cell cycle arrest, differentiation, and apoptosis.[9,24,26,28,31,42,48,65] Seven brain tumor pairs consisted of tumors of high grade both at presentation and at recurrence. The p53 mutation was found in four of the recurrent high-grade tumors. In three of these malignant gliomas, the same p53 missense mutation was found in both the recurrent tumor and the primary tumor. Three brain tumor pairs consisted of low-grade tumors that had progressed to a higher grade. In the tumors that had progressed, cells in the high-grade neoplasm were enriched for the same p53 mutations present in a subpopulation of cells present in the low-grade tumor. Sidransky et al concluded that astrocytic tumor progression was associated with a clonal expansion of cells with a p53 mutation that provided them with a selective growth advantage. Berkman et al[1] used both X chromosome inactivation analysis and somatic mutation analysis of chromosomes 10 and 17 in GBMs. They found that a monoclonal pattern was obtained on X chromosome analysis via RFLP for 10 tumors (eight primary and two recurrent tumors) from nine female patients with GBM. In addition, identical somatic deletions on chromosomes 10 and 17 occurred in all nine GBMs, also supporting a monoclonal composition for these tumors.

Molecular Evidence for Tumor Progression

With increased understanding of the molecular pathogenesis of cancer via oncogenes and tumor suppressor genes, a picture of the molecular changes involved in progression of gliomas has gradually emerged, as it has for other tumor models.[3,6,34] Current models correlating progression with specific genetic changes have been documented in a number of tumors. The retinoblastoma (Rb) tumor suppressor gene has provided a clear picture of how loss of tumor suppressor genes may be directly correlated with tumor progression. In patients with familial retinoblastoma, the patient inherits one mutant inactive copy of the retinoblastoma gene. Subsequent mutation of the remaining retinoblastoma gene leads to development of a retinoblastoma. In patients with sporadic retinoblastoma, no germline mutation is inherited. Therefore, a tumor will develop only after both retinoblastoma genes are inactivated during a patient's lifetime. Thus, patients with a sporadic retinoblastoma are less likely to develop a second tumor after removal of the first retinoblastoma, and their tumors occur later in life than in patients with familial retinoblastoma.[4,5] Vogelstein and Kinzler[58] have constructed an elegant model for the carcinogenesis of colorectal carcinoma, correlating distinct histological changes with molecular events. Several important points are highlighted in the Vogelstein model that may be applied to tumor progression in general. 1) Carcinogenesis is a multi-step process. Multiple "hits," either by loss of tumor suppressor genes or development of oncogenes, are needed before an increase in tumor grade is seen histologically. 2) The overall accumulation of genetic changes is more important in the pathogenesis of cancer than the exact sequence of "hits."

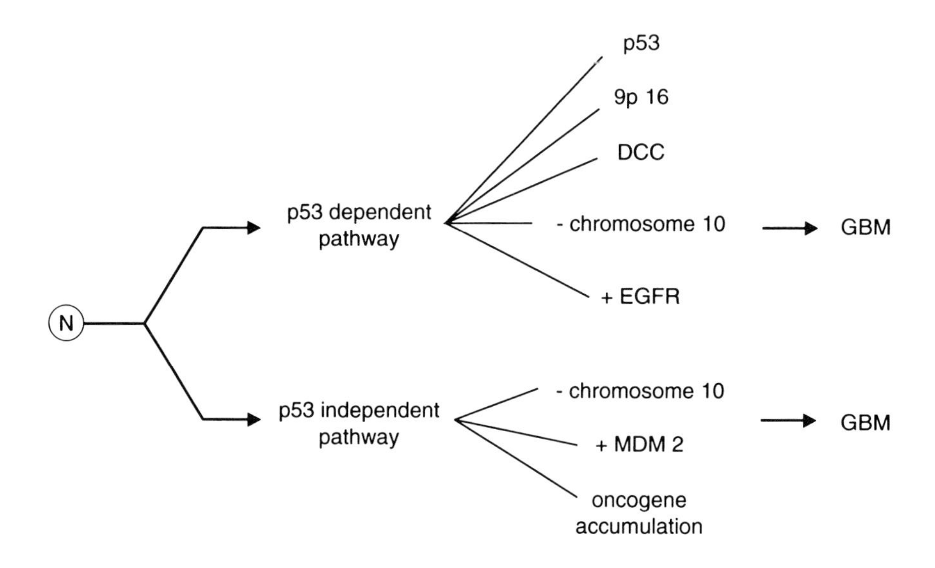

Figure 2: The divergent model of astrocytoma progression showing the orderly progression of the p53-dependent pathway, and the random disorderly changes of the p53-independent pathway, resulting in a GBM developing from an astrocytoma. N = normal cell.

A similar model is now emerging for the pathogenesis of malignant gliomas, explaining the progression from an astrocytoma to a GBM. The preceding chapter by Louis et al[27] addresses in detail the topic of molecular changes in gliomas. The present chapter will simply illustrate the progression model as we currently understand it in relation to gliomas. There appear to be two independent pathways for glioma progression: p53-dependent or p53-independent[55] (Figure 2). In the p53-dependent pathway, loss of the p53 tumor suppressor gene (chromosome 17p) has been identified at each malignancy stage, suggesting that this may be an early event in the formation of at least a subgroup of astrocytomas.[13,17,50,56,61,64] A mutant p53 gene, usually by a missense or point mutation, results in a dominant negative mutant gene, causing accumulation of the mutant p53 protein complexed to wild-type p53 protein, inactivating it.[21] Using immunohistochemistry, Ellison et al[8] showed that there is an increased accumulation of p53 protein with increasing malignancy in gliomas. Del Arco et al[7] have demonstrated that low-grade gliomas are heterozygous for p53 mutations, but high-grade gliomas are homozygous for p53 mutations. Makos et al[29] found that DNA hypermethylation is present in chromosome 17p, suggesting that it may predispose to genetic instability leading to loss of the p53 gene. Other chromosomal changes associated with astrocytoma progression involve chromosomes 13 (Rb gene), 22, 6, and 1.[2,18,23,25,47,56,64] After the initial loss of the p53 gene, later changes include loss of the newly identified tumor suppressor gene at chromosome 9p16 (multiple tumor suppressor 1-MTS1), which may also predispose an astrocytoma to progress to a malignant glioma.[19,20,32] Von Deimling et al[60,63] found that chromosome 19q deletions are restricted to anaplastic astrocytoma and GBM, suggesting that its deletion may predispose to progression to a malignant glioma. Recently, loss of the DCC gene (chromosome 18q) has been reported for GBMs as well.[49] Subsequent deletion of chromosome 10 (found only in GBMs) may be necessary for epidermal growth factor receptor (EGFR) gene amplification.[62]

Some tumors may progress to a GBM from an astrocytoma in an erratic and unpredictable manner, independent of p53, by direct loss of

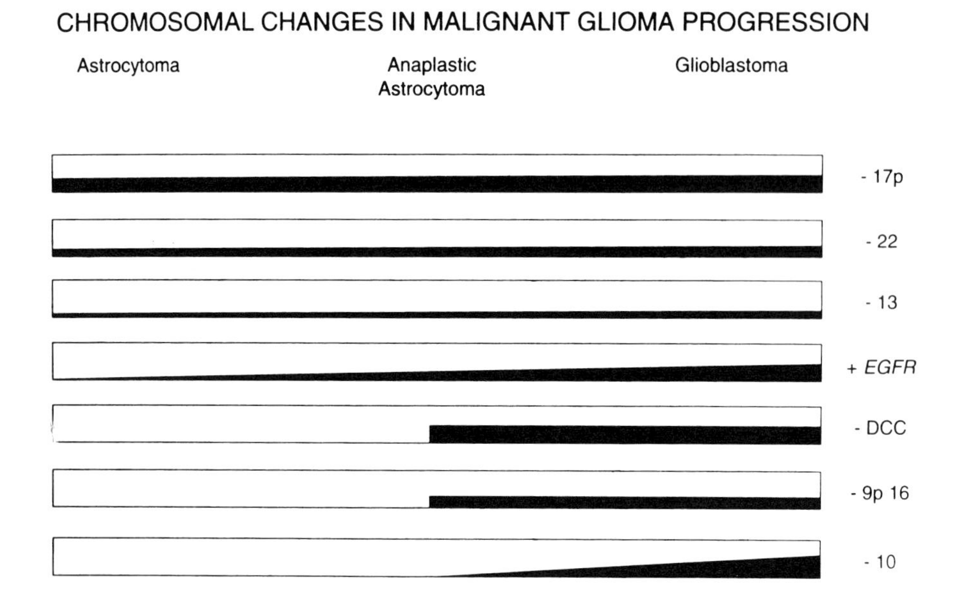

Figure 3: Diagram of the genetic changes seen in glioma progression. The location of the genetic change depicted is only a rough guideline of where the mutation occurs in the progression of an astrocytoma to a GBM. Note that the predominant changes are alterations in tumor suppressor genes. The oncogene EGFR, although present in astrocytomas, is predominantly present in anaplastic astrocytomas and GBMs.

chromosome 10.[16,18] Recently, overexpression of the MDM2 (murine double minute 2, chromosome 12q13-14) gene has been found in human malignant gliomas without p53 mutations.[46] Moreover, accumulation of oncogenes (i.e., c-*erb* B1, c-*myc*, Ha-*ras*, c-*fos*) may be p53-independent.[43,44] The overall genetic changes are summarized in Figure 3. Again, emphasis must be placed on the accumulation and the type of genetic change, not on its exact sequence.

Clinical Implications

Given the fact that a number of clinical series and molecular studies suggest that astrocytomas appear to progress to malignant gliomas over time, what implications can we draw for the treatment of patients with astrocytomas? Although several studies have not found a survival advantage with radiation therapy or radical surgery for astrocytomas, the fact remains that an astrocytoma left in the brain will likely progress to a more malignant tumor.[36] Therefore, should radical surgery with cytoreduction be performed early in order to remove the tumor burden and decrease the chance of tumor progression? The answer is probably yes; however, several detailed studies need to be performed.

First, a molecular profile should be obtained on patients with astrocytomas, documenting the baseline genetic changes (i.e., p53 mutation) that have occurred. The patients may subsequently be treated with cytoreductive surgery, irradiation, or chemotherapy. If the tumor recurs, then a subsequent molecular profile can be obtained. If additional genetic changes have occurred (i.e., deletions in chromosomes 9 or 10, or EGFR amplication), this provides another method for documenting progression independent of the histological grade. Second, we need a more sensitive method of detecting tumor boundaries. Currently, tumor resection margins are determined by the ability to distinguish normal from abnormal tissue on histological study. This problem is accentuated in low-grade gliomas, as they may be difficult to distinguish from normal brain both histologically and intraoperatively. An in situ hybridization or immunohistochemical technique to examine a chromosomal change or the mutant protein produced may be useful in determining whether a complete tumor resection may ever be achieved in patients with low-grade gliomas. If a clean margin cannot be obtained, total resection at the risk of increased neurological deficits should not be attempted in patients with astrocytomas. Third, large randomized prospective studies should be performed to examine early aggressive cytoreductive treatment of astrocytomas versus conservative treatment with biopsy alone, with serial radiological follow-up. Fourth, factors that may affect progression (i.e., age, nutrition, therapeutic protocols) need to be identified and optimized.

As the majority of astrocytomas occur in young, neurologically intact patients, it is imperative that we aggressively seek out answers to the etiology of molecular progression in gliomas.

REFERENCES

1. Berkman RA, Clark WC, Saxena A, et al: Clonal composition of glioblastoma multiforme. **J Neurosurg** 77:432-437, 1992
2. Bigner SH, Mark J, Burger PC, et al: Specific chromosomal abnormalities in malignant human gliomas. **Cancer Res 48**:405-411, 1988
3. Cavenee WK: Accumulation of genetic defects during astrocytoma progression. **Cancer 70**:1788-1793, 1992
4. Cavenee WK, Dryja P, Phillips RA, et al: Expression of recessive alleles by chromosomal mechanisms in retinoblastoma. **Nature 305**:779-784, 1983
5. Cavenee WK, Murphree AL, Shull MM, et al: Prediction of familial predisposition to retinoblastoma. **N Engl J Med 314**:1201-1207, 1986
6. Cavenee WK, Scrable HJ, James CD: Molecular genetics of human cancer predisposition and progression. **Mutat Res 247**:199-202, 1991
7. del Arco A, Garcia J, Arribas C, et al: Timing of p53 mutations during astrocytoma tumorigenesis. **Hum Mol Genet 2**:1687-1690, 1993
8. Ellison DW, Gatter KC, Steart PV, et al: Expression of the p53 protein in a spectrum of astrocytic tumours. **J Pathol 168**:383-386, 1992
9. Finlay CA, Hinds PW, Levine AJ: The p53 proto-oncogene can act as a suppressor of transformation. **Cell 57**:1083-1093, 1989
10. Foulds L: The natural history of cancer. **J Chron Dis 8**:2-37, 1958
11. Foulds L: Tumor progression. **Cancer Res 17**: 355-356, 1957
12. Friend SH, Dryja TP, Weinberg RA: Oncogenes and tumor-suppressing genes. **N Engl J Med 318**: 618-622, 1988
13. Fults D, Tippets RH, Thomas GA, et al: Loss of heterozygosity for loci on chromosome 17p in human malignant astrocytoma. **Cancer Res 49**:6572-6577, 1989
14. Heim S, Mandahl N, Mitelman F: Genetic convergence and divergence in tumor progression. **Cancer Res 48**:5911-5916, 1988
15. Jacoby LB. Clonal origin of nervous system tumors, in Levine AJ, Schmidek HH (eds): **Molecular Genetics of Nervous System Tumors.** New York: Wiley-Liss, 1993, pp 209-217
16. James CD, Carlbom E, Dumanski JP, et al. Clonal genomic alterations in glioma malignancy stages. **Cancer Res 48**:5546-5551, 1988
17. James CD, Carlbom E, Nordenskjold M, et al: Mitotic recombination of chromosome 17 in astrocytomas. **Proc Natl Acad Sci USA 86**:2858-2862, 1989
18. James CD, Collins VP: Glial tumors, in Levine AJ, Schmidek HH (eds): **Molecular Genetics of Nervous System Tumors.** New York: Wiley-Liss, 1993, pp 241-249
19. James CD, He J, Carlbom E, et al: Chromosome 9 deletion mapping reveals interferon a and interferon B-1 gene deletions in human glial tumors. **Cancer Res 51**:1684-1688, 1991
20. Kamb A, Gruis NA, Weaver-Feldhaus J, et al: A cell cycle regulator potentially involved in genesis of many tumor types. **Science 264**:436-439, 1994
21. Lang FF, Miller DC, Pisharody S, et al: High frequency of p53 protein accumulation without p53 mutation in human juvenile pilocytic, low grade and anaplastic astrocytomas. **Oncogene 9**:949-954, 1994
22. Laws ER Jr, Taylor WF, Clifton MB, et al: Neurosurgical management of low-grade astrocytoma of the cerebral hemispheres. **J Neurosurg 61**:665-673, 1984
23. Leon SP, Zhu J, Black PM: Genetic aberrations in human brain tumors. **Neurosurgery 34**:708-722, 1994
24. Levine AJ, Momand J, Finlay CA: The p53 tumour suppressor gene. **Nature 351**:453-456, 1991
25. Liang BC, Ross DA, Greenberg HS, et al: Evidence of allelic imbalance of chromosome 6 in human astrocytomas. **Neurology 44**:533-536, 1994
26. Livingstone LR, White A, Sprouse J, et al: Altered cell cycle arrest and gene amplification potential accompany loss of wild-type p53. **Cell 70**:923-935, 1992
27. Louis DN, Seizinger BR, Cavenee WK: Molecular genetic basis of cerebral gliomas, in Apuzzo MLJ (ed): **Benign Cerebral Glioma. Neurosurgical Topics Series.** Park Ridge, Ill: American Association Neurological Surgeons, 1995, pp 163-180
28. Louis DN, von Deimling A, Chung RY, et al: Comparative study of p53 gene and protein alterations in human astrocytic tumors. **J Neuropathol Exp Neurol 52**:31-38, 1993
29. Makos M, Nelkin BD, Chazin VR, et al: DNA hypermethylation is associated with 17p allelic loss in neural tumors. **Cancer Res 53**:2715-2718, 1993

30. Marsa GW, Goffinet DR, Rubinstein LJ, et al: Megavoltage irradiation in the treatment of gliomas of the brain and spinal cord. **Cancer 36**:1681-1689, 1975
31. Marx J: How p53 suppresses cell growth. **Science 262**:1644-1645, 1993
32. Marx J: New tumor suppressor may rival p53. **Science 264**:344-345, 1994
33. McCormack BM, Miller DC, Budzilovich GN, et al: Treatment and survival of low-grade astrocytoma in adults—1977-1988. **Neurosurgery 31**:636-642, 1992
34. Mikkelsen T, Cairncross JG, Cavenee WK: Genetics of the malignant progression of astrocytoma. **J Cell Biochem 46**:3-8, 1991
35. Morantz RA. The management of low-grade cerebral astrocytomas. **Perspect Neurol Surg 1**:1-23, 1990
36. Morantz RA: The management of the patient with a low-grade cerebral astrocytoma, in Morantz RA, Walsh JW (eds): **Brain Tumors: A Comprehensive Text.** New York: Marcel Dekker, 1994, pp 387-415
37. Müller W, Afra D, Schröder R: Supratentorial recurrences of gliomas. Morphological studies in relation to time intervals with astrocytomas. **Acta Neurochir 37**:75-91, 1977
38. Nicolson GL: Tumor cell instability, diversification, and progression to the metastatic phenotype: from oncogene to oncofetal expression. **Cancer Res 47**:1473-1487, 1987
39. Nowell PC: Chromosomal and molecular clues to tumor progression. **Semin Oncol 16**:116-127, 1989
40. Nowell PC: The clonal evolution of tumor cell populations. Acquired genetic lability permits stepwise selection of variant sublines and underlies tumor progression. **Science 194**:23-28, 1976
41. Nowell PC: Mechanisms of tumor progression. **Cancer Res 46**:2203-2207, 1986
42. Ohgaki H, Eibl RH, Schwab M, et al: Mutations of the p53 tumor suppressor gene in neoplasms of the human nervous system. **Mol Carcinogenet 8**:74-80, 1993
43. Orian JM, Vasilopoulos K, Yoshida S, et al: Overexpression of multiple oncogenes related to histological grade of astrocytic glioma. **Br J Cancer 66**:106-112, 1992
44. Patt S, Thiel G, Maas S, et al: Chromosomal changes and correspondingly altered proto-oncogene expression in human gliomas. Value of combined cytogenetic and molecular genetic analysis. **Anticancer Res 13**:113-118, 1993
45. Piepmeier JM: Observations on the current treatment of low-grade astrocytic tumors of the cerebral hemispheres. **J Neurosurg 67**:177-181, 1987
46. Reifenberger G, Liu L, Ichimura K, et al: Amplification and overexpression of the mdm2 gene in a subset of human malignant gliomas without p53 mutations. **Cancer Res 53**:2736-2739, 1993
47. Rey JA, Bello MJ, Jiménez-Lara AM, et al: Loss of heterozygosity for distal markers on 22q in human gliomas. **Int J Cancer 51**:703-706, 1992
48. Rubio MP, von Deimling A, Yandell DW, et al: Accumulation of wild type p53 protein in human astrocytomas. **Cancer Res 53**:3465-3467, 1993
49. Scheck AC, Coons SW: Expression of the tumor suppressor gene **DCC** in human gliomas. **Cancer Res 53**:5605-5609, 1993
50. Schmidek HH: Molecular genetic events in some primary human brain tumors, in Morantz RA, Walsh JW (eds): **Brain Tumors: A Comprehensive Text.** New York: Marcel Dekker, 1994, pp 173-181
51. Sidransky D, Mikkelsen T, Schwechheimer K, et al: Clonal expansion of p53 mutant cells is associated with brain tumour progression. **Nature 355**:846-847, 1992
52. Soffietti R, Chio A, Giordana MT, et al: Prognostic factors in well-differentiated cerebral astrocytomas in the adult. **Neurosurgery 24**:686-692, 1989
53. Steiger HJ, Markwalder RV, Seiler RW, et al: Early prognosis of supratentorial grade 2 astrocytomas in adult patients after resection or stereotactic biopsy. **Acta Neurochir 106**:99-105, 1990
54. Van de Kelft E, de Boulle K, Willems P, et al: Loss of constitutional heterozygosity in human astrocytomas. **Acta Neurochir 117**:172-177, 1992
55. van Meir EG, Kikuchi T, Tada M, et al: Analysis of the p53 gene and its expression in human glioblastoma cells. **Cancer Res 54**:649-652, 1994
56. Venter DJ, Thomas DGT: Multiple sequential molecular abnormalities in the evolution of human gliomas. **Br J Cancer 63**:753-757, 1991
57. Vertosick FT, Selker RG, Arena VC: Survival of patients with well-differentiated astrocytomas diagnosed in the era of computed tomography. **Neurosurgery 28**:496-502, 1991
58. Vogelstein B, Kinzler KW: The multistep nature of cancer. **Trends Genet 9**:138-141, 1993
59. Volpe JPG: Genetic instability of cancer. Why a metastatic tumor is unstable and a benign tumor is stable. **Cancer Genet Cytogenet 34**:125-134,1988
60. von Deimling A, Bender B, Jahnke R, et al: Loci associated with malignant progression in astrocytomas: a candidate on chromosome 19q. **Cancer Res 54**:1397-1401, 1994
61. von Deimling A, Eibl RH, Ohgaki H, et al: p53 mutations are associated with 17p allelic loss in grade II and grade III astrocytoma. **Cancer Res 52**:2987-2990, 1992
62. von Deimling A, Louis DN, von Ammon K, et al: Association of epidermal growth factor receptor gene amplification with loss of chromosome 10 in human glioblastoma multiforme. **J Neurosurg 77**:295-301, 1992
63. von Deimling A, Louis DN, von Ammon K, et al: Evidence for a tumor suppressor gene on chromosome 19q associated with human astrocytomas, oligodendrogliomas, and mixed gliomas. **Cancer Res 52**:4277-4279, 1992
64. Wu JK, Ye Z, Darras BT: Frequency of p53 tumor suppressor gene mutations in human primary brain tumors. **Neurosurgery 33**:824-831, 1993
65. Yin Y, Tainsky MA, Bischoff FZ, et al. Wild-type p53 restores cell cycle control and inhibits gene amplification in cells with mutant p53 alleles. **Cell 70**: 937-948, 1992

QUESTIONS FOR *Benign Cerebral Glioma, Volume I*

The following questions have been provided to give physicians the option of testing their comprehension of the material provided in *Benign Cerebral Glioma, Volume I.* The test is to be self-scored. Answers may be found in the back of this book. A Continuing Medical Education (CME) certificate will be mailed upon the return of the enclosed test evaluation/feedback card along with a $25 administrative fee. Telephone 708-692-9500 to order additional evaluation/feedback cards or information about other CME products from the American Association of Neurological Surgeons.

After reading this book, a physician should be able to:

- comprehend the current prevailing classification schema of intrinsic glial tumors
- comprehend tumor growth patterns as a relative substrate for treatment effort
- comprehend selected aspects molecular biology as applied to intrinsic glial tumors
- comprehend current theory related to malignant progression in "benign" gliomas

CHAPTER 2

THE DEVELOPMENTAL BIOLOGY OF GLIAL CELLS AND ITS RELATION TO THE STUDY OF GLIOMA BIOLOGY

1. Which of the following statements is *false*?
   (A) Growth factors and their second messenger intracellular pathways provide a key link between cellular proliferation, cellular differentiation, cell survival, and glial oncogenesis.
   (B) Differentiation agents are a heterogeneous class of pharmacological agents that could theoretically prove useful in the treatment of patients with "low-grade" gliomas.
   (C) Most patients with "low-grade" astrocytomas (excluding subependymal giant cell astrocytomas, pilocytic astrocytomas, gangliogliomas, and pure oligodendrogliomas) die from progressive growth of their glioma.
   (D) Radiation therapy and chemotherapy mainly exploit a difference in proliferation rate between neoplastic and normal cells for their effectiveness.
   (E) Many transplacental nitrosourea-induced rat glioma cell lines appear to be of oligodendrocyte-type-2 astrocyte (O-2A) lineage.

2. Ways of exploiting information and techniques learned from developmental glial biology to improve the study of glioma biology include all of the following *except*:
   (A) Exploring the potential role of synergistic cooperation of growth factors in glioma biology.
   (B) Performing primary glioma cell culture in serum-free, type-1 astrocyte (T1A)-conditioned media rather than media containing animal serum, in order to better approximate the actual extracellular conditions present in vivo.
   (C) Beginning to apply glial lineage analysis to the diagnosis, prognosis, and response to therapy of human gliomas.
   (D) Ignoring the potential contribution of three-dimensional embryonic glial reaggregation culture for providing in vitro substrates for studying glioma-brain interactions, including central nervous system invasion.
   (E) Exploring the use of ^{1}H nuclear magnetic resonance (NMR) spectroscopy to provide lineage analysis of human gliomas in vivo.

3. The five zones of the developing neural tube are:
   (A) the primitive ependyma, the subependymal layer, the mantle layer, the cortical plate, and the marginal zone.
   (B) the ventricular zone, the subventricular zone, the intermediate zone, the cortical plate, and the marginal zone.
   (C) the ventricular zone, the subependymal germinal matrix, the intermediate zone, the cortical plate, and the marginal zone.
   (D) the matrix layer, the subventricular zone, the intermediate zone, the cortical plate, and the marginal zone.
   (E) the medulloepithelial layer, the subependymal germinal matrix, the mantle layer, the cortical plate, and the marginal zone.

4. Which of the following statements is *true*?
   (A) Morphological criteria alone are sufficient to identify and distinguish neuroglial precursor cells by light microscopy in in vivo tissue sections.
   (B) Gangliosides, sulfatides, and cerebrosides (which are useful cell-surface antigens for studying glial lineage and stage of maturation) can be readily studied on formalin-fixed, paraffin-embedded tissue specimens.
   (C) The ultimate advancement in developmental glial biology required the development of new scientific tools based on advances in already established fields, as well as the development of whole new fields of science including in vitro cellular biology, immunology, and molecular biology.
   (D) Growing cells in vitro in media containing animal serum provides a good model for approximating the in vivo extracellular environment in the central nervous system.
   (E) A medulloblast is a well-defined and readily identifiable cell which can give rise to either astrocytes or oligodendrocytes.

5. The cellular fate of progeny of a single cell of interest can best be determined by:
   (A) time-lapse cinemicroscopy in vitro and immunohistochemistry in vivo.
   (B) clonal analysis in vitro and in situ hybridization techniques in vivo.
   (C) dissociated cell suspension culture in vitro and retroviral gene transfer techniques in vivo.
   (D) time-lapse cinemicroscopy in vitro and in situ hybridization techniques in vivo.
   (E) clonal analysis in vitro and retroviral gene transfer techniques in vivo.

6-10: For each question number, answer:

A: if only statements 1, 2, and 3 are correct

B: if only statements 1 and 3 are correct

C: if only statements 2 and 4 are correct

D: if only statement 4 is correct

E: if all four statements are correct

6.1. The most extensively studied mammalian system for developmental glial biology is the rat.
  2. The optic nerve is the simplest model for studying glial developmental biology.
  3. Structural radial glia persist into adulthood in non-mammalian cortex but appear to transform into cortical astrocytes in mammalian cortex.
  4. Type-1 astrocytes (T1As) and type-2 astrocytes (T2As) can be unambiguously distinguished by morphological criteria.

7.1. The O-2A lineage includes perinatal O-2A progenitor cells, oligodendrocytes, T2As, and radial glia.
  2. Using ^{1}H NMR spectra to examine cellular metabolites, O-2A progenitor cells can be distinguished from oligodendrocytes and T1As by the presence of high concentrations of N-acetyl-aspartate, and can be distinguished from neurons by the almost complete absence of β-hydroxybutyrate.

3. Once perinatal O-2A progenitor cells express monoclonal antibody O4, they are committed oligodendrocytes and are no longer capable of differentiating into T2As.
4. Macroglia have been shown to possess both voltage-dependent ion channels (Na^+, K^+, Cl^-, and Ca^{++}) and neurotransmitter-gated ion channels in their plasma membranes.

8.1. The T1A lineage includes T1A precursor cells and mature T1As, which are both monoclonal antibody A2B5$^-$.
2. T1A precursor cells appear to migrate into the optic nerve from an adjacent subventricular zone.
3. T1As have been shown to proliferate in response to epidermal growth factor, platelet-derived growth factor (PDGF), basic fibroblast growth factor (bFGF), and to a lesser extent acidic fibroblast growth factor.
4. Mature T1As cease dividing as soon as they begin to express glial fibrillary acidic protein.

9.1. Adult O-2A progenitor cells are true stem cells that persist throughout life in rats, providing a continuing source for oligodendrocytes and their own replenishment through asymmetric division.
2. PDGF used in combination with bFGF will convert adult O-2A progenitor cells into cells with the characteristics of perinatal O-2A progenitor cells in vitro, and may therefore provide a mechanism to rapidly amplify the O-2A progenitor cell population in vivo (in the setting of central nervous system injury or demyelination) in order to facilitate repair mechanisms.
3. Multipotential neuroglial precursor cells, which can give rise to both neurons and macroglia, have been identified in vitro and in vivo.
4. In vitro perinatal O-2A progenitor cells proliferate in response to PDGF and to a lesser extent bFGF alone, while the combination of PDGF and bFGF or PDGF and neurotrophin-3 will promote perinatal O-2A progenitor cell proliferation beyond the point when they would otherwise have differentiated into oligodendrocytes.

10. 1. Oligodendrocytes, like neurons, are normally overproduced during development in vivo and redundant cells subsequently undergo a process of programmed cell death (apoptosis).
2. Oligodendrocyte apoptosis appears to be triggered by the limited availability of critical growth factors such as insulin-like growth factor (IGF)-1, IFG-2, insulin, ciliary neurotrophic factor, neurotrophin-3, and leukemia inhibitory factor.
3. The ventricular and subventricular zones (which are comprised of a population of multipotential neuroglial precursor cells, neuronal precursor cells, and perinatal oligodendrocyte-T2A precursor cells) appear to be heterogeneous on both a cellular and a regional basis.
4. T2As have been conclusively shown to exist both in vitro and in vivo.

CHAPTER 3

THE PATHOLOGY OF BENIGN CEREBRAL ASTROCYTOMAS

1. Which of the following features influences prognosis in patients with pilocytic astrocytoma?
   (A) the presence of cytological atypia
   (B) the presence of macrocysts
   (C) local leptomeningeal infiltration
   (D) gross total excision
   (E) all of the above

2. Pleomorphic xanthoastrocytoma:
   (A) commonly presents with seizures.
   (B) is usually periventricular in location.
   (C) is usually nonenhancing on computed tomography (CT) scans.
   (D) may contain foci of necrosis.
   (E) most commonly presents in the first decade.

3. Subependymal giant cell astrocytomas are:
   (A) common in the fourth ventricle.
   (B) rich in reticulin fibers.
   (C) common in patients with von Recklinghausen's disease.
   (D) immunoreactive for glial fibrillary acidic protein.
   (E) usually nonenhancing on CT scans.

4. Spindle-shaped cells may be found in:
   (A) juvenile pilocytic astrocytomas.
   (B) pleomorphic xanthoastrocytomas.
   (C) subependymal giant cell astrocytomas.
   (D) all of the above.
   (E) none of the above.

5. Neurofilament protein immunoreactivity has been described in:
   (A) pilocytic astrocytoma.
   (B) subependymal giant cell astrocytoma.
   (C) desmoplastic ganglioglioma of infancy.
   (D) gliofibroma.
   (E) all of the above.

6. Features used to grade astrocytomas using the new World Health Organization system (1993) include:
   (A) cellularity.
   (B) endothelial proliferation.
   (C) leptomeningeal infiltration.
   (D) proliferating cell nuclear antigen or Ki-67 labeling index.
   (E) the presence or absence of gemistocytes.

7. Cerebral pilocytic astrocytomas:
   (A) are usually diagnosed in the first decade.
   (B) are usually well circumscribed.
   (C) are diploid by flow cytometry in >75% of cases.
   (D) have a significantly worse prognosis than cerebellar pilocytic astrocytomas.
   (E) may be reticulin rich.

8. Rosenthal fibers are:
   (A) immunoreactive for α-1-antichymotrypsin.
   (B) usually found in pleomorphic xanthoastrocytoma.
   (C) extracellular collections of amorphous granular material.
   (D) immunoreactive for glial fibrillary acidic protein.
   (E) immunoreactive for αβ-crystallin.

9. Desmoplastic cerebral astrocytoma of infancy:
   (A) is usually found in the temporal lobe.
   (B) is usually solid.
   (C) may appear predominantly extracerebral.
   (D) contains numerous giant cells.
   (E) contains numerous fibroblasts.

10. Gliofibroma:
   (A) contains distinct populations of astrocytes and fibroblasts.
   (B) contains pericellular reticulin but no fibrous tissue.
   (C) is usually cystic.
   (D) shares ultrastructural features with subpial astrocytes.
   (E) occurs most commonly in the elderly.

CHAPTER 4

THE PATHOLOGY OF OLIGODENDROGLIOMAS

1-3. Which of the following describe:

1. the typical computed tomography and/or magnetic resonance imaging aspects of oligodendrogliomas.
   (A) hypodensity, low signal intensity on noncontrast studies
   (B) cortical sparing
   (C) demarcation
   (D) edema-associated
   (E) calcification in the minority of tumors

2. the immunohistochemical features of oligodendrogliomas.
   (A) GFAP and "minigemistocytes"
   (B) Leu- 7 immunostaining
   (C) S-100 immunoreactivity
   (D) myelin basic protein immunoreaction
   (E) vimentin immunoreaction

3. the typical ultrastructural features of oligodendrogliomas.
   (A) long, broad cytoplasmic processes
   (B) neurosecretory granules
   (C) desmosomal junctions
   (D) microvilli-containing extracellular spaces
   (E) none of the above

4. The typical hematoxylin-eosin appearance of oligodendroglioma includes:
   (A) cellular and nuclear pleomorphism.
   (B) lack of perinuclear halos in specimens subject to delayed fixation.
   (C) mitotic activity ≥1/high power ($\times$ 400) microscopic field.
   (D) endothelial proliferation.
   (E) occasional presence of "minigemistocytes."

5. Clinicopathologically, oligodendrogliomas differ from dysembryoplastic neuroepithelial tumors in that the latter:
   (A) are almost exclusively cortical in location.
   (B) exhibit the formation of patterned nodules composed of oligodendrocyte-like cells as well as an internodular mucin-rich matrix containing "floating" neurons.
   (C) tend not to be seizure-associated.
   (D) require aggressive adjuvant therapy.
   (E) occur primarily in older adults.

6. Oligodendrogliomas are distinguished from central neurocytomas in that the latter:
   - (A) are intraventricular in location.
   - (B) do not show clear cell formation.
   - (C) contain neurosecretory granules.
   - (D) do not exhibit calcification.
   - (E) are synaptophysin immunoreactive.

7. In relation to the molecular genetic profile of oligodendrogliomas,
   - (A) the majority present with deletion and/or abnormalities on chromosome 22.
   - (B) similar to astrocytic tumors, oligodendrogliomas exhibit amplification of the epidermal growth factor receptor gene.
   - (C) allelic deletions on chromosome 19 have been demonstrated in great numbers of oligodendrogliomas.
   - (D) point mutations of the p53 tumor suppression gene are more common in oligodendrogliomas than in astrocytomas.

8. Select the *incorrect* statement.
   - (A) Oligodendrogliomas most frequently affect the cerebral hemispheres.
   - (B) Involvement of multiple lobes and bilaterality are common findings in oligodendrogliomas.
   - (C) Cystic degeneration and areas of necrosis are commonly seen at gross inspection of low-grade oligodendrogliomas.
   - (D) Calcification and foci of hemorrhage are commonly seen at gross inspection of low-grade oligodendrogliomas.

9. Select the *correct* statement.
   - (A) Oligodendrogliomas are common in children and adolescents, with a peak incidence in the second decade.
   - (B) The majority of oligodendrogliomas are associated with a long history of seizures.
   - (C) The spinal cord and cerebral hemispheres are equally involved by oligodendrogliomas.
   - (D) A 2:1 to 3:2 female-to-male predominance is seen in oligodendrogliomas.

10. Select the *incorrect* statement.
    - (A) Anaplastic oligodendrogliomas are characterized by cellular pleomorphism, increased mitotic activity, and endothelial proliferation.
    - (B) The great majority of oligodendrogliomas progress to more anaplastic forms.
    - (C) GFAP-immunoreactive cells tend to increase in number with anaplastic progression.
    - (D) Mitotic index and proliferative activity assessed by S-phase fraction appear to be associated with survival in oligodendrogliomas.

CHAPTER 5

THE PATHOLOGY OF BENIGN EPENDYMOMAS

1. Embryologically, ependymomas are tumors derived from which of the following cell precursors?
   (A) astrocytes
   (B) neuroblasts
   (C) ependymoglia
   (D) radial glia
   (E) endoderm

2. Select the most consistent cellular components of ependymomas.
   (A) neurons, astrocytes, and fibroblasts
   (B) oligodendrocytes, astrocytes, and calcifications
   (C) astrocytes, oligodendrocytes, and microcysts
   (D) epithelial cells and astrocytes
   (E) epithelial cells with blepharoplasts lining fibrovascular cores

3. The following are histological criteria for the diagnosis of ependymoma, *except:*
   (A) ependymal rosettes, tubules, and clefts.
   (B) astrocytic component.
   (C) perivascular pseudorosettes.
   (D) sheets of ependymal cells.
   (E) necrosis and palisading of tumor cells.

4. According to the World Health Organization classification of brain tumors, benign ependymomas are a heterogeneous group that includes all of the following types *except:*
   (A) a papillary variant.
   (B) ependymoblastoma.
   (C) a cellular variant.
   (D) a myxopapillary variant.
   (E) subependymoma.

5. Ependymomas are more common in the pediatric population. What is the proportion of all tumors in this age group?
   (A) 0.5% - 1.3%
   (B) 2% - 6%
   (C) 4% - 7%
   (D) 9% - 11%
   (E) 10% - 15%

6. Although ependymomas may originate from any portion of the ventricular system and occasionally from rests buried deep in the white matter, which is their most common location?
   (A) stria terminali
   (B) temporal horns
   (C) fourth ventricle
   (D) intraspinal
   (E) cauda equina

7. The macroscopic feature(s) of ependymomas that sets them apart surgically from most other brain tumors:
   (A) is color.
   (B) are the sharp margins.
   (C) are calcifications.
   (D) is consistency.
   (E) is cyst formation.

8. Prognosis of ependymomas depends upon consideration of the following variables, *except:*
   (A) location.
   (B) association with von Recklinghausen's disease.
   (C) extent of surgical resection.
   (D) histological diagnosis.
   (E) patient age.

9. Occasionally reported as an incidental finding, which of the following tumors occurs in a characteristic location and has a predominant astrocytic component?
   (A) ependymoblastoma
   (B) myxopapillary ependymoma
   (C) subependymoma
   (D) anaplastic ependymoma
   (E) papillary ependymoma

10. The following are characteristics of myxopapillary ependymomas, *except:*
    (A) they are hypovascular.
    (B) they are almost restricted to the cauda equina.
    (C) perivascular pseudorosettes exhibit microcyst formation.
    (D) notably, they have a gelatinous appearance.
    (E) metastasis is rare.

CHAPTER 6

THE PATHOLOGY OF GANGLION CELL TUMORS

1. Desmoplastic infantile gangliogliomas tend to be:
   (A) small, solid tumors.
   (B) diffuse, infiltrative tumors.
   (C) massive cystic tumors.
   (D) all of the above.

2. Desmoplastic infantile gangliogliomas may:
   (A) infiltrate the leptomeninges and dura.
   (B) contain dense reticulin deposition.
   (C) contain primitive neuroepithelial cells.
   (D) all of the above.

3. Histologically, desmoplastic infantile gangliogliomas may resemble:
   (A) a dysembryoplastic neuroepithelial tumor.
   (B) a gliosarcoma.
   (C) a desmoplastic cerebral astrocytoma.
   (D) all of the above.

4. Histologically, central neurocytomas may resemble:
   (A) an oligodendroglioma.
   (B) a choroid plexus papilloma.
   (C) a neuroblastoma.
   (D) all of the above.

5. At low magnification, central neurocytomas are:
   (A) uniform.
   (B) cystic.
   (C) anaplastic.
   (D) all of the above.

6. The definitive diagnosis of central neurocytoma usually requires:
   (A) flow cytometry.
   (B) histochemical stains.
   (C) electron microscopy.
   (D) all of the above.

7. Histologically, dysembryoplastic neuroepithelial tumors may resemble:
   (A) astrocytomas.
   (B) oligoastrocytomas.
   (C) neurocytomas.
   (D) all of the above.

8. A histological hallmark of the dysembyroplastic neuroepithelial tumor is:
   (A) desmoplasia.
   (B) binucleate ganglion cells.
   (C) specific glioneuronal elements.
   (D) all of the above.

9. Complex dysembryoplastic neuroepithelial tumors may contain:
   (A) nodular astrocytic components.
   (B) cortical components.
   (C) nodular oligodendroglial components.
   (D) all of the above.

10. A histological hallmark of ganglion cell tumors is:
   (A) dysplastic or binucleate ganglion cell tumors.
   (B) microcysts.
   (C) calcification.
   (D) all of the above.

CHAPTER 7

Patterns of Tumor Growth and Problems Associated with Histological Typing of Low-Grade Gliomas

1. All but one of the following are *true* concerning the structure type of gliomas:
   (A) Structure type I tumors consist only of solid tumor tissue.
   (B) Structure type II tumors consist of solid tumor tissue and isolated tumor cells.
   (C) Structure type III tumors consist of isolated tumor cells only.
   (D) Structure type III tumors consist of isolated tumors cells in association with small foci of tumor tissue.

2. Which one of the following tumors often adopts a structure type III?
   (A) low-grade oligodendrogliomas
   (B) pilocytic astrocytomas
   (C) low-grade ordinary astrocytomas
   (D) dysembryoplastic neuroepithelial tumors (DNTs)
   (E) high-grade ordinary astrocytomas

3. Surgical removal can be performed without a resultant deficit in all but one of the following instances:
   (A) Structure type I gliomas in eloquent brain structure.
   (B) Structure type I tumors situated in noneloquent brain area.
   (C) Structure type III gliomas in eloquent brain area.
   (D) Structure type III gliomas in nonessential brain structure.
   (E) The solid part of a structure type II tumor.

4. Which of the following is *true* with regard to contrast enhancement in gliomas? Contrast enhancement is:
   (A) absent in structure type I gliomas.
   (B) not always present in structure type III gliomas.
   (C) constant in structure type III gliomas.
   (D) strongly correlated with the degree of tumor microvascularity.
   (E) usually located within isolated tumor cells.

5. Structure type I is commonly observed in which one of the following histological tumor types?
   (A) pilocytic astrocytomas
   (B) ordinary oligodendrogliomas
   (C) oligoastrocytomas
   (D) grade 4 astrocytomas (glioblastomas)
   (E) oligodendrogliomas

6. Which of the following is *not* true concerning the pattern of growth of oligodendrogliomas?
   (A) Oligodendrogliomas often adopt a structure type I.
   (B) About two of three oligodendrogliomas are of structure type III.
   (C) Contrast enhancement is not seen in low-grade structure type III tumors.
   (D) Oligodendrogliomas of structure type III usually involve both the cortex and the white matter.
   (E) On T2-weighted magnetic resonance images, oligodendrogliomas of structure type III are usually seen as a well-delineated increased signal.

7. Which of the following is *false*?
   (A) DNTs are carcinogenically stable lesions.
   (B) DNTs are usually associated with phacomatosis.
   (C) DNTs may resemble pilocytic astrocytomas.
   (D) DNTs may resemble ordinary oligodendrogliomas.
   (E) DNTs may show multinodular architecture.

8. In the setting of DNTs located in elo quent brain area, which of the following would be appropriate therapy?
   (A) avoid surgical removal
   (B) surgical removal as complete as possible
   (C) partial removal plus radiotherapy
   (D) radiotherapy only

9. Which of the following is *not* true concerning the histology of DNTs?
   (A) The tumor may not show specific morphological features allowing distinction from conventional categories of gliomas.
   (B) Foci of cortical dysplasia are often associated with DNTs.
   (C) Presence of a specific glioneuronal element is required for the diagnosis of DNTs.
   (D) Mitosis and necrosis may be seen in DNTs.
   (E) Kinetic markers such as MIB1 or Ki-67 may disclose growth fractions as high as those seen in malignant gliomas.

10. Which of the following is *not* used as a criterion for distinguishing DNTs from ordinary gliomas?
    (A) absence of mitotic activity
    (B) partial seizures with or without secondary generalization
    (C) no neurological deficit or stable congenital deficit
    (D) onset of symptoms before the age of 20 years
    (E) cortical topography of the lesion

CHAPTER 8

GROWTH FACTORS AND PROLIFERATION POTENTIAL

1. Which of the following is *not* an angiogenic factor?
   (A) vascular endothelial growth factor (VEGF)
   (B) basic fibroblast growth factor (bFGF)
   (C) platelet-derived growth factor (PDGF)
   (D) transforming growth factor (TGF)-β
   (E) p53

2. Which of the following proliferation markers is limited in distribution to S-phase?
   (A) Ki-67
   (B) MIB1
   (C) proliferating cell nuclear antigen (PCNA)
   (D) bromodeoxyuridine
   (E) statin

3. Which of the following statements about proliferative labeling indices in benign (grade I) gliomas is *true?*
   (A) There is a wide range of labeling indices which do not, in general, correlate with prognosis.
   (B) There is a strong correlation between labeling index and survival.
   (C) Tumors with high labeling indices must be considered malignant.
   (D) Pleomorphic xanthoastrocytomas never contain mitotic figures.

4. Which of the following tests for proliferative potential may *not* be reliably performed on paraffin-embedded material?
   (A) Ki-67 labeling with Ki-67 antibody
   (B) Ki-67 labeling with MIB1 antibody
   (C) PCNA
   (D) flow cytometry
   (E) identification of incorporated bromodeoxyuridine

5. Which of the following cytokines/growth factors may be secreted by glial cells?
   (A) TNF-α
   (B) TGF-β
   (C) PDGF
   (D) VEGF
   (E) interferon-γ

6. Which of the following is *true* about the differentiation of reactive gliosis from low-grade glioma?
   (A) Gliotic astrocytes are not labeled by Ki-67.
   (B) In reactive gliosis, you may find mitotic activity.
   (C) Silver-staining nucleolar organizer region counting may help in the differentation of gliosis from low-grade astrocytoma.
   (D) PCNA labeling easily distinguishes gliosis from low-grade glioma.

7. Which of the following have been suggested as autocrine loops for potential growth mechanisms in malignant glioma cells?
   (A) PDGF/PDGF receptor
   (B) epidermal growth factor (EGF)/EGF receptor
   (C) bFGF/FGF receptor
   (D) VEGF/VEGF receptor

8. Which of the following statements about the differentiation of necrosis from apoptosis are *true?*
   (A) Apoptosis is usually associated with inflammation.
   (B) Apoptosis may be initiated by a signal from tumor necrosis factor (TNF)-α or *fas.*
   (C) Apoptosis is often characterized by digestion of deoxyribonucleic acid (DNA) into oligonucleosomal fragments.
   (D) Although common in development, apoptosis is rare in tumors.

9. During the cell cycle, which of the following are *true?*
   (A) The longest phase is the M phase.
   (B) Normal G1 phase contains diploid (2C) DNA content.
   (C) Normal S phase contains tetraploid (4C) DNA content.
   (D) PCNA is synthesized in S phase.

10. A stereotactic biopsy of a supratentorial glial tumor shows a MIB1 labeling index of 5%. Which of the following are *true?*
   (A) The labeling index indicates a high proliferative potential.
   (B) The tumor is enlarging at a rapid rate.
   (C) The tumor must be anaplastic in behavior.
   (D) The rate of cell death can be directly correlated with the proliferation rate.
   (E) The index should be interpreted in conjunction with the tumor histology, clinical presentation, and radiological characteristics.

CHAPTER 9

MOLECULAR GENETIC BASIS OF CEREBRAL GLIOMAS

1. The formation of low-grade astrocytoma may involve one or more of the following genetic alterations:
   (A) p53 mutation
   (B) loss of chromosome 17p
   (C) epidermal growth factor receptor (EGFR) gene amplification
   (D) loss of chromosome 10

2. Tumor suppressor genes on which one or more of the following chromosomes may be involved in the transition to anaplastic astrocytoma?
   (A) chromosome 9p
   (B) chromosome 10
   (C) chromosome 13q
   (D) chromosome 19q

3. The transition to glioblastoma multiforme may involve which of the following genetic alterations?
   (A) loss of chromosome 22q
   (B) loss of chromosome 17p
   (C) EGFR gene amplification
   (D) loss of chromosome 10

4. EGFR gene amplification occurs in tumors that have:
   (A) p53 gene mutations.
   (B) lost chromosome 17p.
   (C) lost chromosome 10.
   (D) an overexpression of PDGF receptors.

5. Which of the following genetic alterations may be alternative events and may define subsets of glioblastoma multiforme?
   (A) platelet-derived growth factor-α -receptor overexpression and chromosome 17p loss
   (B) p53 mutation and chromosome 17p loss
   (C) loss of the first and second alleles of chromosome 9p
   (D) chromosome 17p loss and EGFR gene amplification

6. p53 mutations are common in which of the following gliomas?
   (A) diffuse, fibrillary astrocytomas
   (B) pediatric brain stem gliomas
   (C) pilocytic astrocytomas
   (D) oligodendrogliomas

7. In addition to p53, which one of the following tumor suppressor genes has been implicated in astrocytoma progression?
   (A) neurofibromatosis 2
   (B) retinoblastoma susceptibility
   (C) familial adenomatous polyposis
   (D) tuberous sclerosis

8. A tumor suppressor gene involved in oligodendroglioma tumorigenesis may reside on:
   (A) chromosome 9p
   (B) chromosome 17p
   (C) chromosome 19q
   (D) chromosome 22q

9. Ependymomas often show loss of:
   (A) chromosome 9p
   (B) chromosome 10
   (C) chromosome 19q
   (D) chromosome 22q

10. Subependymal giant cell astrocytomas may be expected to show abnormalities in a tumor suppressor gene on:
   (A) chromosome 1p
   (B) chromosome 9q
   (C) chromosome 16q
   (D) chromosome 22q

CHAPTER 10

MALIGNANT PROGRESSION IN GLIOMAS

1. Tumor progression:
   (A) occurs in multiple steps.
   (B) is not affected by the host immune system.
   (C) is not preceded by initiation.
   (D) results in tumors with decreased malignancy.

2. The concept of initiation and progression was first described by:
   (A) Peter Nowell.
   (B) Leslie Foulds.
   (C) Stephen Friend.
   (D) Stephen Gould.

3. The initial definition of progression was based on:
   (A) histological changes only.
   (B) alterations of tumor suppressor genes and oncogenes.
   (C) the clonal hypothesis.
   (D) benign tumors only.

4. In the clonal hypothesis,
   (A) neoplasms arise simultaneously from multiple clones.
   (B) neoplasms arise from one clone.
   (C) genetic heterogeneity occurs secondary to survival of the majority of daughter clones.
   (D) all mutant cells are at a growth disadvantage compared to the original tumor.

5. The incidence of documented progression to glioblastoma multiforme in published series is:
   (A) 25%.
   (B) 30%.
   (C) 40%.
   (D) 50%.
   (E) 75%.

6. The two pathways for glioma progression may be p53 dependent or independent.
   (A) true
   (B) false

7. The tumor suppressor gene p53 is located on:
   (A) chromosome 10.
   (B) chromosome 13.
   (C) chromosome 17.
   (D) chromosome 9.
   (E) chromosome 12.

8. A newly identified tumor suppressor gene is located on:
   (A) chromosome 8.
   (B) chromosome 13.
   (C) chromosome 10.
   (D) chromosome 9.
   (E) chromosome 21.

9. X chromosome inactivation may be determined by which of the following markers?
   (A) glucose-6-phosphate dehydrogenase
   (B) restriction fragment length polymorphisms
   (C) loss of heterozygosity
   (D) DNA fingerprinting
   (E) point mutations

10. Models of tumor progression have been documented for:
   (A) colon carcinoma.
   (B) retinoblastoma.
   (C) stomach cancer.
   (D) hepatomas.
   (E) osteosarcoma.

Benign Cerebral Glioma, Volume I
ANSWERS TO CME QUESTIONS

Chapter 2

Answers: 1. C; 2. D; 3. B; 4. C; 5. E; 6. A; 7. C; 8. B; 9. E; 10. A

Chapter 3

Answers: 1. D; 2. A; 3. D; 4. D; 5. D; 6. B; 7. B; 8. E; 9. C; 10. D

Chapter 4

Answers: 1. A, C, E; 2. A, B, C; 3. E; 4. E; 5. A, C, E; 6. A, B; 7. C; 8. C; 9. B; 10. B

Chapter 5

Answers: 1. C; 2. D; 3. E; 4. B; 5. D; 6. C; 7. B; 8. B; 9. C; 10. A

Chapter 6

Answers: 1. C; 2. D; 3. C; 4. A; 5. A; 6. C; 7. B; 8. C; 9. D; 10. A

Chapter 7

Answers: 1. D; 2. A; 3. C; 4. D; 5. A; 6. A; 7. A; 8. C; 9. B; 10. A

Chapter 8

Answers: 1. E; 2. D; 3. A; 4. A; 5. C; 6. B, C; 7. A, B, C; 8. A, B,C,D; 9. B, C, D; 10. A, E

Chapter 9

Answers: 1. A, B; 2. A, C, D; 3. C, D; 4. C; 5. D; 6. A, B; 7. B; 8. C; 9. D; 10. B, C

Chapter 10

Answers: 1. A; 2. B; 3. A; 4. B; 5. D; 6. A; 7. C; 8. D; 9. A; 10. A, B

INDEX
Volumes I and II

Page numbers for figures and tables are in ***boldface italics.***
(1) = entry in Volume I
(2) = entry in Volume II

A

A2B5-immunoreactive cells in oligodendrogliomas, (1) 88
Abl, (1) 39
Ablation, (1) 6-7, ***7,*** 8, ***8, 9***
Acidic fibroblast growth factor (aFGF), (1) 28
Acoustic neuromas as indication for stereotactic radiosurgery, (2) 330
Acquired immune deficiency syndrome (AIDS) and benign cerebral gliomas, (2) 270
Acromegaly as indication for stereotactic radiosurgery, (2) 330
Adenomas sebaceum
 in subependymal giant cell astrocytomas, (2) 260
 in tuberous sclerosis, (2) 237-238
Age, as factor
 in astrocytomas, (2) 215, 216-217, 218, 318, 382
  piloid juvenile, (2) 214-215
 in benign gliomas, (2) 247
 in ependymomas, (1) 96; (2) 224, 418-419, ***419***
 in interpretation of glial tumors, (1) 142
 in malignant transformation, (2) 295
 in oligodendrogliomas, (1) 83; (2) 220, 222
AgNOR technique
 in diagnosing pleomorphic xanthoastrocytoma, (1) 67
 in differentiating between gliosis and low-grade fibrillary astrocytomas, (1) 156
AIDS (acquired immune deficiency syndrome) and benign cerebral gliomas, (2) 270
Alleles, (1) 180
Allelic chromosomal loss in identifying tumor suppressor genes, (1) 164
Amalgam, (1) 5-6
American College of Surgeons (ACS) Study, survival rate in, (2) 218
Amnesia, bitemporal lesions in, (2) 351
Amplification, (1) 163
Amygdalohippocampectomy, (2) 365, 374
Amytal test for lateralization of language, (2) 351
Anaplastic astrocytomas
 progression to, (1) 168-170, ***170***
 recurrence of, (2) 217, 218
Anaplastic ependymomas, (1) 96
 diagnosis of, (1) 106-109, 110
 distinguishing between ependymoblastomas and, (1) 109
 histolic structure of, (2) 416
Anaplastic oligodendrogliomas
 characteristics of, (1) ***89***
 pathological features of, (2) 399, ***399***
 progression of, (1) 89-90
 vimentin expression in, (1) 88
Anesthesia, cortical simulation under local, (2) 352
Angiofibromas, cutaneous, (1) 71
Angiogenesis, (1) 157
Angiogenic factors, (1) 157-159
 basic fibroblast growth factor, (1) 158
 cytokines, (1) 159
 epidermal growth receptor factor, (1) 90-91, 158-159, 166, ***167,*** 171
 platelet-derived growth factor, (1) 28, 29, 90, 157, 158, 166

transforming growth factor-β, (1) 90, 157-158
vascular endothelial growth factor, (1) 157, 158
Angiography, (1) 2
in determining resectability, (2) 351
in diagnosing
astrocytomas, (2) 384
central neurocytomas, (2) 428
ganglion cell tumors, (2) 427, ***428***
Von Hippel-Lindau syndrome, (2) 241,***242***
in stereotactic radiosurgery, (2) 329
Angiomatosis, retinal, (2) 240
Angiomyolipomas, renal, (1) 71; (2) 239
Antibodies, (1) 21. *See also specific antibodies*
α-1-Antichymotrypsin, (1) 75
in pleomorphic xanthoastrocytoma, (1) 66
Antigenic phenotype, (1) 17, 24
α-1-Antitrypsin in pleomorphic xanthoastrocytoma, (1) 66
Aphasia, partial, as complication in particle beam radiosurgery, (2) 332
Apoptosis, (1) 150
Apraxia in ependymomas, (2) 415
Arc-mounted stereotactic retractor system, (2) 277
Argyrophilic method, (1) 153
Arteriovenous malformation (AVM)
radiosurgery for, (2) 329, 330-331, 332
gamma knife, (2) 335
stereotactic, (2) 329, 330
Artificial nucleotides, (1) 21
Ash-leaf spots in diagnosing tuberous sclerosis, (2) 237-238
Astroblasts, (1) 17
Astrocytes, (1) 17, 21-22, 83
fibrous, (1) 15
neoplastic, (1) 115, 116
protoplasmic, (1) 15
reactive, (1) 86
type-1, (1), 22-23, 28, 83
type-2, (2), 23-24, ***29,*** 33-34, 83
Astrocytomas, (2) 213. *See also* Low-grade gliomas
adjuncts to surgical management, (2) 391-392
anaplastic, (2) 218, 382
assessment of surgical results, (2) 390-391
benign behavior of, (2) 213
benign cerebellar, (1) 143-144, ***145,*** 146
brain stem, (2) 259, ***260, 261,*** 388
pediatric, (1) 173
cerebellar, (2) 214, 255, 257-259, ***259***
clinical presentations of, (2) 383
cystic, (2) 382
dedifferentiation of, (2) 372
desmoplastic cerebral, of infancy, (1) 72-74, 155-156, 174
diffuse fibrillary, molecular genetics of, (1) 166, ***167***
ependymomas, (1) 175
formation of low-grade, (1) 166-168
oligoastrocytomas, (1) 174-175
oligodendrogliomas, (1) 174-175
progression to anaplastic, (1) 168-170, ***170***
progression to glioblastoma multiforme, (1) ***170,*** 171
subsets of glioblastoma multiforme, (1) 172-173, ***172***
epidermal growth factor receptor gene amplification in, (1) 91
fibrillary, (1) 131; (2) 372
low-grade, (1) 156-157
in frontal lobe gliomas, (2) 370, ***370***
future prospects and therapeutic horizons, (2) 394
gangliogliomas, (1) 174
gemistocytic variant of, (1) 72; (2) 218, 372, 382, 392-393
general considerations, (2) 382-383
imaging features of, (2) 252, ***253,*** 254-255, ***254, 255, 256, 257,*** 381-394, ***383-385***
incidence of, (1) 181; (2) 214, 247
in children, (2) 213
malignant dedifferentiation of low-grade, into high-grade, (2) 247, ***248***
ordinary, (2) 215-220, ***216, 218***
pediatric, (2) 382
brain stem gliomas, (1) 173
pilocytic, (1) 91, 129-131, 149, 173; (2) 254, 289-290
juvenile, (2) 416
proliferation-related markers in, (1) 155, ***155***
piloid juvenile, (2) 214-215
pleomorphic xanthoastrocytomas, (1) 156, 173
prognosis following surgery, (2) 392-394, ***393***
protoplasmic, (2) ***370,*** 371
radiotherapy for low-grade, (2) 318-321, ***320, 321***
structural classification of, (1) 127
subependymal giant cell, (1) 149, 174; (2) 238-240, 260-261, ***262***
supratentorial, (2) 391
surgical treatment
adjuncts to, (2) 391-392
assessment of, (2) 390-391
goals of, (2) 387-388

indications for, (2) 385-387
prognosis following, (2) 392-394, ***393***
strategies in, (2) 388-389
technical aspects of, (2) 389-390
in temporal lobe gliomas, (2) 368, ***369***
true pilocytic, (1) 144
tumor tissue in, (1) 127
in World Health Organization (WHO) classification, (1) 55-57, ***56;*** (2) ***309,*** 381, 382
Astrogliosis, chronic, (1) 132
Ataxia
in ependymomas, (2) 413, 414
in ganglion cell tumors, (2) 436
Autocrine hypotheses, and growth factors, (1) 37-38
Autografts, (1) 8
Automated protein sequencers and synthesizers, (1) 17
Axillary freckling in diagnosis of von Recklinghausen's disease, (2) 231, ***231***
AZQ (diaziquone) for oligodendrogliomas, (2) 408, 409

B

Basic fibroblast growth factor (bFGF), (1) 28, 153, 157, 158
α-B-crystallin in pilocytic astrocytomas, (1) 62
BCNU (carmustine) for oligodendrogliomas, (2) 408, 409
Behavioral change in ependymomas, (2) 415
Benign
application of term, to glial tumors, (2) 231
as term, (2) 309
Benign cerebellar astrocytomas versus dysembryoplastic neuroepithelial tumors, (1) 143-144, ***145,*** 146
Benign ependymomas. *See* Ependymomas
Benign gliomas. *See also* Glioma(s); Low-grade gliomas
congenital syndromes associated with, (2) 231-243
neurofibromatosis type 1
diagnosis of, (2) 231, ***231***
genetics in, (2) 232
imaging in, (2) 232-233, ***232, 233, 234***
optic glioma, (2) 233-237
tumors in, (2) 233, 237
definition of, (1) 125
and epilepsy. *See* Epilepsy
imaging features of
astrocytoma, (2) 252, ***253,*** 254-255, ***254, 255, 256, 257***
brain stem astrocytoma, (2) 259, ***260, 261***
cerebellar astrocytoma, (2) 255, 257-259, ***259***
choroid plexus papilloma, (2) 266-267, ***266, 267***
ependymoma, (2) 263-264, ***264***
gangliocytoma, (2) 267-268, ***268***
ganglioglioma, (2) 267-268, ***268***
gliomatosis cerebri, (2) 267
infratentorial ependymoma, (2) 265-266, ***265***
oligodendroglioma, (2) 262-263, ***263***
positron emission tomography, (2) 268-270
single-photon emission computed tomography, (2) 270-272
subependymal giant cell astrocytoma, (2) 260-261, ***262***
use of proliferation markers in biopsy analysis of, (1) 154-157
in World Health Organization (WHO) classification, (1) 57
Benign mixed glial mesenchymal tumors, rarity of, (1) 75
Bergmann glial cells, (1) 8, 15
Biochemistry, advances in, (1) 17
Biology. *See also* Glioma biology
advances in molecular, (1) 21
cell cycle in, (1) 149-150
in vitro cellular, (1) 19, ***20***
Biopsy
proliferation markers in, for benign gliomas, (1) 154-157
stereotactic, (2) 275, 389-390
in diagnosing
astrocytomas, (2) 387, 388
of ganglion cell tumors, (2) 430-431
procedures in, (2) 278-279, 389-390
serial, (2) 286-288
Bitemporal lesions in amnesia, (2) 351
Blepharoplasts, (1) 98, 104; (2) 416
Blood-brain barrier of pilocytic astrocytomas, (1) 58
Blood type as factor in oligodendrogliomas, (2) 222
Brachytherapy with stereotactically placed sealed radioactive isotopes for low-grade gliomas, (2) 314-315
Bragg peak absorption, (1) 6; (2) 331
Brain necrosis
laboratory studies of post-radiation, (2) 325, ***325***
documentation of focal, following radiotherapy, (2) 324
Brain stem
astrocytomas in, (2) 213, 259, ***260, 261,*** 320, 388
gliomas in, (2) 233, 237, 242

pediatric, (1) 173
survival rate of, (2) 215
hemangioblastoma tumors in, (2) 242
Brain tumor, incidence of epilepsy as symptom of, (2) 347-348
Broca's area, (2) 301
Bromodeoxyuridine (BUdR), (1) 142, 151-152, ***151***
in biopsy analysis of gliomas, (1) 154
in diagnosing pilocytic astrocytomas, (1) 62
in labeling pilocytic tumors, (2) 214, 217

C

Café-au-lait spots in diagnosis of von Recklinghausen's disease, (2) 231, ***231***
Calcification
in astrocytomas, (2) 252, 254, 384
in brain stem, (2) 259
subependymal giant cell, (2) 260
in choroid plexus papilloma, (2) 266
in ependymomas, (2) 415
infratentorial, (2) 265-266
in gangliocytomas, (2) 268
in gangliogliomas, (2) 268
in gradient-echo imaging, (2) 251
in oligodendrogliomas, (2) 252, 263, 397
Calcospherites in oligodendrogliomas, (2) 398
cAMP analogs, (1) 31-32
Cancer genes, oncogenic alterations in, (1) 179
Cancer genetics. *See also* Genetics
glossary of, (1) 179-180
Candle gutterings, (1) 71, 174
Carbohydrate moieties, (1) 21
Carbon-11-labeled methionine in imaging cerebral gliomas, (2) 270
Carbon-11-labeled thymidine in imaging cerebral gliomas, (2) 270
Carboplatinum, (2) 424
Carcinogenesis, (1) 184
Carcinoma, renal cell, (2) 241
Carmustine (BCNU) for oligodendrogliomas, (2) 408, 409
Cardiac rhabdomyomas, (2) 239
Carotid-cavernous fistulae as indication for stereotactic radiosurgery, (2) 330
CCNU (lomustine)
for oligodendrogliomas, (2) 408
for optic gliomas, (2) 236
CD68, (1) 75
Cell
Bergmann glial, (1) 8, 15
dysplastic, neuronal identity of, (1) 115
ependymal, (1) 15, 27, 96
ependymoglial, (1) 95
genetically modified, (1) 8
glia, (1) 15, 27-28
isolated tumor, (1) ***126,*** 127, 129
Müller, (1) 15
precursor, (1) 16
specialized glia, (1) 15, 27-28
Cell-cell adhesion, (1) 36
Cell-cell interactions, (1) 19
Cell cycle
definition of, (1) 149
phases of, (1) 149-150
Cell cycle biology, (1) 149-150
Cell density in oligodendrogliomas, (2) 220, 221, 399
Cell kinetics mathematics, (1) 154
Cell loss, (1) 150-151
determination of, (1) 153
methods of measuring, (1) 151-154, ***151***
Cell proliferation, (1) 17
methods of measuring, (1) 151-154, ***151***
Cellular neurosurgery, (1) 8
Cellular pleomorphism
in oligodendrogliomas, (2) 220
in piloid juvenile astrocytoma, (2) 214
Central area, gliomas of, (2) 371, ***372***
Central nervous system (CNS)
antibodies for distinguishing cell types in, (1) ***19***
hemangioblastoma in, (2) 242
histogenesis in, (1) 14-16, ***15***
impact of fractionated doses of radiotherapy on, (2) 325-326
mechanisms of cellular migration in, (1) 36-37
neoplasms in, (1) 115
organogenesis in, (1) 14
reactions to radiotherapy, (2) 324-325
toxicity in, (1) 13
Central neurocytomas
clinical presentation of, (2) 427-428, ***429***
as mimic of oligodendroglioma, (1) 92
Central tumors, resection method for, (2) 358-362, ***358, 359, 361, 362***
C-erb B1, (1) 186
Cerebellar astrocytomas
association with neurofibromatosis 1, (2) 233, 237
benign, (1) 143-144, ***145,*** 146; (2) 255, 257-259, ***259***
in children, (2) 255
incidence of, (2) 213, 214
magnetic resonance imaging of, (2) 258, ***259***

Cerebellar Bergmann glial cells, (1) 27
Cerebellar hemangioblastomas, (2) 241, 242
Cerebral aneurysms as indication for stereotactic radiosurgery, (2) 330
Cerebral astrocytomas
  desmoplastic, of infancy, (1) 118, 155-156
    clinical features of, (1) 72
    cytogenetic studies of, (1) 73
    differential diagnosis of, (1) 73-74
    pathological findings of, (1) 72-73
    prognosis of, (1) 73
  gliofibroma, (1) 74-75
  grading systems, (1) 55-57, ***56***
  outcome of treatment for, (2) 310, ***311***
  pilocytic
    clinical features of, (1) 57-58
    cytogenetic studies of, (1) 62-63
    neuroimaging features of, (1) 58
    pathological findings of, (1) 58-62, ***59, 60, 61, 62***
    prognosis of, (1) 63-65
  pleomorphic xanthoastrocytoma, (1) 65
    cytogenetic studies of, (1) 67
    differential diagnosis of, (1) 68-69
    neuroimaging features of, (1) 65
    pathological findings of, (1) 65-67, ***66***
    prognosis of, (1) 67
  subependymal giant cell
    clinical features of, (1) 69
    differential diagnosis of, (1) 71-72
    pathological findings of, (1) 69-71, ***70, 71***
Cerebral fungus, (2) 381
Cerebral gliomas
  as indication for stereotactic radiosurgery, (2) 330
  molecular genetic basis of, (1) 163
    desmoplastic infantile gliomas, (1) 174
    diffuse fibrillary astrocytomas, (1) 166, ***167***
      formation of low-grade gliomas, (1) 166-168
      oncogenes and tumor suppressor genes in, (1) 163-165
      progression to anaplastic, (1) 168-170, ***170***
      progression to glioblastoma multiforme, (1) 171
      subsets of glioblastoma multiforme, (1) 172-173, ***172***
    ependymomas, (1) 175
    gangliogliomas, (1) 174
    neurological tumor syndromes, (1) 165-166
    oligoastrocytomas, (1) 174-175
    oligodendrogliomas, (1) 174-175
    pediatric brain stem gliomas, (1) 173
    pilocytic astrocytomas, (1) 173
    pleomorphic xanthoastrocytomas, (1) 173
    subependymal giant astrocytomas, (1) 174
Cerebral glucose utilization as measure of cerebral energy metabolism, (2) 269
Cerebral imaging. *See also specific imaging technique*
  functional definition, (1) 2-3
  structural definition, (1) 2, 3
Cerebral navigation and localization, (1) 3-4
  stereotaxy, (1) 4-6, ***5***
Cerebral peduncles in pilocytic astrocytomas, (1) 64
Cerebral piloid astrocytomas, survival rate for, (2) 215
Cerebral struma, (2) 381
Cerebral surgery, milieus and developments in, (1) 1-2, ***1***
Cerebrosides, (1) 21
Cerebrospinal fluid (CSF) dissemination, (2) 214
Cerebrospinal fluid (CSF) seeding, incidence of, in ependymomas, (2) 322
Cervical-hindbrain junction, (1) 14
C-fos, (1) 186
Chemotherapy
  for ependymomas, (2) 423
  for ganglion cell tumors, (2) 438-439
  for low-grade astrocytomas, (2) 392
  for oligodendrogliomas, (2) 408-410
  for optic gliomas, (2) 236-237
Chiasmatic gliomas, survival rates for, (2) 215
Childhood Brain Tumor Consortium (CBTC) database, (1) 96, 97, 101-102, 110
  surgical appearance of ependymomas in, (1) ***98***
Children. *See also* Age
  astrocytomas in, (2) 213, 214-215, 294, 382, 416
  brain stem gliomas in, (1) 173
  glial tumors in, (1) 142-143
  supratentorial tumors in, (2) 247
Choline:aspartate ratio, (1) ***17***
Choline:glumate ratio, (1) ***17***
Choline:glycine ratio, (1) ***17***
Chordomas as indication for stereotactic radiosurgery, (2) 330
Choroid plexus papillomas
  characteristics of, (1) 102
  imaging of, (2) 266-267, ***266, 267,*** 416
  incidence of, (2) 247
Chromogen X-gal, (1) 21
Chromogranin A, (1) 116
Chromosomal loci, (1) 180
Chromosome, (1) 180

Chromosome 1, (1) 185
Chromosome 6, (1) 185
Chromosome 9, (1) 186
Chromosome 9p, (1) 169-170, 174
Chromosome 9q, (1) 174
Chromosome 10, (1) 63, 186
 deletion of, (1) 90, 185
 loss of heterozygosity, (1) 41
Chromosome 10q, (1) ***170,*** 171, 174-175
Chromosome 11, (1) 103
Chromosome 13, (1) 185
Chromosome 13q, (1) 168-169
Chromosome 16p, (1) 174
Chromosome 17, (1) 63, 184
Chromosome 17p, (1) 166-167, 172. *See also* p53 tumor suppression gene
 presence of deoxyribonucleic acid hypermethylation in, (1) 185
Chromosome 18q, (1) 166-167, 172, 185
Chromosome 19, (1) 63
Chromosome 19q, (1) 90, 169, ***170,*** 174, 175, 185
Chromosome 22, (1) 185
Chromosome 22q, (1) 103, 168, 175
Ciliary neurotrophic factor (CNTF), (1) 32
Cisplatin
 for ependymomas, (2) 423, 424
 for oligodendrogliomas, (2) 408
C-jun, (1) 150
^{11}C-labeled methionine in imaging cerebral gliomas, (2) 270
Clear cell ependymoma, (1) 92, 118
Clonal analysis, (1) 19
Clonal hypothesis, (1) 181-183, ***182***
C-myc, (1) 150, 154, 159, 171, 186
CNP, (1) 31-32
Collimator size, (1) 6, ***8***
Collins' law for congenital tumors, (2) 214
COMPASS stereotactic system, (2) 276, 280
Computed tomography (CT) scans, (1) 2
 in diagnosing
  astrocytomas, (2) 252, ***254,*** 255, 383-385, ***384, 385, 386, 387, 388, 389, 390***
   brain stem, (2) 259
   cerebellar, (2) 258
   pilocytic, (1) 58
  benign gliomas, (2) 249, 251, 268
  choroid plexus papilloma, (2) 266-267, ***266***
  dysembryoplastic neuroepithelial tumors, (1) 139
  ependymomas, (2) 264, 415, ***415***
  ganglion cell tumors, (2) 427, ***428***
  gliomatosis cerebri, (2) 267
  intracranial tumors, (2) 248
  low-grade gliomas, (2) 285-286, ***287,*** 288-290, ***288, 289, 290,*** 293-294, 297, 304, 371
  oligodendrogliomas, (2) 262, ***263,*** 400
  subependymal giant cell, (2) 261
  tuberous sclerosis, (2) 238-239
  volumetric stereotaxis, (2) 275, 278
  xanthoastrocytoma pleomorphic, (1) 65
 sensitivity of, in tumor detection, (2) 350
 in stereotactic radiosurgery, (2) 329
Computer analysis, (1) 1
Congenital syndromes, associated with benign gliomas, (2) 231-243
 neurofibromatosis type 1
  diagnosis of, (2) 231, ***231***
  genetics in, (2) 232
  imaging in, (2) 232-233, ***233, 234***
  optic glioma, (2) 233-237
  other tumors in, (2) 233, 237
 tuberous sclerosis
  diagnosis of, (2) 237-238
  genetics in, (2) 238, 241
  imaging in, (2) 238-239
  tumors in, (2) 239-240
 Von Hippel-Lindau syndrome, (2) 241
  diagnosis of, (2) 240-241
  tumors in, (2) 242-243
Corpus callosum in pilocytic astrocytomas, (1) 64
Cortical dysplasia, (1) 92
 association with dysembryoplastic neuroepithelial tumors, (1) 121
 borderline relationship between tumors and, (2) 358-359, ***358***
 as cause of epilepsy, (2) 373
 tumors associated with, (2) 348
Cortical infiltration in gliomatosis cerebri, (1) 91
Cortical mapping for oligodendrogliomas, (2) 403, ***405***
Cortical plate, (1) 15
Cortical resection, (2) 353-354
 methods and illustrative cases, (2) 354-367
Cortical stimulation, (2) 352, 353
 in mapping speech and motor function, (2) 390
Corticectomy, (2) 351, 352
 peritumoral, (2) 354-358, ***355, 356, 357***
Corticosteroids for low-grade astrocytomas, (2) 392
Cranial nerve palsy in ependymomas, (2) 414
Craniectomy, suboccipital, (2) 417
Craniopharyngiomas
 gamma knife radiosurgery for, (2) 335

stereotactic radiosurgery for, (2) 330
Craniospinal radiation
for ependymomas, (2) 225-226
for ganglion cell tumors, (2) 439
Craniotomy
for benign cerebral gliomas, (2) 352-353
for ganglion cell tumors, (2) 431, ***432***
nonstereotactic, (2) 275
^{11}C thymidine in imaging cerebral gliomas, (2) 270
Cushing's disease as indication for stereotactic radiosurgery, (2) 330
Cutaneous angiofibromas in subependymal giant cell astrocytoma, (1) 71
Cutaneous neurofibromas in diagnosis of von Recklinghausen's disease, (2) 231, ***231***
Cyclin A, (1) 159
Cystic astrocytomas, (2) 382
Cystic degeneration
in choroid plexus papilloma, (2) 266
in ependymomas, (2) 264
in oligodendrogliomas, (2) 262, 263
Cystic necrosis in benign gliomas, (2) 249
Cytogenetic alterations in oligodendrocytic tumors, (1) 90
Cytogenetic studies
of desmoplastic cerebral astrocytoma of infancy, (1) 73
of pilocytic astrocytomas, (1) 62-63
of pleomorphic xanthoastrocytomas, (1) 67
Cytokeratin expression in pleomorphic xanthoastrocytomas, (1) 66
Cytokines, (1) 17, 159
Cytoreduction
in low-grade gliomas, (2) 290
as surgical goal in astrocytomas, (2) 388

D

Darwinian genetic selection process, (1) 182
Data acquisition in computer-assisted stereotactic procedures, (2) 277-278, ***278***
Deep tumors, stereotactic procedures for removal of deep, (2) 282-284, ***282, 283***
Deletion mapping studies, (1) 168, 180
Demyelinating disease, (1) 91
Deoxyribonucleic acid (DNA), (1) 21
in cell cycle, (1) 149-150
in choroid plexus tumors, (1) 103
comparison of polymorphisms in normal and tumor, (1) 164
in ependymomas, (1) 103
flow cytometry in analysis of
anaplastic progression, (1) 89-90
cell proliferation and cell loss, (1) 153
cerebellar pilocytic astrocytomas, (1) 63
hypermethylation, (1) 185
ligase I, (1) 169
nucleolar organizer regions of, (1) 153
Deoxyribonucleic acid (DNA) ploidy in diagnosing low-grade gliomas, (2) 295
Dermoids, magnetic resonance imaging identification of, (2) 250
Descriptive morphology and histology
central nervous system histogenesis, (1) 14-16, ***15***
central nervous system organogenesis, (1) 14
Desmoplastic cerebral astrocytoma of infancy
clinical features of, (1) 72
cytogenetic studies of, (1) 73
differential diagnosis of, (1) 73-74
histology of, (1) 118
pathological findings of, (1) 72-73
prognosis of, (1) 73
proliferation markers in biopsy analysis of, (1) 155-156
as subset of glioblastoma multiforme, (1) 174
Desmoplastic change in piloid juvenile astrocytoma, (2) 214-215
Desmoplastic infantile ganglioglioma (DIG), (2) 428-429
clinical presentation of, (2) 428-429
differential diagnosis of, (1) 73
pathology of, (1) 117-118, ***118***
D-glucose in imaging cerebral gliomas, (2) 270
Diabetes insipidus in optic gliomas, (2) 235
Diacylglycerol, (1) 38
Diaziquone (AZQ) for oligodendrogliomas, (2) 408, 409
Dibromodulcitol for optic gliomas, (2) 236
Diencephalic syndrome, (2) 235
Differentiation agents, (1) 41-42
Diffuse chiasmatic tumors, (2) 235
therapy for, (2) 236
Diffuse fibrillary astrocytoma, molecular genetics of, (1) 166-173, ***167, 170, 172***
Diffusion imaging, (2) 252
DIG. *See* Desmoplastic infantile ganglioglioma
Digital angiography (DA) in stereotactic imaging, (2) 276, 278, 280
Dimethyl sulfoxide (DMSO), (1) 41
Dissociated suspension, (1) 19
Dizziness in ependymomas, (2) 413, 414

DNA. *See* Deoxyribonucleic acid (DNA)
DNT. *See* Dysembryoplastic neuroepithelial tumor
Drippings, (1) 71
Dual pathology, (2) 352
Dynamic devices, (1) 6, ***8***
Dynamic susceptibility contrast magnetic resonance imaging, (2) 252
Dysembryoplastic neuroepithelial tumor (DNT), (2) 213, 218
  versus benign cerebellar astrocytomas, (1) 143-144, ***145***, 146
  complex forms of, (1) 134-135, ***135, 136***
  diagnosis of, (1) 120-121, 142
  differentiating oligodendroglioma from, (1) 91-92
  differentiating pilocytic astrocytomas from, (1) 131
  follow-up data on, (1) 139, 142
  histological features of, (1) 86, ***86***, 126
  in interpretation of glial tumors in children, (1) 142-143
  kinetic data on, (1) 142
  neuroimaging appearance of, (1) 139, ***140, 141***
  nonspecific histological forms of, (1) 135, 137, ***138***
  origin of, (1) 134
  proliferation markers in biopsy analysis of, (1) 156
  simple form of, (1) 135
  supratentorial cortical
    clinical presentation of, (1) 137, ***137***
    tumor location of, (1) 137, 139, ***139***
Dysembryoplastic neuroepitheliomas in computed tomography scans, (2) 288
Dysplastic cells, neuronal identity of, (1) 115
Dysplastic cortex in gangliogliomas, (2) 373

E

Echo-planar magnetic resonance imaging, (1) 3; (2) 252
Elderly, incidence of brain tumors in, (2) 214
Electrocorticography (ECoG)
  in defining extent of epileptogenic area, (2) 350, 353, 374
  in enhancing tumor resection, (2) 301
  for ganglion cell tumors, (2) 439
  in seizure control, (2) 299, 300
Electroencephalography (EEG) findings in tumoral epilepsy, (2) 350
Electromagnetic spectrum, (1) 7
Electron microscopy, (1) 17
Electrophysiology, advances in, (1) 17
Endocrine dysfunction in optic gliomas, (2) 235
Endocrinopathy, (2) 235
Endopial resection, (2) 353-354
Ependymal cells, (1) 15, 27, 96
Ependymal rosette, (1) 95, 96, 98, ***99, 100***
Ependymal spongioblast, (1) 95
Ependymal tubules, (1) 102
Ependymoblastomas
  distinguishing between anaplastic ependymoma and, (1) 109
  ependymal differentiation in, (1) 107-109
  leptomeningeal, (1) 108
  as malignant, (1) 96
  subcutaneous, (1) 108
Ependymoglial cell, (1) 95
Ependymomas, (2) 413-424. *See also* Low-grade gliomas
  anaplastic, (1) 106-109, 110; (2) 416
  benign, (1) 109-110
  cells in, (1) 15, 27, 96
  chemotherapy for, (2) 423
  clear cell, (1) 92, 118
  definition of, (1) 95 (2) 413
  demographics in, (2) 413
  distinguishing from neurocytoma, (1) 119
  distinguishing from oligodendrogliomas, (1) 92, 119
  epidemiology of, (2) 213
  genetic studies of, (1) 103
  hemorrhage in, (2) 249
  histology of, (2) 416
  imaging features of, (2) 263-264, ***264***
  immunohistochemical features of, (1) 103
  incidence of, (1) 96; (2) 214, 247, 413
  infratentorial, (1) 97, 107, 110; (2) 265-266, ***265***, 413
  intracranial, (1) 97; (2) 223-226, ***224, 225***, 413, ***414***, 418
  intraspinal, (1) 97
  macroscopic appearance of, (1) 97, ***98***
  microscopic description of, (1) 97-99, ***99, 100***, 101-102, ***102***
  molecular genetic and cytogenetic studies of, (1) 175
  multicompartmental, (1) 97
  myxopapillary, (1) 109
    immunohistochemical features of, (1) 106-109
    location of, (1) 105
    macroscopic appearance of, (1) 105
    microscopic description of, (1) 105

ultrastructure of, (1) 106
neuroimaging of, (2) 415-416, ***415***
nonanaplastic, (1) 106-109
overall management plan, (2) 423-424, ***423, 424***
papillary, (1) 102
pediatric, (2) 413
plastic, (1) 97; (2) 417
posterior fossa, (2) 413
prognostic factors in, (2) ***225***
radiation therapy for, (2) 311
radiotherapy for, (2) 322-323, ***323,*** 422-423
recurrence of, (2) 223
signs and symptoms of, (2) 413-415, ***414***
stroma in, (1) 102
subependymomas, (1) 103-104
incidence of, (1) 104
location of, (1) 104
macroscopic appearance of, (1) 104
microscopic description of, (1) 104-105
ultrastructure of, (1) 105
supratentorial, (1) 97, 110; (2) 413, 418-419
anaplastic, (1) 107
surgical staging system for, (2) 224
surgical therapy for, (2) 417-418, ***417***
survival, (2) 418
curves for, (2) 223, ***224***
extent of tumor resection, (2) 420-421, ***422***
patient age, (2) 418-419, ***419***
tumor grade, (2) 419-420, ***420, 421***
and tumor location, (2) 419
tumor location in, (1) 97
tumor recurrence and pattern of failure, (2) 421-422
types of, (1) 96
ultrastructure of, (1) 103
World Health Organization (WHO) classification of, (2) ***309,*** 420, ***420***
Epidemiology of low-grade gliomas, (2) 213-214
Epidermal growth factor (EGF), (1) 28
Epidermal growth factor receptor (EGFR), (1) 90-91, 158-159, 166, ***167,*** 171
Epidermal growth factor receptor (EGFR) gene amplification, in astrocytomas, (1) 91
Epididymal adenomas, association with Von Hippel-Lindau syndrome, (2) 241
Epilepsy, (2) 347-375. *See also* Seizures
clinical presentation of, (2) 349
determination of resectability, (2) 351
distribution of benign gliomas with seizures, (2) 368, ***368***
of central, parietal, and occipital areas, (2) 371, ***372***
of frontal lobe, (2) 370-371, ***370***
of temporal lobe gliomas, (2) 368-370, ***369***
and tumor recurrences, (2) 371
in gangliocytomas, (2) 268
in gangliogliomas, (2) 268
incidence of, as symptom of brain tumor, (2) 347-348
neuropsychological studies of, (2) 350-351
pathophysiology, (2) 348-349
resection methods and illustrative cases, (2) 354
central tumors, (2) 358-362, ***358, 359, 361, 362***
frontal tumors, (2) 354-358, ***355, 356, 357***
parietal area lesions, (2) 365-367, ***366, 367***
temporal neocortical lesions, (2) 362-365, ***363, 364***
seizure focus identification, (2) 350
surgery for
and identification of dysembryoplastic neuroepithelial tumors, (1) 135, 137, 142
techniques in, (2) 351-352
cortical resection, (2) 353-354
electrocorticography, (2) 353
intraoperative cortical mapping, (2) 353
local or general anesthesia in, (2) 352
scalp incisions and craniotomy, (2) 352-353
tumor diagnosis, (2) 349-350
Epileptogenesis, secondary, (2) 373
Epileptogenic cortex, (2) 299
Erb A, (1) 39
Erb B, (1) 37, 90-91
ERCC1, (1) 169
ERCC2, (1) 169
Ethylnitrosourea in studying glioma biology, (1) 40
Etoposide (VP-16) for ependymomas, (2) 423, 424
Ets, (1) 39
Evoked response testing, (1) 4
Exophytic chiasmatic-hypothalamic gliomas, (2) 235
External beam radiation therapy
for ganglion cell tumors, (2) 439
for oligodendrogliomas, (1) 134
Extracellular methemoglobin, detection of, (2) 249
Extraventricular ependymomas, imaging of, (2) 416
Extraventricular tumors, supratentorial, (2) 416
Ezrin, (1) 166

F

Factor XIIIa immunoreactivity in subependymal giant cell astrocytoma, (1) 71
Failure to thrive, association of, with exophytic chiasmatic-hypothalamic gliomas, (2) 235
Fentanyl, (2) 352
Fetal calf serum (FCS), (1) 19
^{18}F fluorine 2-deoxyglucose (FDG) in positron emission tomography, (2) 269, 270
^{18}F fluorodeoxyglucose positron emission tomography (FDG PET), glucose utilization studies using, (1) 58
Fibrillary astrocytomas
  benign behavior of, (2) 213
  morphological appearance of, (1) 131
  proliferation markers in biopsy analysis of, (1) 156-157
  stereotactic serial biopsy studies of, (2) 289
Fibrous astrocytes, (1) 15
Fibroxanthoma, (1) 68
Fiducials, (1) 5
Fixed collimator system, (1) 6, ***7***
Flow cytometry, (1) 153-154, ***154***
Focal brain necrosis, documentation of, following radiotherapy, (2) 324
Focal hypercellularity, (2) 214
Focal midbrain astrocytomas, (1) 146
Focal neurological deficit in ependymomas, (2) 415
Focused beam radiotherapy, (2) 329-343
  for astrocytomas, (2) 392
  gamma knife radiosurgery, (2) 333-336, ***333, 335, 336***
  particle beam radiosurgery, (2) 331-333, ***331***
  stereotactic radiosurgery, (2) 329-330
    complications of, (2) 343
    indications for, (2) 330
    linear accelerator-based, (2) 336-338, ***336, 337, 338***
      planning in, (2) 338-341, ***339, 340***
    for low-grade gliomas, (2) 342-343
    radiobiological considerations, (2) 330-331
    results in, (2) 341-342, ***342***
Forceps-based orientation system, ***5***
Forebrain, (1) 14
Fos, (1) 39
Frameshift mutations, (1) 179
Free-electron lasers, (1) 6-7
Frontal lobe gliomas
  astrocytoma as, (2) 370, ***370***
  ganglioglioma as, (2) 370, ***370,*** 371
  mixed, (2) ***330,*** 371
  oligodendroglioma as, (2) 370, ***370***
  protoplasmic astrocytoma as, (2) ***370,*** 371
Frontal lobe surgery, incision for, (2) 352-353
Frontal lobe tumors, resection method for, (2) 354-358, ***355, 356, 357***
Functional imaging, (2) 252
  concept of, (1) 2-3
Functional magnetic resonance imaging in determination of respectability, (2) 351
Functional mapping techniques in enhancing tumor resection, (2) 300-301
Functional restoration, (1) 6, 7-8, ***9***
Fungus, cerebral, (2) 381

G

Gait ataxia as complication in particle beam radiosurgery, (2) 332
Galactocerebroside (GalC), (1) 88
Galactocerebroside immunoreactivity, (1) 88
β-galactosidase gene, (1) 21
GalC immunoreactivity, (1) 88
Gamma-aminobutyric acid (GABA) and occurrence of seizures, (2) 348
Gamma aminobutyric acid (GABA)-gated Cl^- channels, (1) 23
Gamma knife, (2) 329
Gamma knife radiosurgery, (2) 333-336, ***333, 335, 336***
  for astrocytomas, (2) 392
Gangliocytomas, (1) 115; (2) 267-268, ***268***
Gangliogliomas, (2) 267-268, ***268***
  association of epilepsy with, (2) 348, 374
  benign behavior, (2) 218
  clinical presentation of, (2) 427, ***428***
  in computed tomography scans, (2) 288
  desmoplastic infantile, (1) 117-118, ***118***
    clinical presentation of, (2) 428-429
  distinguishing from dysembryoplastic neuroepithelial tumors, (1) 121
  dysplastic cortex in, (2) 373
  epidemiology of, (2) 213
  in frontal lobe gliomas, (2) ***370,*** 371
  histological characteristics of, (1) 116
  as subset of glioblastoma multiforme, (1) 174
  surgical treatment of, (2) 352
  in temporal lobe gliomas, (2) 369
  as type 1 tumor, (2) 285
Ganglion cell tumors
  chemotherapy for, (2) 438-439

clinical presentation of
central neurocytomas, (2) 427-428, ***429***
desmoplastic infantile gangliogliomas, (2) 428-429
dysembryoplastic neuroepithelial tumors, (2) 429
gangliogliomas, (2) 427
craniotomy for, (2) 431, ***432***
desmoplastic infantile ganglioglioma, (1) 117-118, ***118***
diagnosis of, (1) 115-116
dysembryoplastic neuroepithelial tumor, (1) 120-121, ***121***
interactive image-guided neurosurgical techniques for, (2) 433-434, ***434, 435, 436***
intraoperative electrocorticography for, (2) 431-433
management principles for, (2) 429-430
neurocytoma, (1) 118-120, ***119, 120***
radiation therapy for, (2) 438-439
site of, (1) 115
stereotactic biopsy of, (2) 430-431
stereotactic radiosurgery for, (2) 434, 436-438, ***437, 438***
treatment paradigm for, (2) 439-440
Gangliosides, (1) 21
Gaze palsy in ependymomas, (2) 414
Gemistocytic astrocytomas
age factors in, (2) 218
differential diagnosis of, (1) 72
prognosis following surgery for, (2) 392-393
Gender, as factor
in astrocytomas, (2) 216
in ependymomas, (1) 96
in oligodendroglioma, (1) 83
Gene amplication, (1) 179
Gene mutation, (1) 179
Genetically modified cells, (1) 8
Genetic information, (1) 8
Genetics, (1) 8
in cerebral gliomas, (1) 163-176
glossary of terms, (1) 179-180
in neoplastic initiation and progression, (1) 182
in tuberous sclerosis, (2) 238
in Von Hippel-Lindau syndrome, (2) 241
Genomic deletion mapping, (1) 169-170
Genomic hybridization in diagnosing astrocytomas, (2) 382
Genomic nucleotides, (1) 21
Gli, (1) 171
Glia, origin of, (1) 16
Glial cell types, (1) 21-22
multipotential neuroglial precursor cells, (1) 28
oligodendrocyte-type-2 astrocyte (O-2A) lineage, (1) ***18,*** 23-24, ***25, 26,*** 27
radial glia, (1) 27-28
specialized glia, (1) 27-28
type 1 astrocyte (T1A) lineage, (1) 22-23
Glial fibrillary acidic protein (GFAP), in diagnosing
choroid plexus tumors, (1) 103
ependymomas, (1) 103
ganglion cell tumors, (1) 116
oligodendrogliomas, (1) 88-89, ***88,*** 131; (2) 398
pilocytic astrocytoma, (1) 61-62
in pleomorphic xanthoastrocytoma, (1) 66
positive cells, (1) 89
in subependymal giant cell astrocytoma, (1) 71
Glial swelling, (1) 3
Glial tumor spatial definition of low-grade gliomas, (2) ***284,*** 285-286, ***285, 286, 287,*** 288-290, ***288, 289, 290, 291***
Glioblastoma multiforme (GBM)
progression to, (1) 149, 181; (2) 200
subsets of, (1) 172-173, ***172***
Glioblastomas
glomerular appearance associated with, (2) 398
hemorrhaging in, (2) 249
incidence of, (2) 215, 247
progression to, (2) 220
recurrence of, (2) 217
Gliocytoma embryonale, (1) 144
Gliofibrillary oligodendrocytes, (1) 88
Gliofibroma, (1) 74-75
Gliogenesis, progression and control of
multipotential neuroglial precursor cells, (1) 35
oligodendrocyte-type 2 astrocyte lineage, (1) 28-34
radial glia, (1) 34-35
timing in vitro versus in vivo, (1) 28
type 1 astrocyte lineage, (1) 28
Glioma(s)
benign. *See* Benign gliomas
brain stem, (2) 237
of central area, (2) 371, ***372***
conservative and nonrestrictive adjunctive surgical care of, (2) 296-297
control of seizures in, (2) 298-300
desmoplastic infantile, (1) 174
frontal lobe, (2) 370-371, ***370***
functional mapping techniques to enhance resection in, (2) 300-301
influence of extent of tumor resection on

outcome, (2) 297
low-grade. *See* Low-grade gliomas
mixed, (1) 174-175
new directions for therapy, (1) 41-44
of occipital area, (2) 371, ***372***
outcome based on quantitative volumetric analysis, (2) ***302-303,*** 304-305
of parental area, (2) 371, ***372***
rationale for surgery, (2) 293-295
resective surgery in diagnosis of, (2) 295-296
stereotypes in management of low-grade intracranial, (2) 275-291
temporal lobe, (2) 368-370, ***369***
timing of surgery, (2) 297-298
tumor progression in, (1) 181
clinical implications of, (1) 186-187
clinical series of, (1) 183, ***183***
clonal hypothesis in, (1) 181-182
clonal origin of malignant, (1) 183-184
molecular evidence for, (1) 184-186, ***185***
Glioma biology, (1) 13-14
confirmation of nonprimate mammalian data in humans, (1) 37
descriptive morphology and histology, (1) 14
central nervous system histogenesis, (1) 14-16, ***15***
central nervous system organogenesis, (1) 14
glial cell types in, (1) 21-28
implications for neuro-oncology, (1) 37-44
improved methods for in vitro study of, (1) ***20,*** 39-41, ***40***
modern tools for study of, (1) 16-21
biochemistry, (1) 17
electrophysiology, (1) 17
immunology, (1) ***19,*** 21
molecular, (1) 21
physical chemistry, (1) 17, ***17, 18***
physics, (1) 17
in vitro cellular, (1) 19, ***20***
progression and control of gliogenesis, (1) 28-35
subventricular zone heterogeneity and precursor migration, (1) 35-37
Glioma therapy
differentiation agents in, (1) 41-44
potential for specifically targeted therapies, (1) 42-44
Gliomatosis cerebri
cortical infiltration and nuclear regularity in, (1) 91
imaging features of, (2) 267
Glioneuronal elements, uniqueness of, in dysembryoplastic neuroepithelial tumors, (1) 135
Gliosarcomas, distinguishing ependymomas from, (1) 95
Glomus jugular tumors as indication for stereotactic radiosurgery, (2) 330
Glucose-6-phosphate dehydrogenase (GPD), (1) 184
Glucose utilization studies using fluorine-18 fluorodeoxyglucose positron emission tomography (FDG PET), (1) 58
Glycine, ***17***
Gradient-echo imaging in detection of intracranial hemorrhage, (2) 251
Grading systems. *See also* St. Anne/Mayo classification system; World Health Organization (WHO) classification system
for astrocytomas, (1) 55-57, ***56***
Granular bodies in pilocytic astrocytomas, (1) 62, 64
Growth factors, (1) 17
angiogenic factors
basic fibroblast factor, (1) 158
cytokines, (1) 159
epidermal growth factor receptor, (1) 158-159
platelet-derived factor, (1) 158, 168
transforming growth factor-beta, (1) 157-158
vascular endothelial growth factor, (1) 158
and autocrine hypotheses, (1) 37-38
expression of, (1) 157-159, ***157,*** 163
methods to measure cell proliferation and cell loss, (1) 151, ***151***
bromodeoxyuridine, (1) 151-152
cell loss determination, (1) 153
cell nuclear antigen, (1) 152-153
flow cytometry, (1) 153-154, ***154***
^{3}H-thymidine, (1) 151
Ki-67 antibody, (1) 152
mitotic index, (1) 151
in oligodendrocytic tumors, (1) 90-91
and proliferation potential, (1) 149
cell cycle biology, (1) 149-150
cell kinetics mathematics, (1) 154
cell loss, (1) 150-151
silver-staining nucleolar organizer regions, (1) 153
statin, (1) 153
use of markers in biopsy analysis of benign gliomas, (1) 154
desmoplastic cerebral astrocytomas of infancy, (1) 155-156
dysembryoplastic neuroepithelial tumors, (1) 156
low-grade fibrillary astrocytomas, (1) 156-157

pilocytic astrocytomas, (1) 155, ***155***
pleomorphic xanthoastrocytomas, (1) 156
Guanosine diphosphate (GDP), (2) 232
Guanosine triphosphate (GTP), (2) 232

H

HAM-56, (1) 91
Hamartomas
definition of, (1) 72
in subependymal giant cell astrocytomas, (2) 260-261
in temporal lobe gliomas, (2) ***369,*** 370
Ha-*ras,* (1) 186
Headache
in ependymomas, (2) 413, 414, 415
in piloid juvenile astrocytomas, (2) 215
Headholder in stereotactic frame, (2) 276
Heads-up display in stereotaxis, (2) 277, ***277,*** 280
Heidelberg, University of, stereotactic radiosurgery at, (2) 342
Hemangioblastomas
cerebellar, (2) 242
as indication for stereotactic radiosurgery, (2) 330
in Von Hippel-Lindau syndrome, (2) 242
Hemiparesis
as complication in particle beam radiosurgery, (2) 332
in ependymomas, (2) 413, 414, 415
Hemorrhage
in brain stem astrocytomas, (2) 259
in diagnosis of astrocytomas, (2) 383-384
in ependymomas, (2) 264
in infratentorial ependymomas, (2) 266
magnetic resonance imaging of, (2) 250-251
in oligodendrogliomas, (2) 263
Hemosiderin in chronic hemorrhage, (2) 249-250
Heterogeneous signal intensity, (2) 250
Heterozygosity studies, loss of, (1) 164, 180
Hexamethylene bisacetamide (HMBA), (1) 41
Hindbrain, (1) 14
Hippocampal sclerosis, (2) 374
Histogenesis in central nervous system, (1) 14-16, ***15***
Histological typing, patterns of tumor growth associated with low-grade gliomas, (1) 125-146
dysembryoplastic neuroepithelial tumor, (1) 134
versus benign cerebellar astrocytomas, (1) 143-144, ***145,*** 146
complex forms of, (1) 134-135, ***135,*** 136
diagnosis of, (1) 142
follow-up data, (1) 139, 142
and interpretation of glial tumors in children, (1) 142
kinetic data, (1) 142
neuroimaging appearance of, (1) 139, ***140, 141***
nonspecific histological forms of, (1) 135, 137, ***138***
simple forms of, (1) 135
supratentorial cortical, (1) 137, ***137,*** 139, ***139***
growth patterns
histological assessment, (1) ***126,*** 127, ***128***
structural classification, (1) 127, 129
oligodendrogliomas, structural types and histological diagnosis, (1) ***128, 130,*** 131-134, ***132, 133***
pilocytic astrocytomas, (1) 129-131
HNK-1, (1) 88, 103
^{1}H NMR spectra, (1) 23
in analyzing cell metabolites in vitro, (1) ***17, 18,*** 27
Homer Wright rosettes, (1) 118
^{3}H-thymidine, (1) 151, ***151,*** 154
in autoradiography, (1) 17
Hydrocephalus
in choroid plexus papilloma, (2) 266-267
in ependymomas, (2) 413
in infratentorial ependymomas, (2) 265
obstructive, in astrocytomas, (2) 383
in optic glioma, (2) 233
preoperative shunting for, (2) 417
ventriculoperitoneal shunting for, (2) 431
β-Hydroxybutyrate, (1) ***17,*** 27
Hypercellularity
focal, (2) 214
in grading astrocytomas, (2) 217
Hypothalamic syndrome as complication in particle beam radiosurgery, (2) 332
Hypothalamus, astrocytomas in, (2) 213
Hypothermia for astrocytomas, (2) 392

I

Imaging
of benign gliomas, (2) 247-272, ***248, 249, 250, 251***
astrocytomas, (2) 252, ***253,*** 254-255, ***254, 255, 256, 257***
brain stem, (2) 259, ***260, 261***
cerebellar, (2) 255, 257-259, ***259***
subependymal giant cell, (2) 260-261, ***262***
choroid plexus papilloma, (2) 266-267, ***266, 267***

ependymoma, (2) 263-264, ***264***
gangliocytoma, (2) 267-268, ***268***
ganglioglioma, (2) 267-268, ***268***
gliomatosis cerebri, (2) 267
infratentorial ependymoma, (2) 265-266, ***265***
oligodendroglioma, (2) 262-263, ***263***
positron emission tomography in, (2) 268-270
single-photon emission computed tomography in, (2) 270-272
of tuberous sclerosis, (2) 238-239
of Von Hippel-Lindau syndrome, (2) 241
Immunoblot analysis of Ki-67 antibodies, (1) 152
Immunocytology, (1) 21
Immunoelectron microscopy, (1) 21
Immunohistology, (1) 21
Immunology, advances in, (1) ***19,*** 21
Immunotherapy, (2) 394
for astrocytomas, (2) 392
Increased intracranial pressure from astrocytoma, (2) 391
Infrared light-emitting diodes (IREDs), (2) 434
Infratentorial ependymomas, (2) 265-266, ***265***
age as factor in, (2) 413
in children, (2) 247
histological features of, (1) 107
incidence of, (1) 97
operative mortality for, (1) 110
Inositol triphosphate ($InsP_3$), (1) 38
In situ hybridization, (1) 21
In situ nick translation methods, (1) 153
Insulin-like growth factor 1 (IGF-1), (1) 90
Int-2, (1) 37
Intellectual impairment in ependymomas, (2) 415
Interactive image-guided neurosurgical techniques for ganglion cell tumors, (2) 433-434, ***434, 435, 436***
Interleukin (IL), (1) 157
Interleukin-1, (1) 159
Interleukin-6, (1) 159
Intermediate zone, (1) 15
Internal capsule in pilocytic astrocytomas, (1) 64
Interphase cytogenetics in diagnosing astrocytomas, (2) 382
Interstitial brachytherapy with iodine-125, (2) 215
Intracellular proteins, (1) 21
Intracellular second-messenger pathways, (1) 38-39
Intracranial approach for optic gliomas, (2) 235-236
Intracranial ependymomas, (1) 97; (2) 265, 413, ***414,*** 418
Intracytoplasmic blepharoplasts, (1) 95
Intraoperative cortical mapping, (2) 353
Intraoperative electrocorticography for ganglion cell tumors, (2) 431-433
Intraoperative localization device (ILD) attachments, (2) 434
Intraoperative mapping techniques for ganglion cell tumors, (2) 432
Intraspinal ependymomas, (1) 97; (2) 265
Intravascular dyes, utilization of, (1) 7
Intraventricular supratentorial tumors, (2) 416
Intrinsic gliomas of cervicomedullary junction, (1) 146
In vitro cellular biology, (1) 19, ***20***
In vitro morphology, (1) 24
In vitro studies of glioma biology, (1) ***20,*** 39-41, ***40***
In vivo type-2 astrocyte controversy, (1) 34
Ionic currents, flow of, (1) 3
Isoelectric focusing, (1) 17
Isolated tumor cells (ITCs), (1) ***126,*** 127, 129

J

Japan Brain Tumor Registry, (2) 219
Jet Propulsion Laboratory, (1) 1, 9
Jun, (1) 39
Juvenile pilocytic astrocytomas, (2) 214-215. *See also* Pilocytic astrocytomas
imaging of, (2) 416
radical resection of, (2) 294

K

Karnofsky Performance Scale (KPS) scores, (2) 218, 219, 402
Karolinska Institute, development of gamma knife at, (2) 333, 335
Karoytype analysis of pleomorphic xanthoastrocytomas, (1) 67
Kernohan grading system survival rate for
grade I tumors, (2) 216
grade II tumor, (2) 216
in tumor classification, (2) 215, 217, 399
Ki-67 antigen, (1) ***151***
in biopsy analysis of gliomas, (1) 154
in diagnosing
astrocytomas, (1) 56; (2) 383
pilocytic, (1) 62, 155
ependymomas, (1) 110
low-grade gliomas, (1) 142; (2) 295-296
pleomorphic xanthoastrocytomas, (1) 67
immunoblot analysis of, (1) 152
in measuring growth factor, (1) 153, 154

Kidney, angiomyolipoma in, (2) 239
KP-1, (1) 91
K-*ras*, (1) 171

L

L428 cells, (1) 152
Labeling index (LI)
  for bromodeoxyuridine, (2) 214
  definition of, (1) 154
  and growth rate, (2) 295
  for Ki-67, (1) 155
Language, Amytal test for lateralization of, (2) 351
Lasers
  free-electron, (1) 6-7
  medical, (1) 6
Lawrence Berkeley Laboratory, particle beam radiotherapy at, (2) 331
Leksell gamma unit, (1) 6
Leptomeningeal dissemination in pilocytic astrocytomas, (1) 63
Leptomeningeal ependymoblastoma, (1) 108
Leptomeningeal infiltration, (1) 86
Leptomeningeal xanthosarcoma, (1) 68
Lesionectomy, (2) 351, 352, 354, 374
Lethargy in ependymomas, (2) 415
Leu-7, (1) 88, 103
  immunoreactivity in oligodendrogliomas, (1) 120
Leukemia inhibitory factor (LIF), (1) 32
Leukemia in neurofibromatosis 1, (2) 233
Lhermitte-Duclos disease, (1) 117
Li-Fraumeni cancer syndrome, (1) 165, 166
Linear accelerator-based stereotactic radiosurgery, (2) 336-338
  planning in, (2) 338-341, ***339, 340***
  results in, (2) 341-342, ***342***
Linkage studies, (1) 165-166, 180
Lipomas, magnetic resonance imaging identification of, (2) 250
Lisch nodules in diagnosis of von Recklinghausen's disease, (2) 231, ***231***
Lomustine (CCNU)
  for oligodendrogliomas, (2) 408
  for optic gliomas, (2) 236
Loss of heterozygosity (LOH) studies, (1) 164, 180
Low-grade astrocytomas
  fibrillary, (1) 156-157
    proliferation markers in biopsy analysis of, (1) 156-157
  formation of, (1) 166-168
Low-grade gliomas, (2) 213-226. *See also* Benign gliomas; Glioma(s)
  biological variability of, (2) 213
  dysembryoplastic neuroepithelial tumors, (1) 134
    application of, in interpretation of glial tumors in children, (1) 142-143
    versus benign cerebellar astrocytomas, (1) 143-144, ***145,*** 146
    complex forms of, (1) 134-135, ***135, 136***
    diagnosis of, (1) 142
    follow-up data, (1) 139, 142
    kinetic data, (1) 142
    neuroimaging appearance of, (1) 139, ***140, 141***
    nonspecific histological form, (1) 135, 137, ***138***
    simple form of, (1) 135
    supratentorial cortical, (1) 137, ***137,*** 139, ***139***
  ependymomas, (2) 223-226, ***224, 225***
    prognostic factors in, (2) ***225***
    survival curves for, (2) 223, ***224***
  epidemiology in, (2) 213-214
  growth pattern of
    histological assessment, (1) ***126,*** 127, ***128***
    structural classification, (1) 127
  imaging correlations, (1) 129
  indications for radiotherapy in, (2) 311-312
  oligodendroglioma, (2) 220-223, ***221, 222***
  ordinary astrocytoma, (2) 215-220, ***216***
  patterns of tumor growth and problems associated with histological typing of, (1) 125-146
    dysembryoplastic neuroepithelial tumors, (1) 134-135, ***135, 136,*** 137, ***137, 138,*** 139, ***139, 40, 141,*** 142-144, ***143, 145,*** 146
    gliomas, (1) 127, ***128,*** 129
    oligodendrogliomas, (1) ***128, 130,*** 131-134, ***132, 133***
    pilocytic astrocytomas, (1) 129-131
    piloid juvenile astrocytoma, (2) 214-215
    radiation therapy for, (2) 310-311, ***311***
    stereotactic radiosurgery for, (2) 342-343
    structural types of, (1) 129
    surgical decision-making, (1) 129
    survival rate for, (2) 213
    treatment of, (2) 310
    with tumor progression, (2) ***302-303***
    World Health Organization (WHO) classification of, (2) 309, ***309***
  slow-growing structure type III, (1) 132-134, ***133***
  stereotactic radiosurgery for, (2) 330
  structural types and histological diagnosis, (1) ***128, 130,*** 131-132, ***132***
Lumen, (1) 14

M

Macrocephaly, association of, with exophytic chiasmatic-hypothalamic gliomas, (2) 235
Macroglial cells, (1) 15
 development of, (1) 83-84
Magnetic flux, changes in, (1) 3
Magnetic resonance imaging (MRI), (1) 2, 4
 in diagnosing
  astrocytomas, (2) 252, ***253, 254,*** 383-385, ***384, 385, 386,*** 387, ***387, 388, 389, 390***
  benign gliomas, (2) 249-252, 268
  brain stem astrocytomas, (2) 259
  central neurocytomas, (2) 428
  cerebellar astrocytomas, (2) 258
  dysembryoplastic neuroepithelial tumors, (1) 139
  ependymomas, (2) 264, ***264,*** 415, ***415***
  ganglion cell tumors, (2) 427, ***428,*** 439
  gliomatosis cerebri, (2) 267
  infratentorial ependymoma, (2) ***265,*** 266
  low-grade gliomas, (2) 286, ***286,*** 288-290, 293-294, 296, ***298,*** 304
  neurofibromatosis type 1, (2) 232-233, ***232, 233, 234***
  oligodendrogliomas, (2) 401
  optic system gliomas, (2) 233, ***233, 234***
  pilocytic astrocytoma, (1) 58
  posterior fossa pilocytic astrocytomas, (2) 258-259, ***259***
  subependymal giant cell, (2) 261, ***262***
  tuberous sclerosis, (2) 238-239
  tumor in epileptic suspect, (2) 349-350, 373
  Von Hippel-Lindau syndrome, (2) 241
  xanthoastrocytoma pleomorphic, (1) 65
 echo-planar, (1) 3
 and management of brain tumors and epilepsy, (2) 375
 sensitivity of, in tumor detection, (2) 350
 in stereotactic radiosurgery, (2) 329
Magnetic resonance spectroscopy, (2) 252
 in differential diagnosis of tumor, (2) 350
Magnetic source imaging, (1) 3, ***4***
 in determination of respectability, (2) 351
Magnetoencephalographic imaging, (1) 2, 4
Malignant astrocytoma glioblastoma multiforme, (2) 382
Manned space flight, contributions from achievements in, (1) 1-2
Mantle layer, (1) 15
MAP-2, (1) 150
Marginal zone, (1) 15
Mars Expedition, (1) 1-2
Massachusetts General Hospital, particle beam radiotherapy at, (2) 331
Mass effect
 in ependymomas, (2) 415
 and occurrence of seizures, (2) 348
Maternal layer, (1) 15
Matrix layer, (1) 15
Mayfield head holder, (2) 403
McGill University, stereotactic radiotherapy at, (2) 337, 342
MDM2 gene amplification, (1) 167, 171, 186
Medical lasers, (1) 6
Medulloblastomas, (1) 16; (2) 266
 chromosome 17p in, (1) 167
 neuroimaging of, (2) 416
Medulloepithelial layer, (1) 15
Melphalan for oligodendrogliomas, (2) 408
Meningeal sarcoma, (1) 73
Meningiomas, (2) 254
 gamma knife radiosurgery for, (2) 335
 imaging of, (2) 416
 as indication for stereotactic radiosurgery, (2) 330
Mental retardation
 in gangliocytomas, (2) 268
 in gangliogliomas, (2) 268
 in subependymal giant cell astrocytomas, (2) 260
 in tuberous sclerosis, (2) 237, 238
Merlin, (1) 165-166
Mesencephalon, (1) 14
Mesial temporal sclerosis, (2) 374
Met-enkephalin, (1) 116
Methemoglobin, (2) 249
Methylthioadenosine phosphorylase (MTAP), (1) 169-170
MIB-1 immunostaining, (1) ***151,*** 152; (2) 272
 in studying growth of dysembryoplastic neuroepithelial tumors, (1) 142
Microcysts
 in oligodendrogliomas, (2) 221
 in pilocytic astrocytomas, (1) 64
Microelectrophysiology, (1) 17
Microsatellite polymorphisms, (1) 164
Midbrain-forebrain junction, (1) 14
Missense mutations, (1) 179
Mitotic activity in oligodendrogliomas, (2) 399
Mitotic figures in grading astrocytomas, (2) 214, 217
Mitotic index, (1) 151
Mixed gliomas. *See also* Oligoastrocytomas
 in frontal lobe, (2) ***330,*** 371

molecular genetic basis of, (1) 174-175
in temporal lobe, (2) 369, ***369***
Moesin, (1) 166
Molecular biology, advances in, (1) 21
Molecular neurosurgery, (1) 6, 8
Monstrocellular sarcoma, (1) 68
Mos, (1) 39
Mucin deposition, (1) 86
Müller cells, (1) 15
Multichanneled recording devices, (1) 3
Multicompartmental ependymomas, (1) 97
Multiple-arc stereotactic treatment, (2) 337
Multiple imaging plane slices, (1) 4
Multipotential neuroglial precursor cells, (1) 28
Mutations
frameshift, (1) 179
missense, (1) 179
nonsense, (1) 179
of p53 tumor suppression cells, (1) 90, 167, 184
point, (1), 90, 179
somatic, (1) 184
Myb, (1) 39, 171
Myc, (1) 39
Myelin-associated glycoprotein, (1) 87
Myelin basic protein (MBP), (1) 87
Myelography, in diagnosing
ependymomas, (2) 415-416
oligodendrogliomas, (2) 400
Myxopapillary ependymomas
immunohistochemical features of, (1) 106-109
location of, (1) 105
macroscopic appearance of, (1) 105
microscopic description of, (1) 105
ultrastructure of, (1) 106

N

N-acetyl-aspartate (NAA), (1) ***17***, 27
Nausea in ependymomas, (2) 413, 414, 415
Neck pain in ependymomas, (2) 413, 414
Necrosis
in astrocytomas, (2) 214, 217, 383-384
and cell loss, (1) 150-151
cystic, in benign gliomas, (2) 249
documentation of focal brain, following radiotherapy, (2) 324
effects of, on MRI signal intensity, (2) ***251***
in ependymomas, (2) 264
laboratory studies of post-radiation, (2) 325, ***325***
in oligodendrogliomas, (2) 221, 262, 399
radiation, (2) 255
Nelson's disease as indication for stereotactic radiosurgery, (2) 330
Neoplasia, role of apoptosis in, (1) 150
Neoplastic astrocytes, (1) 115, 116
Neoplastic transformation, (1) 163
Neovascularization in grading astrocytomas, (2) 217
Nerve palsies as complication in particle beam radiosurgery, (2) 332
Neu, (1) 37
Neural cell adhesion molecule (N-CAM), (1) 27
Neural tube lumen, (1) 14
Neurocutaneous syndromes, (1) 165
Neurocytomas
central, (1) 92, 118
clinical presentation of, (2) 427
identification of glial markers in, (1) 119
pathology of, (1) 118-120, ***119, 120***
Neurodiagnostic imaging
of central neurocytomas, (2) 428
of desmoplastic infantile gangliogliomas, (2) 429
of ganglion cell tumors, (2) 427, ***428***
of pilocytic astrocytomas, (1) 58
of pleomorphic xanthoastrocytomas, (1) 65
Neuroectoderm, (1) 14
Neuroepithelial layer, (1) 15
Neurofibromas, malignant degeneration of, into neurofibrosarcoma, (2) 233
Neurofibromatosis
conservative management of, (2) 296
survival rate of, (2) 215
Neurofibromatosis type 1 (NF1) gene, (2) 232, 235, 237
diagnosis of, (2) 231, ***231***
genetics in, (2) 232
imaging in, (2) 232-233, ***232, 233, 234***
optic glioma, (2) 233-237
in pilocytic astrocytoma, (1) 57
tumors in, (2) 233, 237
Neurofibromatosis type 2 (NF2) gene, (1) 165, 168, 175
Neurofibromin, (1) 165; (2) 232
Neurofibrosarcoma, malignant degeneration of neurofibroma, (2) 233
Neurofilament, (1) 117
Neuroleptanalgesia, (2) 352
Neurological surgery, historical analysis of, (1) 2
Neurological tumor syndromes, (1) 165-166
Neuromas, acoustic, as indication for stereotactic radiosurgery, (2) 330
Neuronal-glial malignancies, (1) 16, ***16***
Neuronavigator, (1) 5

Neurons, origin of, (1) 16
Neuron-specific enolase (NSE), (1) 117
Neuro-oncology, (1) 37-44
  autocrine hypotheses in, (1) 37-38
  glioma therapy in, (1) 41-44
  growth factors in, (1) 37-38
  intracellular second-messenger pathways in, (1) 38-39
  in vitro study of glioma biology in, (1) ***20,*** 39-41, ***40***
Neuropsychological studies of epileptic tumor suspect, (2) 350-351
Neuroradiological imaging studies in diagnosis of intracranial tumors, (2) 248
Neurosurgery. *See also* Surgery
  cellular, (1) 8
  molecular, (1) 8
Neurotensin, (1) 116
Neurotransmitter-gated ion channels, (1) 22
Neurulation, (1) 14
"New Windows on the Human Brain," (1) 9, ***9***
Nitrosourea in studying glioma biology, (1) 40
N-*myc* gene amplification in neurofibromatosis, (1) 165, 171
Nonanaplastic ependymomas, (1) 106-109
Nonlinkage stereotaxy, (1) 4-5, ***5***
Nonprimate mammalian data, confirmation of, in humans, (1) 37
Nonsense mutations, (1) 179
Nonstereotactic craniotomy, (2) 275
Northern blotting, (1) 21
Nuclear pleomorphism in grading astrocytomas, (2) 217
Nuclear protein, (1) 152-153
Nuclear regularity in gliomatosis cerebri, (1) 91
Nucleotides
  artificial, (1) 21
  genomic, (1) 21
Number counting, stimulation-induced blocking of, (2) 301
Nystagmus in ependymomas, (2) 414

O

Occipital area
  gliomas of, (2) 371, ***372***
  seizures associated with tumors in, (2) 365
Oligoastrocytomas
  distinguishing from dysembryoplastic neuroepithelial tumors, (1) 121
  epidemiology of, (2) 213
  molecular genetic studies of, (1) 174-175
  stereotactic serial biopsy studies of, (2) 289
  structural classification of, (1) 127
Oligodendroblastomas, (2) 399
Oligodendroblasts, (1) 17
Oligodendrocytes, (1) 15, 17, 21-22, 23, 30-32, 83
  lack of visible cytoplasm in, (1) 127, ***128***
  role of, (2) 397
  type-2 astrocyte lineage, (1) ***18,*** 23-24, ***25, 26,*** 27, 28-34, 88
    adult O-2A progenitor cells, (1) 32-33
    antigenic phenotype and in vitro morphology, (1) 24
    distinguishing features, (1) 24, 27
    oligodendrocytes, (1) 30-32
    perinatal, (1) 23, 28-30, 35-36
    perinatal O-2A progenitor cells, (1) 28-30
    type-2 astrocytes, (1) ***29,*** 33-34
    in vivo controversy, (1) 34
Oligodendrocytic tumors
  cytogenetic alterations in, (1) 90
  growth factors in, (1) 90-91
Oligodendrogliomas, (2) 213, 220-223, 397-410. *See also* Low-grade gliomas
  age as factor in, (2) 222
  anaplastic, (1) 88, 89-90, ***89;*** (2) 399, ***399***
  appearance of, (2) 398
  benign behavior of, (2) 213
  blood type as factor in, (2) 222
  chemosensitivity of, (2) 222
  chemotherapy for, (2) 408-410
  components of, (2) 398, ***398***
  in computed tomography scans, (2) 288
  cytogenetic alterations in tumors, (1) 90
  definition of, (2) 397-399
  description of, (1) 83-84
    cytological considerations in, (1) 87, ***87***
    histopathological features of, (1) 83
    immunohistochemical features of, (1) 87-89, ***88***
    pathological features of, (1) 85-86, ***85, 86, 87***
      macroscopic appearance, (1) 84-85, ***84***
  differential diagnosis of, (1) 91-92, ***92,*** 119
  distinguishing from dysembryoplastic neuroepithelial tumor, (1) 91-92
  in frontal lobe gliomas, (2) 370, ***370***
  future prospects for, (2) 410
  grading schemes for, (2) 220
  growth factors in, (1) 90-91
  hemorrhaging in, (2) 249

histological assessment of, (1) 127, ***128;*** (2) 398-399
imaging of, (2) 262-263, ***263***
incidence of, (2) 214, 247
influence of surgery on survival of patients with, (2) 221
Leu-7 immunoreactivity in, (1) 120
molecular genetic studies of, (1) 174-175
natural history of, (2) 399-400
pathological features of, (2) ***398, 399***
prognosis for, (2) 410, ***410***
prognostic factors in, (2) ***222***
radiation therapy for, (2) 311, 321-322, 404-408, ***406***
slow-growing structure type-III, (1) 132-134, ***133***
stereotactic serial biopsy studies of, (2) 289
structural classification of, (1) 127, ***128, 130,*** 131-132, ***132***
supratentorial, (2) 401
surgery for, (2) 400-403, ***401, 404***
survival rate for, (2) 220, ***221,*** 297
in temporal lobe gliomas, (2) 368-369, ***369***
treatment of, (1) 134
as type 1 tumor, (2) 285
World Health Organization (WHO) classification of, (2) ***309***
Oligonucleotide probe, (1) 21
Ki-67 antigen-specific antisense, (1) 152
Ommaya reservoir, (2) 296
Oncogenes, (1) 163-165, 179
Oncogenic alterations in cancer genes, (1) 179
Oncology, autocrine hypothesis of, (1) 37-38
Operating room, (1) 10
Operative corridors, minimization of, (1) 2
Operative trauma. *See also* Surgery
reduction of, (1) 2
Operative venue, (1) 8-10, ***10,*** 12
Ophthalmoplegia in ependymomas, (2) 415
Optical imaging, (1) 3
Optic gliomas
conservative management of, (2) 296
magnetic resonance imaging of, (2) 233, ***233, 234***
in neurofibromatosis type 1, (1) 57; (2) 233-237
prognosis for, (2) 320-321
Optic nerve/chiasm, astrocytomas in, (2) 213, 320
Optic nerve tumors, survival time for, (2) 215
Ordinary astrocytomas, (2) 215-220, ***216***
prognostic factors in, (2) ***218***
Organogenesis, central nervous system, (1) 14
Oxygen delivery, (1) 3

P

p53 tumor suppression gene, (1) 166-167, 174-175. *See also* Chromosome 17p
abnormalities in breast carcinoma, (1) 165
dependent pathway for, (1) 185
independent pathway for, (1) 186
mutations of, (1) 90, 167, 184
Palsy
gaze, in ependymomas, (2) 414
nerve, as complication in particle beam radiosurgery, (2) 332
Pancreatic cysts, association with Von Hippel-Lindau syndrome, (2) 241
Pancreatic islet cell tumors, association with Von Hippel-Lindau syndrome, (2) 241
Papillary ependymomas, (1) 101-102
Papilledema in ependymomas, (2) 414, 415
Paragangliomatous components, (1) 98
Parietal area
gliomas of, (2) 371, ***372***
resection method for lesions in, (2) 365-367, ***366, 367***
Parinaud's syndrome in ganglion cell tumors, (2) 436
Particle beam radiosurgery, (2) 331-333, ***331***
Particle radiation, (1) 6, ***6***
Patch clamp techniques, (1) 17
Pathological findings
of desmoplastic cerebral astrocytoma of infancy, (1) 72-73
of pilocytic astrocytomas, (1) 58-62, ***59, 60, 61, 62***
of pleomorphic xanthoastrocytomas, (1) 65-67, ***66***
of subependymal giant cell astrocytomas, (1) 69-71, ***70, 71***
Patient rotation in stereotactic resection procedures, (2) 280
PC10 antibody, (2) 295-296
PCV (procarbazine)
for oligodendrogliomas, (2) 408, 409
for optic gliomas, (2) 236
Pediatric astrocytoma, (2) 213, 214-215, 382
Pediatric brain stem gliomas, (1) 173
Perinatal O-2A progenitor cells, (1) 23, 28-30, 35-36
Perineuronal satellitosis, (1) 86
Perinuclear halos, (1) 91
Peritumoral corticectomy, (2) 354-358, ***355, 356, 357***
Peritumoral edema in ependymomas, (2) 264
Perivascular pseudorosettes, (1) 86, 92, 95, 98-99, ***100***
Pheochromocytoma
in neurofibromatosis 1, (2) 233

risk in developing, (2) 240
Phosphatidyl-inositol-biphosphate (PIP_2), (1) 38
Phospholipase C (PLC), (1) 38
Phosphorus 32 in radiotherapy for astrocytomas, (2) 392
Phosphotungstic acid hematoxylin (PTAH) stain, (1) 101
Photodynamic therapy, (1) 7
for astrocytomas, (2) 392
Physical chemistry, advances in, (1) 17, ***17, 18***
Physics, advances in, (1) 17
Pilocytic astrocytomas, (1) 149
clinical features of, (1) 57-58
cytogenetic studies of, (1) 62-63
cytological criteria of, (1) 131
differential diagnosis of, (1) 91
differentiating from dysembryoplastic neuroepithelial tumors, (1) 131
distinction from ordinary, (1) 130
growth pattern of, (1) 129, 131
histological criteria of, (1) 129-131
imaging of, (2) 254, ***254, 255***
incidence of, (2) 214
juvenile, (2) 214-215, 294, 416
magnetic resonance imaging of, (1) 58
neuroimaging features of, (1) 58
pathological findings of, (1) 58-62, ***59, 60, 61, 62***
posterior fossa, (2) 258-259, ***259***
prognosis of, (1) 63-65
proliferation markers in biopsy analysis of, (1) 155, ***155***
radical surgical resection of, (2) 236
radiotherapy for, (1) 63-64
recurrence of, as malignant tumors, (2) 298
stereotactic resection of, (2) 289-290, 389-390
as subset of glioblastoma multiforme, (1) 173
survival rate for, (2) 297, 320
treatment of, (2) 310
true, (1) 144
as type 1 tumor, (2) 285, 286
Pineal glans, pilocytic astrocytomas in, (1) 57
Pineal tumors
gamma knife radiosurgery for, (2) 335
as indication for stereotactic radiosurgery, (2) 330
Pittsburgh, University of, gamma knife radiosurgery at, (2) 334, 335, 336
Pituitary adenomas, as indication for stereotactic radiosurgery, (2) 330
Plastic ependymomas, (1) 97; (2) 417
Platelet-derived growth factor (PDGF), (1) 28, 29, 90, 153, 157, 158, 166
Platelet-derived growth factor (PDGF)-AA, (1) 168
Platelet-derived growth factor (PDGF)-a receptors, (1) 168, 171
overexpression, (1) 168
Platelet-derived growth factor (PDGF)-BB, (1) 168
Platelet-derived growth factor (PDGF)-β receptors, (1) 168
Pleomorphic xanthoastrocytomas (PXA), (1) 73
cytogenetic studies of, (1) 67
differential diagnosis of, (1) 68-69
neuroimaging features of, (1) 65
pathological findings for, (1) 65-67, ***66***
post operative irradiation in patients with, (2) 320
prognosis of, (1) 67
proliferation markers in biopsy analysis of, (1) 156
as subset of glioblastoma multiforme, (1) 173
Pleomorphism in oligodendrogliomas, (2) 221
Point mutations
definition of, (1) 179
of p53 tumor suppression gene, (1) 90
Polar-apolar compounds, (1) 41
Polar ependymoglioblast, (1) 95
Polymerase chain reaction technology, (1) 21
Polymorphisms, (1) 180
Positron emission tomography (PET), (1) 2; (2) 252
^{18}F fluorine 2-deoxyglucose (FDG), (1) 58; (2) 269-270
in determination of resectability, (2) 351
in diagnosing
astrocytomas, (2) 384
benign cerebral glioma, (2) 268-270
ganglion cell tumors, (2) 436
Posterior fossa
ependymomas in, (2) 413
pilocytic astrocytomas in, (2) 258-259, ***259***
Potassium accumulation, blood volume changes for, (1) 3
Precursor cells, (1) 16
Preschiasmatic optic nerve tumors, (2) 235
Primitive ependyma, (1) 15
Primitive neuroectodermal tumors (PNETs), (1) 108
Procarbazine (PCV)
for oligodendrogliomas, (2) 408, 409
for optic gliomas, (2) 236
Prolactinoma as indication for stereotactic radiosurgery, (2) 330
Proliferating cell nuclear antigen (PCNA), (1) ***151,*** 152-153
in diagnosing
astrocytomas, (2) 383
low-grade gliomas, (1) 62; (2) 295-296

Proliferation markers in biopsy analysis of benign gliomas, (1) 154-157
Prophylactic bilateral nephrectomy, (2) 241
Propofol, (2) 352
Prosencephalon, (1) 14
Protein kinases in cell cycle regulation, (1) 150
Proteolipid protein, (1) 87
Proton beam radiotherapy in diagnosing low-grade gliomas, (2) 314, 331-332
Proton nuclear magnetic resonance (^{1}H NMR), (1) 17, ***17, 18***
Proto-oncogenes, (1) 163, 179, 182
Protoplasmic astrocytes, (1) 15
Protoplasmic astrocytomas
  benign behavior of, (2) 213
  in frontal lobe gliomas, (2) ***370,*** 371
  as type 1 tumor, (2) 285
Pseudorosettes, perivascular, (1) 86, 92, 95, 98-99, ***100***
Pseudostratified columnar epithelium, (1) 14-15
Pterional approach for suprasellar tumors, (2) 236
Puberty, precocious, in optic gliomas, (2) 235

Q

Quality-of-life assessment, in patients with
  astrocytomas, (2) 391
  low-grade gliomas, (2) 323-326, ***325***
Quantitative volumetric analysis, surgical outcome based on, (2) 301, ***302-303,*** 304-305
Question mark incision, (2) 352

R

Radial glia, (1) 27-28, 34-35
Radiation
  particle, (1) 6, ***6***
  craniospinal
    for ependymomas, (2) 225-226
    for ganglion cell tumors, (2) 439
Radiation dosimetry in stereotactic radiosurgery, (2) 337
Radiation necrosis, (2) 255
Radiation therapy, (2) 309-326. *See also* Radiotherapy
  central nervous system reactions to, (2) 324-325
  for ependymomas, (2) 322-323, ***323,*** 422-423
  for ganglion cell tumors, (2) 438-439
  for low-grade astrocytomas, (2) 219, 318-321, ***320, 321***
  for low-grade gliomas, (2) 310-311, ***311***
    contemporary, (2) 311-312
    techniques for, (2) 312-313, ***313, 314, 315, 316, 317, 318***
  for oligodendrogliomas, (2) 221-222, 321-322, 401-402, 404-408, ***406***
  for optic gliomas, (2) 236
  quality-of-life postradiation and toxicity of, (2) 323-326, ***325***
Radioactive isotopes in treating brain tumors, (2) 314-315
Radiotherapy. *See also* Focused beam radiotherapy; Radiation therapy
  for low-grade astrocytomas, (2) 318-320, 391-392
  for low-grade infiltrative gliomas, (1) 129
  for oligodendrogliomas, (2) 407
  for pilocytic astrocytomas, (1) 63-64
Radixin, (1) 166
Raf, (1) 39
Ras, (1) 39, 150
  as tumor suppressor gene, (2) 232
Ras/raf-1, (1) 39
Rb protein (pRb) expression, (1) 159, 169
Reactive astrocytes, (1) 86
Rel, (1) 39
Renal angiomyolipomas in subependymal giant cell astrocytoma, (1) 71
Renal cell carcinoma, (2) 241
Renal cysts, (2) 241
Repeat polymorphisms, (1) 180
Restriction fragment length polymorphisms (RFLP), (1) 164, 180, 184
Reticulin fibers in pleomorphic xanthoastrocytoma, (1) 66
Retinal angiomatosis, (2) 240
Retinal Müller cells, (1) 27
Retinoblastoma (Rb)
  susceptibility gene, (1) 168-169
  tumor suppressor gene, (1) 166, 184
Retinoic acid, (1) 41, 42
Retroviral gene transfer techniques, (1) 21
Rhabdomyomas, cardiac, (2) 239
Rhabdomyosarcoma in neurofibromatosis 1, (2) 233
Rhabdomyosarcomatous components, (1) 98
Rhombencephalon, (1) 14
Ribonucleic acid (RNA), (1) 21
Robotics, (1) 1
Roentgenography in diagnosing oligodendrogliomas, (2) 262
Ros, (1) 37
Rosenthal fibers
  in pilocytic astrocytomas, (1) 61-62, 64
  in piloid juvenile astrocytomas, (2) 215

in subependymal giant cell astrocytoma, (1) 69
Rosettes
ependymal, (1) 95, 96, 98, ***99, 100***
Homer Wright, (1) 118
pseudo-, perivascular, (1) 86, 92, 95, 98-99, ***100***
true, (1) 98, ***100***

S

S100 protein, reactivity of oligodendrogliomas to, (1) 92
St. Anne/Mayo classification system, (2) 399
for astrocytomas, (1) 56-57, ***56***
Sclerosis
hippocampal, (2) 374
mesial temporal, (2) 374
temporomesial, (2) 352, 374
tuberous, (1) 165
association of subependymal giant cell astrocytoma with, (1) 69; (2) 260
conservative management of, (2) 296
diagnosis of, (2) 237-238
genetics in, (2) 238, 241
imaging in, (2) 238-239
intracerebral lesions in patients with, (2) 260-261
tumors in, (2) 239-240
Seizures. *See also* Epilepsy
in astrocytomas, (2) 383
in dysembryoplastic neuroepithelial tumors, (1) 120
in ependymomas, (2) 415
in low-grade gliomas, (2) 294, 298-300
in patients with hemispheric tumors, (2) 427
in tuberous sclerosis, (2) 237, 238
Shagreen patches in diagnosing tuberous sclerosis, (2) 238
Sharplan 1100 CO_2 laser system, (2) 277
Short-chain fatty acids, (1) 41
Signal amplification competency, (1) 1
Signal processing, (1) 1
Signal transmission, (1) 1
Silver-staining nucleolar organizer regions, (1) 153
Single-photon emission computed tomography (SPECT) scans of benign glioma, (2) 270-272
Sis, (1) 37
Sodium butyrate, (1) 41, 42
Software development, (1) 10, 12
Solid tumor tissue, (1) 127
Somatic mutations, (1) 184
Sonic digitizers, (1) 5
Southern blotting, (1) 21
Southern California, University of (USC)
development of operating site at, (1) 8-10, ***9, 10, 11,*** 12
linear accelerator-based stereotactic radiosurgery at, (2) 338-341
Specialized glia cells, (1) 15, 27-28
Speech therapy, cortical mapping protocol in, (2) ***405***
Spinal cord, hemangioblastoma tumors in, (2) 242-243
Spinal subarachnoid seeding in ependymomas, (2) 224-225
Spin-echo imaging in detection of intracranial hemorrhage, (2) 251
Spongioblastoma polare, (1) 86
Src, (1) 39
Statin, (1) ***151,*** 153
Stereoscopic angiography in determination of resectability, (2) 351
Stereotactically delivered linear accelerator teletherapy for astrocytomas, (2) 392
Stereotactic biopsy, (2) 275, 389-390
in diagnosing
astrocytomas, (2) 387, 388
of ganglion cell tumors, (2) 430-431
procedures in, (2) 278-279, 389-390
serial, (2) 286-288
Stereotactic frame, (2) 276-277
Stereotactic radiosurgery, (1) 6; (2) 329-330. *See also* Surgery
complications of, (2) 343
for ganglion cell tumors, (2) 434, 436-438, ***437, 438***
indications for, (2) 330
linear accelerator-based, (2) 336-338, ***336, 337, 338***
planning in, (2) 338-341, ***339, 340***
results in, (2) 341-342, ***342***
for low-grade gliomas, (2) 342-343
data acquisition in, (2) 277-278, ***278***
glial tumor spatial definition of, (2) ***284,*** 285-286, ***285, 286, 287,*** 288-290, ***288, 289, 290, 291***
instrumentation in, (2) 276-277, ***276, 277***
multidisciplinary team in, (2) 330
patient selection for resection, (2) 285
radiobiological considerations in, (2) 330-331
resection procedures in, (2) 279-280
serial biopsy procedures in, (2) 278-279

surgical procedures
for deep tumors, (2) 282-284, ***282, 283***
for superficial lesions, (2) 280-282, ***281***
Stereotactic serial biopsy, (2) 286-288
Stereotaxy, (1) 4-6, ***5***
evolution of, (1) 3-4
nonlinkage, (1) 4-5, ***5***
"point"-oriented method of, (1) 4
"volume"-oriented mode of, (1) 4
Steroid therapy for astrocytomas, (2) 392
Structural substrate, (1) 2
Subcutaneous ependymoblastoma, (1) 108
Subependymal germinal matrix, (1) 15
Subependymal giant cell astrocytoma
clinical features of, (1) 69
conservative management of, (2) 296
differential diagnosis of, (1) 71-72
pathological findings of, (1) 69-71, ***70, 71***
as subset of glioblastoma multiforme, (1) 174
and tuberous sclerosis, (2) 238-239
Subependymal glomerate astrocytoma, (1) 109
Subependymal layer, (1) 15
Subependymomas, (1) 103-104, 109
incidence of, (1) 104
location of, (1) 104
macroscopic appearance of, (1) 104
microscopic description of, (1) 104-105, ***104***
ultrastructure of, (1) 105
Subfrontal approach for optic gliomas, (2) 235-236
Suboccipital craniectomy for ependymomas, (2) 417
Subpial dissection, (2) 354
Subungual fibromas in diagnosing tuberous sclerosis, (2) 238
Subventricular zone, (1) 15, 35-36
heterogeneity and precursor migration, (1) 35-37
mechanisms of migration, (1) 36-37
Sulfatides, (1) 21
SUN SPARC 10 computer system, (2) 276
Suprasellar tumors, pterional approach for, (2) 236
Supratentorial astrocytomas
histological features useful in grading, (2) 217
therapy for, (2) 391
Supratentorial dysembryoplastic neuroepithelial tumor (DNT), (1) 146
clinical presentation of, (1) 137, ***137***
tumor location, (1) 137, 139, ***139***
Supratentorial ependymomas, (1) 97
age as factor in, (2) 418-419
anaplastic, (1) 107
operative mortality for, (1) 110
Supratentorial extraventricular tumors, imaging of, (2) 416
Supratentorial oligodendrogliomas, treatment of, (2) 401
Supratentorial tumors in children, (2) 247
Surgery. *See also* Stereotactic radiosurgery
for astrocytomas
adjuncts to, (2) 391-392
assessment of, (2) 390-391
goals of, (2) 387-388
indication for, (2) 385-387
prognosis following, (2) 392-394, ***393***
strategies for, (2) 388-389
technical aspects of, (2) 389-390
conservative and nonresective adjunctive care, (2) 296-297
in control of seizures, (2) 298-300
for ependymomas, (2) 417-418
functional mapping techniques to enhance tumor resection, (2) 300-301
influence of extent of tumor resection on outcome, (2) 297
for oligodendrogliomas, (2) 400-403, ***401, 404***
influence of, on survival in patients with, (2) 221
for optic gliomas, (2) 235-236
quantitative volumetric analysis in, (2) 301, ***302-303,*** 304-305
rationale for, (2) 293-295
role of resective, in diagnosis, (2) 295-296
timing of, (2) 297-298
Surveillance, Epidemiology, and End Result (SEER) Study of the National Cancer Institute, (1) 143
Synaptophysin, (1) 117
immunohistochemical reactivity for, (1) 92
immunoreactivity, (1) 116
in neurocytomas, (1) 119
Syringomyelia, association of ependymomas with, (1) 97

T

Tanycytes, (1) 27, 95
Target point action, (1) 6
ablation, (1) 6-7, ***7, 8***
functional restoration, (1) 7-8, ***9***
Tau, (1) 150
Technetium-99m MIBI (methoxyisobutylisonitile), for SPECT imaging, (2) 272
Tectal plate gliomas, conservative management of, (2) 296

Teletherapy for low-grade gliomas, (2) 314
Temporal lobe gliomas, (2) 368-370
  astrocytoma as, (2) 368, ***369***
  ganglioglioma as, (2) 369
  hamartoma as, (2) ***369,*** 370
  mixed, (2) 369, ***369***
  oligodendroglioma as, (2) 368-369, ***369***
  xanthoastrocytoma as, (2) 369
Temporal lobe lesions, (2) 352-353
Temporal neocortical lesions, resection method for, (2) 362-365, ***363, 364***
Temporomesial sclerosis, (2) 352, 374
Teratomas, magnetic resonance imaging identification of, (2) 250
Thallium-201, in tumor imaging, (2) 270-272
Thallium uptake index, (2) 272
Therapeutic index, (1) 13
6-Thioguanine for optic gliomas, (2) 236
Thiotepa for oligodendrogliomas, (2) 408
Three-dimensional (3-D) digital subtraction angiograms, (2) 351
  in determining resectability, (2) 351
Three-dimensional digitizers, (1) 5, ***5***
Three-dimensional MRI reconstruction, (2) 351
Three-dimensional radiation dosimetry, (2) 314
Three-dimensional tumor image reconstruction, (2) 311-312
Todd-Wells stereotactic frame, (2) 276
Transependymal dorsally exophytic brain stem gliomas, (1) 146
Transforming growth factor-β (TGF-β), (1) 90, 157-158, 159
Translocation, (1) 163, 179
Treatment planning in computer-assisted stereotac tic procedures, (2) 278-279
Trk, (1) 37
True rosettes, (1) 98, ***100***
Tuberous sclerosis (TS), (1) 165
  association of subependymal giant cell astrocytoma with, (1) 69; (2) 260
  conservative management of, (2) 296
  diagnosis of, (2) 237-238
  genetics in, (2) 238, 241
  imaging in, (2) 238-239
  intracerebral lesions in patients with, (2) 260-261
  tumors in, (2) 239-240
β-Tubulin, (1) 117
Tumor(s)
  borderline relationship between cortical dysplasias and, (2) 358-359, ***358***
  enhancement of, (1) 58
  functional mapping techniques in, (2) 300-301
  in neurofibromatosis type 1, (2) 233
  stereotactic procedures for removal of deep, (2) 282-284, ***282, 283***
  in tuberous sclerosis, (2) 239-240
  in visual system, (2) 233-237
  in Von Hippel-Lindau syndrome, (2) 242-243
  Wilm's, (2) 233
Tumor growth, patterns of, associated with histological typing of low-grade gliomas, (1) 125-146
  in dysembryoplastic neuroepithelial tumors, (1) 134-135, ***135, 136,*** 137, ***137, 138,*** 139, ***139, 140, 141,*** 142-144, ***143, 145,*** 146
  in gliomas, (1) 127, ***128,*** 129
  in oligodendrogliomas, (1) ***128, 130,*** 131-134, ***132, 133***
  in pilocytic astrocytomas, (1) 129-131
Tumor necrosis, effects of, on magnetic resonance intensity, (2) ***251***
Tumor necrosis factor (TNF), (1) 150
Tumor necrosis factor-α (TNF-α), (1) 157, 159
Tumor progression
  clinical implications, (1) 186-187
  clinical series, (1) 183, ***183***
  clonal hypothesis for, (1) 181-183, ***182***
  clonal origin in, (1) 183-184
  in gliomas, (1) 183, ***183***
  molecular evidence for, (1) 184-186, ***185, 186***
Tumor suppressor genes, (1) 179, 182
Turcot's syndrome, (1) 165
Type-1 astrocytes (T1As), (1) 22-23, 28, 83
  antigenic phenotype and in vitro morphology, (1) 22
  distinguishing features, (1) 22-23
Type-2 astrocytes (T2As), (1) 23-24, ***29,*** 33-34, 83
Tyrosine hydroxylase, (1) 116

U

Ultrasonography in surgical resection of optic nerve gliomas, (2) 236
Urokinase plasminogen activator (uPA), (1) 157

V

Vascular endothelial growth factor (VEGF), (1) 157, 158
Vasoactive intestinal polypeptide, (1) 116
Ventricular zone, (1) 15, 35-36

Vimentin
in ependymomas, (1) 103
in oligodendrogliomas, (1) 88
in pilocytic astrocytomas, (1) 62
Vincristine
for oligodendrogliomas, (2) 408
for optic gliomas, (2) 236
Virchow-Robin spaces, (1) 72
Visual complications, radiation in, (2) 326
Visual disturbances in ependymomas, (2) 413, 414
Visual field loss in ependymomas, (2) 415
Visualization, (1) 9-10, ***10, 11***
Visualization/rehearsal laboratory, (1) 10
Visual loss, association of, with exophytic chiasmatic-hypothalamic gliomas, (2) 235
Visual system, tumors of, (2) 233-237
Vitamin derivatives, (1) 41
Voltage-dependent ion channels, (1) 22
Vomiting in ependymomas, (2) 415
Von Hippel-Lindau syndrome
diagnosis of, (2) 240-241
imaging in, (2) 241
tumors in, (2) 242-243
von Recklinghausen's disease
association of ependymomas in, (1) 97
diagnosis of, (2) 231, ***231***
genetics in, (2) 232
imaging in, (2) 232-233, ***232, 233, 234***
tumors in, (2) 233-237
VP-16 for ependymomas, (2) 423, 424

W

Western blot techniques, (1) 17
Wilm's tumor in neurofibromatosis, (1) 1; (2) 233
World Health Organization (WHO) classification system
of anaplastic ependymomas, (1) 106-107
of astrocytomas, (1) 55-57, ***56;*** (2) ***309,*** 381, 382
of benign gliomas in, (1) 57
of dysembryoplastic neuroepithelial tumors, (1) 135
of ependymoblastomas, (1) 107
of ependymomas, (1) 95, 96, 109; (2) 420, ***420***
of low-grade gliomas, (2) 309, ***309***
of oligodendrogliomas, (1) 131

X

Xanthoastrocytomas
pleomorphic, (1) 149, 156
cytogenetic studies, (1) 67
differential diagnosis of, (1) 68-69
neuroimaging, (1) 65
pathological findings, (1) 65-67, ***66***
prognosis, (1) 67
in temporal lobe gliomas, (2) 369
as type 1 tumor, (2) 285
X chromosome inactivation, (1) 183-184
XRCC, (1) 169

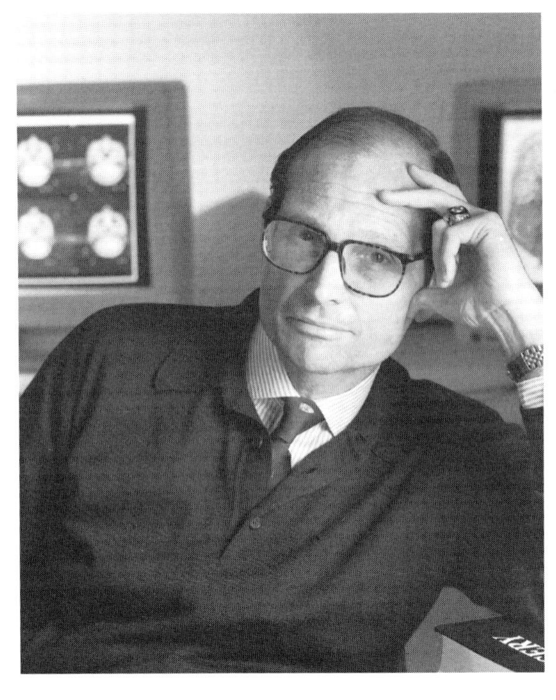

Dr. Apuzzo is the Edwin M. Todd/Trent H. Wells Jr Professor of Neurological Surgery and Professor of Radiation Oncology Biology and Physics at the University of Southern California School of Medicine in Los Angeles. An internationally noted surgeon, neuro-oncologist, scientist, author, and editor, he has made multiple contributions to the field with particular emphasis on innovative methodologies for and scientific applications to cerebral surgery.

This two-volume set is Dr. Apuzzo's fourth contribution to this series.

Publications Office
Patti Lawson
Joanne B. Needham
Gay Palazzo
Lebanon, New Hampshire

Compositor
Barbara Homeyer

Indexer
Sandi Schroeder